Health AND Fitness
An Elementary Teacher's Guide

Scott Melville

Copyright © 2010 Scott Melville
All rights reserved.

ISBN: 1-4392-6873-8
ISBN-13: 9781439268735

Dedicated to my wife Julie.
Her abiding love is all to me.

In life's rough and tumble
You're the crumble on my apple crumble
And the fairy on my Christmas tree!

"Who dares to teach must never cease to learn."
~ John Cotton Dana

[TABLE OF CONTENTS]

[PREFACE] XIII

[CHAPTER 1] 1
   THE IMPORTANCE OF YOUR TEACHING HEALTH & FITNESS
      THE IMPORTANCE OF HEALTH AND FITNESS 2
         Immediate Quality of Life
         Quality of Life as We Age
         Length of Life
      EXERCISE & HEALTH PRACTICES OF AMERICANS 7
         Exercise
         Nutrition
         Sleep
         Brushing and Flossing
         Sun Exposure
         Smoking Tobacco
      HOW YOU CAN PLAY A CRUCIAL ROLE 16
         The Classroom Teacher
         The Specialist
      CHAPTER COMPREHENSION CHECK 22

[CHAPTER 2] 25
   MODELS FOR PHYSICAL ACTIVITY AND NUTRITION
      MODELS FOR PHYSICAL ACTIVITY 27
         The Activity Pyramid
      MODELS FOR NUTRITION 32
         The Healthy Eating Pyramid
         The Vegetarian Pyramid
         Health Reasons
         Environmental Reasons
         Ethical Reasons
      CHAPTER COMPREHENSION CHECK 43

[CHAPTER 3] 45
   EXERCISE PHYSIOLOGY: WHAT YOU NEED TO KNOW
      WHAT IS PHYSICAL FITNESS 47
         Component of Cardio-Respiratory Fitness
         Component of Dynamic Flexibility Fitness
         Component of Muscular Fitness
         Component of Body Composition Fitness

HOW TO DEVELOP AND MAINTAIN THE COMPONENTS OF FITNESS 51
  (F)requency (I)ntensity (T)ime Principle
  F.I.T. Principle Applied to Improving Cardio-Respiratory Fitness (Aerobic)
  F.I.T. Principle Applied to Improving Cardio-Respiratory Fitness (Anaerobic)
  F.I.T Principle Applied to Improving Dynamic Flexibility Fitness
  F.I.T. Principle Applied to Improving Muscular Fitness
  F.I.T. Principle Applied to Reducing Body Composition Fitness
  Qualification of the F.I.T. Principle
  Overuse Principle
  Reversibility Principle
  Readiness/Trainability Principle
  Warm-up and Cool-down Principle
CHAPTER COMPREHENSION CHECK 72

[CHAPTER 4] 75
NUTRITION: WHAT YOU NEED TO KNOW
CARBOHYDRATES 78
FATS AND CHOLESTEROL 79
  Unsaturated Fat
  Saturated Fat
  Trans-Fat
PROTEINS 88
FIBER 90
WATER AND BEVERAGES 91
  Soda
  Juice and Fruit Drinks
  Tea and Coffee
VITAMINS 96
MINERALS 97
  Calcium
  Salt
OMEGA-3 FATTY ACIDS 100
CALORIC BALANCE 101
  Anorexia
CHAPTER COMPREHENSION CHECK 103

[CHAPTER 5] 107
INSTILLING HEALTHY BEHAVIORS
INSTILLING HEALTHY BEHAVIORS 109
  Teaching Self-Responsibility
  Selecting the Behavior
  Recognizing the Benefits of the Behavior
  Doing the Behavior in School
  Tracking/Reinforcing Beyond Class Behavior
  Going Multidisciplinary

  Changing Nutritional Practices
 INSTILLING AFFECTIVE BEHAVIORS   127
  Awareness Talks
  Reflection Times
 CHAPTER COMPREHENSION CHECK   133

[CHAPTER 6]   135
GETTING CHILDREN TO ENJOY PHYSICAL ACTIVITIES & CONDITIONING EXERCISES
 ENJOYMENT OF PHYSICAL ACTIVITIES   138
  Exposure to a Wide Variety of Activities
  Facilitating Successful Perceptions
  Teaching Perseverance
 ENJOYMENT OF CONDITIONING EXERCISES   146
  Sanctioning All Intensity Levels
  Setting Self-Performance & Process Goals
 CHAPTER COMPREHENSION CHECK   150

[CHAPTER 7]   151
MANAGEMENT TECHNIQUES
 ESTABLISHING CLASS RULES   154
 STARTING CLASS   156
 OTHER MANAGEMENT TECHNIQUES   158
  Communication Styles
  Passive Communication
  Aggressive Communication
  Assertive Communication
 MANAGEMENT GAMES   161
 CORRECTING MISBEHAVIOR   164
  Removal of Positive Consequences
  Six-Step Discipline Plan
  Exercise as Punishment
  Group Punishment
 CHAPTER COMPREHENSION CHECK   169

[CHAPTER 8]   171
TECHNIQUES FOR TEACHING MOVEMENT SKILLS
 INTRODUCTORY INSTRUCTIONS & DEMONSTRATIONS   174
  PRACTICE
  FEEDBACK
  REVIEW
 CHAPTER COMPREHENSION CHECK   186

[CHAPTER 9] 189
MAKING GAMES & SPORTS FUN & EDUCATIONAL
MAKING GAMES FUN AND EDUCATIONAL 191
- Introducing Games
- SOS Principle Revisited
- Safety
- On-Task Activity
- Successful

MAKING SPORTS FUN AND EDUCATIONAL 199
- Changing the Rules
- Matching Competitors
- Changing Equipment and Facilities
- Adjusting the Contextual Aspects of Sports
- Traditional vs. Games Approach to Teaching Sport Skills
- Beyond Traditional Sports

CHAPTER COMPREHENSION CHECK 227

[CHAPTER 10] 229
ASSESSMENT OF THE PSYCHOMOTOR DOMAIN
EVALUATION OF PHYSICAL ACTIVITY 232
- Physical Activity Assessment Instruments
- Self-Report Logs
- Pedometers
- Heart-Rate Monitors

EVALUATION OF PHYSICAL FITNESS 238
- What Does a Physical Fitness Test Tell?
- Three Approaches to Physical Fitness Testing
- The Traditional Approach
- The Personal Approach
- The Challenge Approach
- Selecting a Physical Fitness Test
- The President's Challenge
- Fitnessgram
- Grading of Physical Fitness

EVALUATION OF MOTOR SKILLS 246
- Formal vs. Informal Evaluation
- Process vs. Product Evaluation
- Authentic Evaluation
- Holistic Evaluation

REPORTING & GRADING OF THE PSYCOMOTOR DOMAIN 262
- Reporting
- Grading

CHAPTER COMPREHENSION CHECK 265

[CHAPTER 11] 267
OFTEN ASKED QUESTIONS
- WHAT IS AND ISN'T APPROPRIATE TOUCHING IN THE ACTIVITY ENVIRONMENT?
- HOW CAN I ACCOMMODATE STUDENTS WITH SPECIAL NEEDS?
- HOW CAN I TEACH MOVEMENT ACTIVITIES IN THE CLASSROOM?
- WHAT ARE MY SAFETY & LEGAL RESPONSIBILITIES?
- WHAT EQUIPMENT WILL I NEED & HOW MIGHT I ACQUIRE IT?
- WHEN SHOULD & SHOULDN'T BOYS & GIRLS PLAY TOGETHER?
- I HAVE BEEN URGENTLY ASKED TO COACH YOUTH SPORTS. WHAT DO I DO?
- WHAT ARE APPROPRIATE PHYSICAL ACTIVITIES & TEACHING METHODS FOR THE PRE-SCHOOL CHILD?
- CHAPTER COMPREHENSION CHECK — 286

[CHAPTER 12] 287
ACTIVITIES TO HELP YOU START
- BEANBAG ACTIVITIES — 289
- CLASSROOM BASED ACTIVITIES — 290
- COOL-DOWNS — 295
- COOPERATIVE/NEW GAMES — 296
- DANCE — 298
  - Golden Oldies
  - Folk Dance
  - Square Dance
- GENERAL GAMES — 303
- HULA-HOOP ACTIVITIES — 305
- MUSIC ACTIVITIES — 307
- PARACHUTE ACTIVITIES — 308
- RELAYS — 312
- ROPE ACTIVITIES — 313
- TAG GAMES — 318
- STUNTS (INDIVIDUAL CHALLENGES) — 316
- STUNTS (PARTNER CHALLENGES) — 317
- WALK/RUN ACTIVITIES — 320

[ANNOTATED RESOURCES] 327
[NUTRITIONAL VALUES APPENDIX] 331
[ABOUT THE AUTHOR] 343

[PREFACE]

Without good health we are diminished, enjoyment of life is compromised and our personal and social accomplishments are limited. In this book it will become clear that despite our growing wealth, technological achievements, and advances in medicine, America is encountering major health problems as a consequence of our lifestyles. We are much less active than in the past; our diets contain more calories and are less nutritious (dangerous diets and bulimia /anorexia disorders are common); we are finding less time in our stress-filled days for restorative leisure pursuits and sleep; drug abuse and violent behaviors persist; and various health care problems remain (excessive sun exposure, unsafe sexual practices, failure to take prudent measures to minimize accidents and injuries, etc.). As a consequence, American adults are encountering high rates of disabilities such as heart attack, stroke, cancer, diabetes, obesity, depression, arthritis, emphysema, osteoporosis, fatigue, back pain, sexually transmitted diseases and trauma injuries.

Our children are facing these same lifestyle challenges and research data leads to the conclusion that they are a generation at particular risk to the adult health problems listed above. The number of children classified as overweight or obese has risen to around 30 percent (more than double what it was two decades ago). Type II diabetes – once called "adult-onset diabetes" – has increased nine-fold and is now being diagnosed more and more frequently in adolescents. Like adults, the average young person is getting much less physical activity than did past generations and his/her diet is less nutritious and higher in calories. Additionally, there are many other disturbing health practices affecting the young such as violent behaviors (perpetrated on and by them), early smoking and drug usage, excessive sun exposure, and careless sexual practices.

Given the seriousness of the above health profile of our children, action needs to be taken. Establishing sound wellness practices is an integral part of a liberal education. If lifestyles are to be changed, schools must exert a concerted effort and both the health/fitness specialist and the classroom teacher must play symbiotic roles. Regardless of how well a physical education specialist carries out his/her duties, those visits are not going to be sufficient to affect the major lifestyle changes that are necessary. Most schools will have specialist visits of only once or twice a week, and significant numbers of schools do not have any specialist. The average physical education specialist might be servicing as many as 600-800 students and the trend is towards schools supporting yet fewer specialists in the future. Clearly, the specialist will be just one rather ineffectual voice crying in the wilderness unless his/her message is supported and supplemented by the other teachers, the staff, and the administration. Because of the close bonds that will be formed between the classroom teacher and the students over a year's time, he/she naturally becomes a primary influential player. His/her modeling and advice will be critical.

In 2004 the Federal Government passed the *Child Nutrition and WIC Reauthorization Act.* Its intent is to ensure that schools are doing everything possible to promote school-wide wellness practices. The law requires every school district that participates in the federal school meal programs (that includes most parochial and well as public schools) to establish a wellness policy. It states that a committee must set yearly wellness goals and assessment procedures. Besides ensuring that a healthy food environment is created, and that comprehensive nutrition instruction is occurring throughout the curriculum, the schools are responsible for pursuing various means of promoting regular physical activity. The schools are specifically charged with seeing to the following:

1. Students are given opportunities for physical activity during the school day through physical education classes, daily recess periods for elementary school students, and the integration of physical activity into the academic curriculum.

2. Students are given opportunities for physical activity through a range of before and/or after-school programs including, but not limited to, intramurals, interscholastic athletics, and physical activity clubs.

3. Schools work with the community to create ways for students to walk, bike, and rollerblade or skateboard safely to and from school.

4. Schools encourage parents and guardians to support their children's participation in physical activity, to be physically active role models, and to include physical activity in family events.

5. Schools provide training to enable teachers, and other school staff to promote enjoyable, lifelong physical activity among students.

Just because quality health and fitness is now mandated by the federal government it does not mean that each individual school will fulfill it. It ultimately is up to the teachers and the administration to see that it is implemented. If is going to happen in your school the responsibilities of the physical education specialist must extend well beyond the gym class. He/she will need to be working with the administration, classroom teachers and staff to see that these school-wide activities are being carried out. And it means that the classroom teachers must be supporting daily physical activity opportunities, infusing health instruction into their lessons, and modeling good health behaviors. If the classroom teachers do not become actively involved in these school wellness committees the law's intent will not be fully accomplished.

In this book you will be given ideas of how the health and fitness specialists and classroom teachers can work with each other, the administration, parents, and community members to produce health changes in children. You will be presented a few specific overriding goals around which you can focus your planning and instruction. You will learn the basic physiological principles of exercise and the pedagogical principles of teaching motor skills. You will learn the basics of sound nutrition. You will be given simple ideas of how to effectively manage your classes in the gym or playing field environment. You will be given many new physical activities ideas that meet the standard of everyone being active, safe, and successful. You will learn how to select and modify games to make them more enjoyable and educational. You will encounter techniques for affecting behavior changes beyond the school. You will be given feasible assessment ideas for verifying learning and motivating yourself and your students. There is also a chapter on a range of questions commonly asked by classroom teachers about teaching physical activities: how to include special needs children, what are one's safety and legal responsibilities, what are physical activities which can be done in the classroom or other limited space, etc.

An important amount of attention has been directed at the affective domain. If you are like most teachers or prospective teachers, you have a major goal of helping children to become better citizens. Even more than teaching them how to read and write and attain other content skills, you may wish to improve their ability to cooperatively get along with others (regardless of capabilities, gender, social status, or ethnicity), persevere at tasks, be helpful and caring, take responsibility for their actions and their role in the community. These affective behaviors can be well taught through the avenue of physical activities. Practicing individual motor and fitness skills, participating in partner and group cooperative games, and competing in sports activities under effective tutelage can serve as an ideal laboratory for the application of good affective behaviors. You will be given workable guidelines and instructional approaches for achieving them.

Another issue closely dealt with in this text is that of competitive sports. Some of you may have had very positive experiences with sports and are thinking that you would love to offer a similar beneficial experience to your students or to the youth sports teams you may coach. You remember the joy and the excitement, the close camaraderie, and the perseverance and teamwork skills learned. Others of you might have a much different recall of your competitive sports experiences. You might still feel the sting of embarrassment or ridicule that peers, teachers, or coaches may have laid on you or other unfortunates. You remember the inequality of the rewards and the frustration of working towards unattainable targets. Because this author recognizes the potentially powerful influence of competition, careful consideration has been devoted to it throughout much of the book. Many ideas are given to get children focusing on self-improvement-mastery goals and away from social-comparison goals. Also, various suggestions are made to insure that competitive experiences are consistent with a humanistic educational process.

    I hope you enjoy reading this text. May you read it carefully and weigh the concepts and implications they hold for both your personal health practices and teaching career. And finally, may the ideas presented stir you to take an active part in our weekly class discussions. That is the only way to derive full benefit from the course.

[CHAPTER 1]

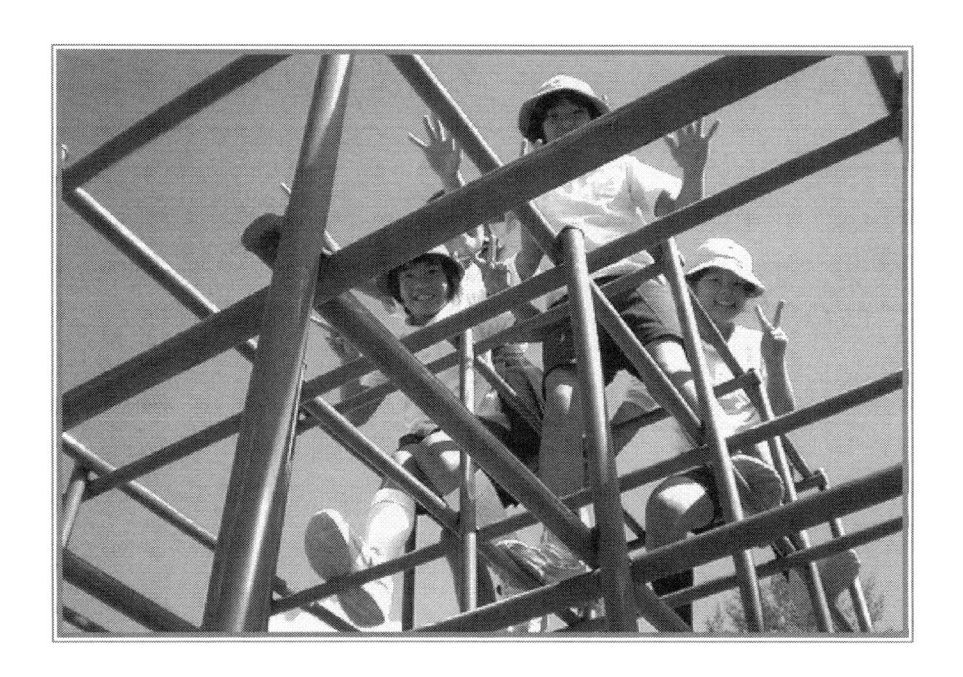

THE IMPORTANCE OF YOUR TEACHING HEALTH & FITNESS

THE IMPORTANCE OF HEALTH AND FITNESS

Immediate Quality of Life
Quality of Life as We Age
Length of Life

EXERCISE & HEALTH PRACTICES OF AMERICANS

Exercise
Nutrition
Sleep
Brushing and Flossing
Sun Exposure
Smoking Tobacco

HOW YOU CAN PLAY A CRUCIAL ROLE

The Classroom Teacher
The Specialist

CHAPTER COMPREHENSION CHECK

> *"When Health is absent, Wisdom cannot reveal itself; Art cannot become manifest; Strength cannot be exerted; Wealth is useless; and Reason is powerless."*
> ~ Herophilus (300 B.C.)

> *"Exercising and recreation are as necessary as reading, I will rather say more necessary because health is worth more than learning."*
> ~ Thomas Jefferson

Before we begin to discuss how you might play a crucial role in the teaching of health the fitness let us first consider the importance of exercise and health. Then we will look at the exercise and health status of the American people. An introductory coverage of these two topics will increase your belief that elementary schools badly need to address this subject.

THE IMPORTANCE OF HEALTH AND FITNESS

"Unless you have health you have nothing!" You probably have heard this or a similar adage spoken many times. Ask anyone and they will agree that good health is your most valuable asset. Anyone who is ill or has been ill in the recent past will certainly agree. Without health a fully enjoyable and productive life is simply not possible. Ralph Waldo Emerson said, "Give me health and a day, and I will make the pomp of emperors ridiculous."

Today's research provides irrefutable evidence of the enormous benefits exercise and sound health habits can have on (1) the immediate quality of life, (2) the quality of life as we age, and (3) the length of life itself. Let us briefly consider each one of these.

Immediate Quality of Life

Most people do not exercise to promote the long-term quality or length of their lives, certainly not many young people. They do it for the very real benefits it can confer here and now. The most common reasons people give for being active is that it is fun, it makes them feel better, it helps them control body fat, and it firms their muscles. But research shows that activity has many other immediate consequences, any one of which would make it well worth doing. Some diverse, clearly documented physiological and psychological benefits of physical activity are: better sleep patterns, higher resistance to infections and more rapid recovery, increased perceptions of energy, better ability to cope with psychological stresses, sharper cognitive processing, improved regularity, better sexual functioning, reduced levels of depression and anxiety, more optimistic outlooks, stronger bones, better flexibility, less arthritic problems, and better overall feelings about physical appearance.

The late George Sheehan was a well-known physician and exercise physiologist. He stated that in the normal course of his medical practice he would have many people come to him for physical check-ups. Invariably, those patients who were not following an active lifestyle would make comments like "What is the matter with me Doc? I feel run down, lethargic, lack energy, depressed." After finding no specific, identifiable ailment he would make this diagnosis, "There is nothing unusual here. Your symptoms are the body's natural response to not exercising. You are suffering from *exercise deficiency*." Sadly, many people may have never experienced, or have forgotten, what it feels like to be vigorously active and physically fit, and they may be unaware of the myriad benefits it can bestow upon one's current quality of life?

Quality of Life As We Age

The second valuable contribution of physical activity and a healthy lifestyle is how these can improve the long-term quality of our lives. I have a good neighbor who likes to make fun of my health conscious practices. On numerous occasions he has made only half in jest comments such as: "Why should I exercise or worry about exercising?" "Why should I follow a low-fat diet or quit smoking?" "I don't want to live longer only to end up in a nursing home and to be a burden on my children," "I'd rather enjoy life and then some day just drop off suddenly." While I respect the opinions of my friend in many things, we need realize that his thesis in this area is not supported by recent studies. The truth is quite the contrary. People who do not exercise regularly, who do not eat properly, or who smoke, will begin to witness clear decreases in their physical and capacities at rather young ages. Aerobic fitness levels begin to decline as soon as the early 20s, flexibility in the mid 20s, bone strength in the mid 30s, muscular strength losses will become apparent in the late 30s to early 40s. It is the gradual, progressive loss of these functions which begins to impinge upon the quality of one's life and limit what a person is capable of doing. Permit me to again personalize and once more pick on my neighbor. Although he is still in his 60s he cannot now do the yard and gardening tasks he used to enjoy. Other of my similarly aged friends who have accustomed themselves to regular robust exercise is not typically experiencing such limitations. These friends not only are doing the likes of yard and garden work, but are in many cases confidently planning long distance bicycling and hiking trips, climbing excursions, and other adventures.

Research indicates that those who remain active can slow the inevitable aging process by something like 20 years. In other words, a 50-year old person who is working to maintain the various components of fitness will likely display similar capacities to that of the inactive 30 year old. If individuals in their twenties remain active, they can expect a natural aging decrease in their abilities of approximately 5 to 10 percent per decade. Although declines of these magnitudes might prevent 40, 60, and 80 year olds from winning races against those in the May-time of their youth, these diminutions are not so great as to severely curtail the activity options of people well into their latter years.

At the Cooper Aerobics Institute in Dallas, Texas, some interesting data has addressed the reality of the nursing home issue. Cooper's records argue that it is those who do not maintain a well balanced, active lifestyle that are the ones in far greater danger of requiring care in their old age. According to him, morbidity (a period of ill health) will be a reality for many of the people who are not following a balanced exercise program. By balanced he meant that the person was exercising not only the aerobic system but was also training for muscular strength and joint flexibility. After all, while. Some people may loose the ability to fully take care of themselves because of various cardiovascular problems, others will encounter difficulties related to functional strength and flexibility. For example, they might not maintain enough strength to get in and out of the bathtub or to carry groceries. Their flexibility might deteriorate to the point where washing their feet is impossible or they cannot turn their head well enough to safely drive a car. Figure 1.1 shows 11.5 years to be the average length of time in which a sedentary person can expect to fall below the level of independence. If poor health habits do not result in an untimely death, more than a decade of dependent living is the expected norm. Notice how this period of morbidity is almost eliminated by adherence to regular exercise. Cooper calls this phenomenon *compressed morbidity*. Those who regularly exercise can generally expect to maintain functional abilities into their final years. Notice how the functional capacity curve of the active/fit individuals is maintained at a high level until pretty much the last months or year of their lives. It is also worth noting that the advances being made in modern medicine might be making this phenomenon of lifestyle compression of morbidity even more important in the future. Evidence suggest that medical care is actually contributing to an opposite trend or expansion of morbidity. Medical improvements have been tending to preserve life more than they have been improving its quality.

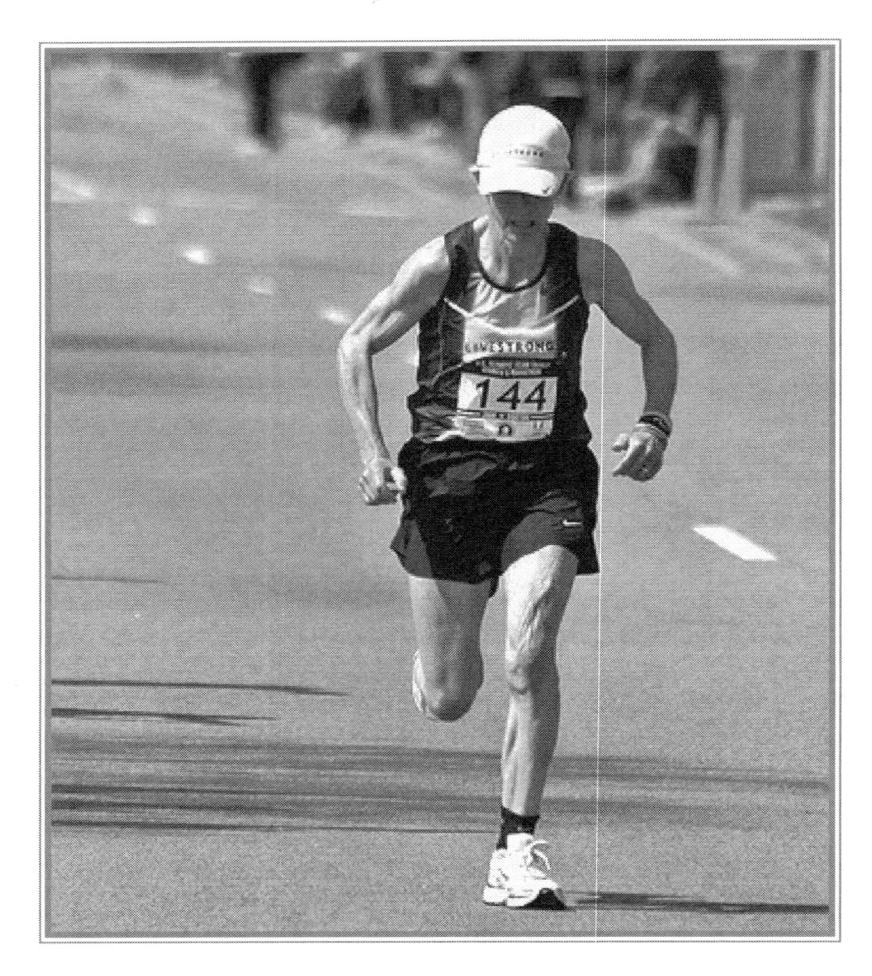

Sometimes I like to determine whether or not research findings really do relate to me. For the last 21 years I have run in the 12K "Bloomsday Race." Over that period of time I maintained a consistent body weight, and conscientiously trained and ran each race to the best of my ability. Here are my times at five-year intervals.

> 40 years old = 43:32 (5:50 per mile pace)
> 45 years old = 45:36 (6:06 per mile pace)
> 50 years old = 47:15 (6:21 per mile pace)
> 55 years old = 46:32 (6.15 per mile pace)
> 60 years old = 50:07 (6:46 per mile pace)

Although specific race times fluctuated due to injuries and weather and such, my long-term performance faithfully surrenders to the projected 5 to 10 percent projected decline across decades; I in fact experienced a 13 percent decline across those two decades. Of course it is always saddening to see aging steal upon us, but maybe there is a bright side. If we don't give up the struggle we just might be chugging along at 80 or 90 – like the woman in the above photo.

Health AND *Fitness* An Elementary Teacher's Guide

A final note needs to be made about the decline in abilities not being limited to bones and muscles and our ability to move. Later in life cognitive declines are also related to lifestyle practices. Both impaired cardiovascular functioning and excess body fat are associated with dementia and the incapacitation of Alzheimer's disease. Researchers have found a strong correlation between body mass index and high levels of beta-amyloid, the sticky protein substance that builds up in the Alzheimer's brain and is through to play a major role in destroying never cells.

Figure 1.1. Exercise and Compressed Morbidity

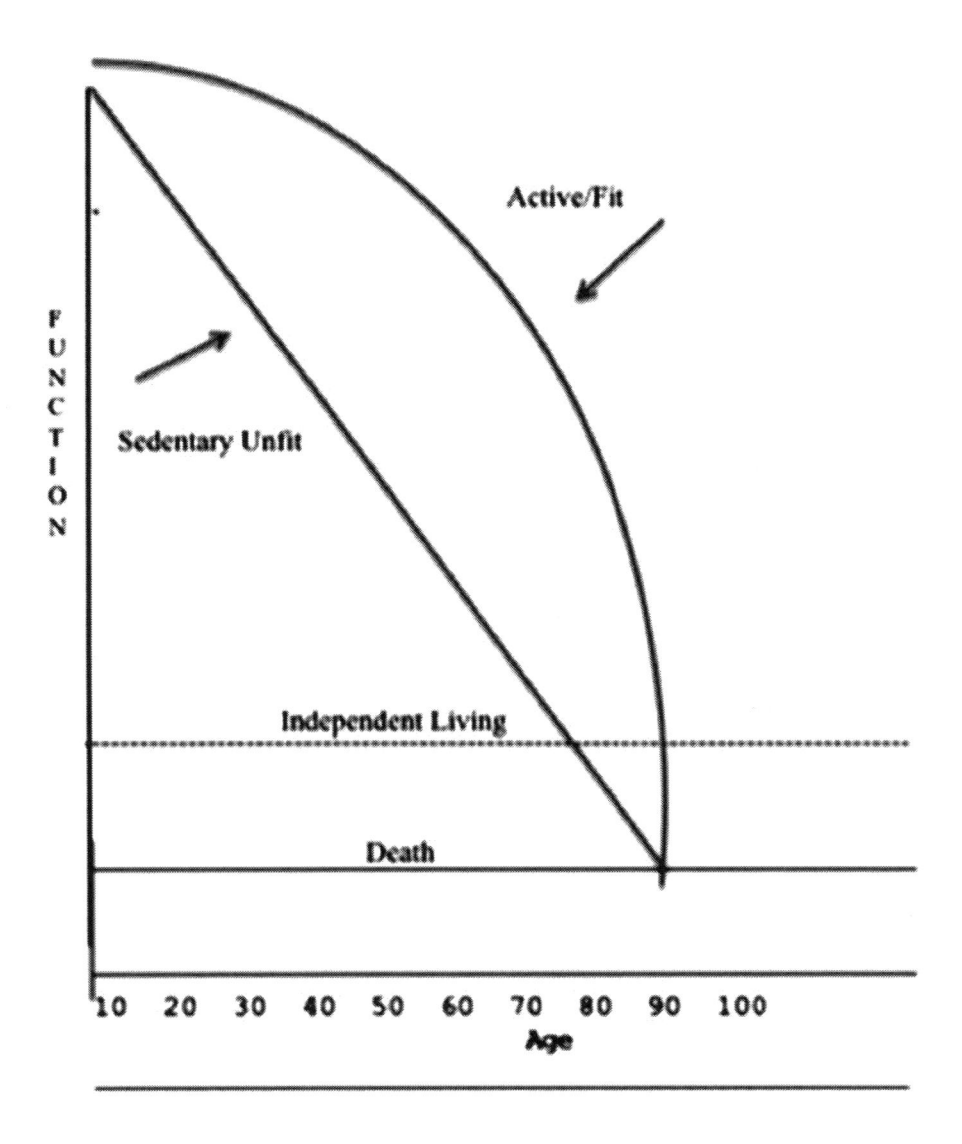

Length of Life

Finally, we need to realize that sound health practices play a big part in length of life. You may have had a friend or family member say something like; "When it's your time to go, it's time to go." "It's all genetics." "Look at that French woman who smoked her entire life and lived to be 120." While genetics obviously plays a role in length of any individual's life, it is foolish to disregard the powerful influence lifestyle contributes. The leading cause of death in both men and women is cardiovascular disease and unhealthy lifestyle practices are the chief cause of these high rates. Cancer is the second leading killer; 65 percent of which are attributable to diet, smoking, and lack of exercise (lung, colon, breast, prostate cancer all correlate with these lifestyle choices). Diabetes rates have soared in recent years and it is now the third leading killer. It is the leading cause of blindness, kidney failure and amputations and dramatically raises the risk of heart attacks. It effects 10 percent of the population and kills 180,000 Americans each year. The Center for Disease Control (CDC) estimates that of all babies born in 2000, one-third will become diabetic sometime in their lives unless they begin eating a lot better and getting a lot more exercise.

For the big picture, consider the overall longevity data; healthy men who do not exercise at all have a 3.44 times greater chance of dying from the three leading causes of death when compared to those who work out vigorously. This figure is even higher, jumping to 4.65 times greater, when sedentary women are compared to vigorously exercising women. When inactive individuals are compared to even lightly active men and women (walking as little as 5 city blocks a day, climbing 5 flights of stairs or engaging in 1/2 hour of vigorous sports on a daily basis) they have a 1.9 times greater chance of dying of these causes. Look at what happens to life span differences when an array of risk factors are added; the average life span is around 85 years for those who get regular exercise, maintain a low level of body fat, don't smoke, keep their blood pressure low, and control their cholesterol levels. On the other hand, those who control none of these risk factors have life expectancies only into the 60s. Of course, life is not always fair and the most fit and health conscientious of individuals could become ill, an invalid, and die young. But such untimely deaths are relatively rare. Untimely deaths are not rare in those who allow time to waste them and hope that genetics will be unusually kind to them.

EXERCISE & HEALTH PRACTICES OF AMERICANS

The opening section of this chapter verified some of the many immediate and long-term benefits sound health practices can yield. Let us now consider how well the United States' population is mining those golden benefits of health. I will state up front that a dispassionate survey of the data forces one to conclude that we are doing abysmally. The numbers in Figure 1.2 represent the percentage of adults who have been, and who now are classified as obese. Obesity is defined as having a BMI (Body Mass Index) of 30 or higher. The numbers are strikingly high and are exhibiting a nearly exponential pattern of increase. When the data is based upon a BMI of 25 or higher (the overweight cut-off) the percentages are doubled. A similar accelerating trend has been occurring in children and today approximately one third are classified as overweight.

Figure 1.2. Age-Adjusted Percentage of Obesity in American Adults Ages 20-71

	1960-62	1971-74	1976-80	1988-94	2001-04
Men	10.7	12.2	12.8	20.6	30.2
Women	15.7	16.8	17.1	26.0	34.0

Studies show that an overweight or obese child has an 80 percent chance of remaining so as an adult. Also, we suffer from much higher rates of cardiovascular disease, cancer and diabetes than is necessary. The Surgeon General has estimated that we could save 300,000 lives a year by eating better and exercising at modest levels (that is more deaths than are caused by infectious disease, firearms, motor vehicles and substance abuse combined). What a colossal tragedy we are permitting; it is equivalent to two loaded 747s crashing everyday of the year. This needlessly high rate of death and disability is even putting the economic future of our nation at risk because of the increasing cost of health care. It is believed that we could save 100 billion dollars yearly if we simply ate better and exercised more. Surely no national health care system will be less than exorbitantly expensive unless we can change our daily behaviors. When looked at from this perspective, taking at least minimal care of our bodies is a demonstration of socially responsible behavior (See Figure 1.3).

We next will survey the data collected on just some health practices. I do not doubt that you will agree that there are many areas in which health practices sorely need changing. Also, it will be obvious that these health habits are normally developed during the school years, usually the elementary years.

Figure 1.3. Causes of Death in the United States 1,120,000 Per Year

1. Tobacco	450,000
2. Diet & Physical Inactivity	300,000
3. Alcohol	100,000
4. Microbial Agents	90,000

5. Toxic Agents	60,000
6. Sexual Behavior	40,000
7. Firearms	35,000
8. Motor Vehicles	25,000
9. Illicit Use of Drugs	20,000

The feature of these statistics that strikes me is the relatively large numbers contributed by the first two categories. The implication to me is that while all of these factors are resulting in tragic numbers that warrant our attention, education regarding smoking prevention and the adoption of good eating and exercise habits is especially critical. Sometimes dramatic instances of such things as a firearm event or drug over-dose can capture our attention and generate preventive school programs, but can we afford to forget about the everyday common life patterns many of our children falling into?

Exercise

Modern research data has been confirming and expanding the diverse health benefits of physically active lifestyles. Inactivity is now considered a leading risk factor and getting Americans to be more active is listed as a major goal for our country. In the age of communication, this message is being constantly sent to the population through the newspapers, popular magazines and media broadcasts. When surveyed, 93 percent of today's American adults agree that regular exercise is one of the best things that can be done to preserve their health. Furthermore, parents are increasingly concerned about their children not getting enough activity. Almost 30 percent of them are somewhat or very concerned about their children's weight. Eighty percent do not want physical education classes in their children's schools reduced for academic classes, and less than half of parents think the schools are doing enough to teach active lifestyles to prevent obesity.

Given the above views it could be expected that adults would be exercising more and schools would be upgrading physical education and health and lifestyle instruction. The reality is otherwise. Less than 25 percent of American adults are classified as regular vigorous exercisers and over 25 percent remain resolutely *sedentary*. Sedentary is defined as not doing any exercise beyond that which is required at work, and of course, most jobs require much less manual labor than in the past. Only about 22 percent are active at a level recommended for any meaningful health benefits by the U.S. Department of Health and Human Services. These figures vary depending on what segment of the population you are considering. People earning less than $25,000 per year are 61 percent inactive while those above $50,000 are 37 percent inactive. Furthermore, current trends are towards less activity. It has been estimated that there has been nearly a 10 percent decline in adult's physical activity over each of the last two decades.

As you might expect, children with their eager supple bodies are more active than are adults. While they don't normally elect to jog or do other steady state aerobic activities for 30 minutes, they tend to be interval trainers, gleefully participating in frequent, short bursts of vigorous activity throughout the day. Young boys accumulate on average 68 minutes of activity a day and girls 59 minutes. However, we should note that the amount of activity children engage in decreases 50 percent across the school years until it is nearly down to the average adult levels by 12th grade. Most parents see their children involved in dance and/or sports lessons when they are 6, 8 or 10 years of age, but big dropouts occur thereafter. Fifty percent quit organized sports by age 12, 70 percent by age 14. Less than 21 percent of high school students are involved in even one school sport.

Probably the best activity generalization that can be made regarding the children you are likely to have in your classroom or gym class is to say that they will be a heterogeneous group. Some of the more athletic students will be taking advantage of expanded youth sport opportunities; they likely will be extremely well trained and skilled. You might also notice that some of these more athletic children are beginning to be tracked into serious pursuit of a single sport at younger and younger ages (we will address some concerns about this phenomenon of early *sport specialization* in a later chapter). At the other extreme, for reasons discussed in the following paragraphs, you will have intermixed in your class a growing segment of children who will be decidedly less active than our society has ever before experienced. For some of them, their fitness levels may already be so low as to be perceptibly impairing their quality of life.

Overall, children's current activity trends are not good. Mirroring the adult population, children have shown a decline of approximately 10 percent over the last couple of decades. I have listed four factors contributing to this drop. The major factor is probably today's ever-present media attractions (television, videos, movies and video games). Sixty-seven percent of children watch at least two hours of television a day, and 26 percent rack up four or more hours. This 25-hour per week average increases to 40 in the summer. Such a large amount of viewing time means the supplanting of much activity. It is interesting to note that a strong positive association exists between the amount of time a child watches television and the percent body fat of the child. For every extra hour averaged above the 25-hour norm, the child's percent body fat normally will be 2 percent higher. Children who watch at least four hours daily have about 20 percent more body fat than kids who watch fewer than two hours.

A second factor limiting children's activity is the reduction in activity during the school day due to less physical education time. Required physical education has been greatly reduced primarily because other expanded curriculum offerings and the pressure to meet state academic standards. The majority of high school students take physical education for only one year between ninth and twelfth grades. In addition, 48 percent of the states allow substitutions for high school physical education. Although elementary schools have experienced smaller decreases in physical education only 8 percent of elementary schools provide daily physical education. There also has been a trend toward fewer recess periods. Currently 71 percent of elementary schools provide regularly scheduled recess for students in all grades kindergarten through fifth.

The structure of our modern society and communities is a third factor that we are beginning to recognize as degrading activity. More working parents mean more school-age children are told to stay indoors until parents come home. Bored and lonely, the children munch, watch television and play video games. More and more children are now living in bigger cities or in suburban environments. Children in the cities might engage in less leisure time sandlot play because conveniently assessable play fields are not commonly available and the areas and surroundings may not be considered safe. For other reasons, neither are the suburban neighborhoods particularly conducive to physical play. These spread-out homes can create an isolating environment that hinders a number of children coming together for games. Also, suburban environments are designed with cars in mind and busy feeder roads can serve as access barriers to any park and recreational areas there may be. The distances between suburban homes and schools/commercial businesses tend to be long and hence so are commuting times. Not many years ago a fourth of all trips were made on foot or bicycle. Now, 90 percent of trips are made by car or bus. In the 1960s one of every two children walked or biked to school; that figure now is only one in ten.

Finally, *labor saving devices* are imperceptibly impacting overall activity levels. I think of these as unnecessary "exercise costing" devices. Each in itself would seem to play an insignificant role but even little things can accumulate over years of daily use. Around the home I am thinking of things such as electric can openers, automatic garage doors, power tools and mowers. In the community there are escalators, elevators, drive-through businesses, automatic doors, people to bag our groceries, etc.

Nutrition

Nutritional practices are now recognized as being far more important than once imagined. In the 1970s the new advocates of aerobics theorized exercise could free you to eat whatever you liked. That is not correct. We now know that eating poorly is a major ingredient in cardiovascular disease, diabetes, and in 60-70 percent of cancers, ranging from colon, to breast, to prostate, to skin.

The diet recommended by the United States Department of Agriculture (USDA), and the other major health organizations, would have no more than 25-30 percent of our calorie consumption coming from fat. Three-fourth of the adults and 5 of 6 school children do not meet that minimal guideline. It also recommends as a minimum that everyone have 5 servings a day of fruits and vegetables. Only 20 percent of children do so. Only 5 percent consume a better 7 per day. One-half eat no fruit during a given day, 25 percent no vegetables, 11 percent get neither. Twenty-five percent of children have a least one vegetable serving a day. Which vegetable do you think is twice as likely to be eaten than any other vegetable? If you guessed broccoli or cauliflower you are in need of a reality check. The correct answer is French-fries. The potato is of course good, but frying has turned it into a high fat food.

These practices result in children's average fiber consumption being approximately 5 grams; the recommended minimal level is 25 grams. You also can expect 19 percent of your children to have skipped breakfast. One-third of adolescent girls will be on a crash diet at any one time. About 1 percent of teen girls are anorexic or bulimic. Researchers say eating disorders appear to be on the rise and are affecting children as young as 8.

Fast food now accounts for more than 40 percent of Americans' food budget. That means they are spending more money on fast food than on higher education, personal computers, computer software, or new cars. That is more spending on fast food than on movies, books, magazines, newspapers, videos, and recorded music combined. The amount of calories in these highly processed foods are much higher than traditional fare and result has been a 6 percent increase in calorie consumption in the last 15 years. Children eating at a fast-food restaurant are almost a daily occurrence. In a typical week there will be a downing of three hamburgers and four orders of French fries. Cookies and other baked sweets, potato chips and other salty treats, candy and gum account for more than half the snacks consumed by kids. During the last three decades children have increased their consumption of these high fat snack foods by 200 percent and are averaging about 300 more calories a day. They are five times more likely to have a carbonated soft drink or sweetened fruit drink than fruit juice for a snack. Also, many foods available to students in school are high in fat, sodium, and added sugars. For example, 62.8 percent of all milk ordered by schools in a typical week is high in fat (whole or 2 percent milk). The common food offerings are soft drinks, sports drinks, or fruit juices that are not 100 percent juice. There are also salty snacks, cookies, and other baked goods that are not low in fat.

Sleep

Getting enough sleep should be considered just as important as eating a healthy diet and exercising. It is recommended the young people get at least nine hours of sleep every night, but only about 15 percent do. A full quarter of them get less than six hours. Nearly 40 percent go to sleep after 11 o'clock on school nights. Every teacher knows that students who do not get adequate sleep do not attend well in class. The data confirms that sleep deprivation is linked to poorer grades. Those deprived of an hour's sleep performed less well on tests for reaction time, recall, and responsiveness, than the children who sleep the extra hour. Of even greater concern is the newer research establishing an association between decreased sleep and dozens of different illnesses and health problems. Among those are heart disease, diabetes, cancer and obesity.

Brushing and Flossing

American Dental Association Guidelines call for adults and children to be brushing their teeth a least twice a day, the optimal times being before going to bed and after breakfast. It is especially important to brush before going to bed because failing to do so gives bacteria as much as 8 to 10 hours to feast on food particles left on the teeth and produce enamel-eating acid. The flow of saliva in the mouth also is lower at night so food is less likely to be washed off the teeth. One in three children are not brushing their teeth before bed and less than half do so after breakfast. Furthermore, two to three minutes of brushing are considered necessary to thoroughly clean the teeth. Most children spend less than a minute. Children need to understand that their dietary practices also affect dental hygiene. Eating lots of fruits and vegetables is desirable. Limiting between meal snacks, especially sugary drinks and sticky sweets, is also good practice. And toothbrushes should be changed every 3 to 4 months.

ADA guidelines state that both adults and children should be flossing at least once each day. Children are generally considered capable of effectively flossing their own teeth by the age of 9 years. The ADA statistics indicate that adults are not modeling this behavior. Only about 12 percent of Americans floss daily, 39 percent floss less than daily, and 49 percent do not floss at all. Many dental professionals view flossing to be just as important as brushing. Most tooth decay and gum problems originate between the teeth and no amount of brushing is able to reach these sites. Furthermore, it is well to remember that more than tooth and gum damage can be the consequence of lax oral care. A substantial link has been made between gum disease and cardiovascular health. Some claim that taking good care of one's teeth is perhaps the most important thing that can be done for care of the cardiovascular system.

Sun Exposure

We all need some sun exposure; it is our primary source of vitamin D, which helps us absorb calcium for stronger healthier bones. It is also important in the regulation of blood pressure and insulin levels. But it does not take much time in the sun for most people to get the vitamin D they need, and unprotected exposure to the sun's ultraviolet rays can cause skin damage, immune system suppression, and even skin cancer. Skin cancer is the most commonly diagnosed cancer in the United States, accounting for as many as half of all cancer diagnoses. About 20 percent of all Americans will develop skin cancer in their lifetime.

Controversy exists among healthcare advisors over whether children should get their vitamin D primarily from supplements or from exposure to sunlight. The Environmental Protection Agency (EPA) advises that all children avoid the sun and take a vitamin supplement providing 100 percent of the Dietary Reference Intake. Other experts contend that brief sun exposure on bare skin (no sunscreen) is the best way to prevent vitamin D deficiency (5 to 15 minutes per day).

Research shows the skin of children to be especially vulnerable to damage from the sun. Most kids rack up between 50 percent and 80 percent of their lifetime sun exposure before age 18, so it is important that they be taught how to enjoy fun in the sun safely. A fundamental guideline for everyone is to avoid being in the sun for prolonged times when it is highest overhead and therefore the strongest (normally from 10:00 AM until 4:00 M in the northern hemisphere). When children are in the sun between these hours they should habitually wear brimmed hats and protective clothing and/or sunscreen (SPF of 15 or more). The sunscreen should be applied 20 minutes before outside sun exposure so that the skin has time to absorb it. It should be applied generously and about every two hours while outdoors. Sweating, swimming, and toweling off will quickly remove a sunscreen's protection, so even water-resistant sunscreens need to be reapplied regularly. These recommendations remain applicable even on cloudy overcast days because Ultra Violet rays travel through the clouds and reflect off sand, water, and even concrete. They also apply to individuals with darker skin color. Although their skin contains more melanin, which provides some protection from the UV rays, any level of tanning or burning is damaging to the skin.

Sun exposure damages the eyes as well as the skin. Cumulative exposure can lead to cataracts later in life (clouding of the eye lens, which results in blindness). The best way to protect eyes is to wear sunglasses. Purchase sunglasses with labels ensuring that they provide 100 percent UV protection.

Smoking Tobacco

Tobacco smoking is perhaps the health habit that has drawn the most attention in recent years and in which major reductions have occurred in the adult population. In the 1950s over half our population smoked and currently that figure has dropped to just under one quarter. However, the snake is only scotched and not killed. Adult rates have shown only slight decreases in recent years despite heightened taxes, restrictions on pro-smoking advertising, and increased anti-smoking messages. Smoking could rightly be considered the worst of health habits. It has disastrous affects on those who continue to smoke (killing 450,000 yearly) and it passively damages many others. Refer again to Figure 1.3 and its unrivaled ranking as a leading cause of death.

Thirty percent of high school seniors said they smoked cigarettes in 1983 and there has been an increase in recent years. Eighty percent of adult smokers started as teenagers and the average starting age has become younger and younger until today it is at 12.5 years of age. This certainly means that it is not too early to begin smoking prevention instruction at the elementary level. Children by definition are immature, and are consequently most foolishly affected by peer pressure to take up the bad habit.

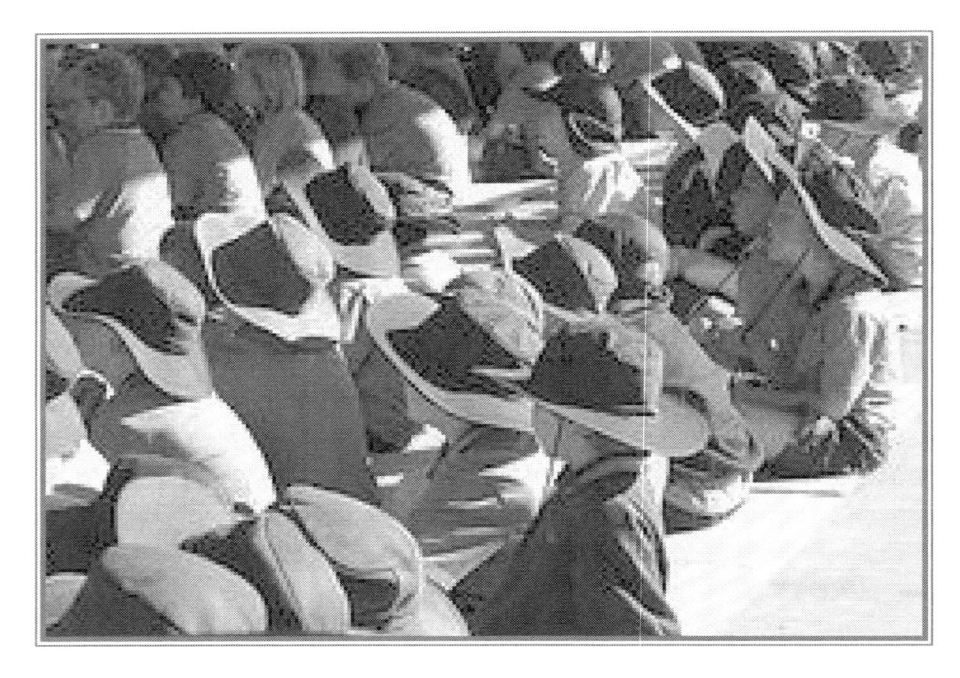

Figure 1.4. Getting Serious About Sun Safety
If a school is serious about teaching sun safety it will require the children and teachers to wear sunhats during recess periods and other outdoor events. When I was teaching in Australia the students and teachers regularly wore uniform wide-brimmed hats similar to those in the above photo. Everyone was happily acculturated to the practice.

HOW YOU CAN PLAY A CRUCIAL ROLE

The prior sections may have reaffirmed your belief that health is important and that something needs to be done to improve the exercise and health practices of Americans. Hopefully, it has also increased your awareness that these habits are more often than not established during the childhood years, and that it is therefore appropriate for elementary schools to address the problem. The question you may be asking yourself is what exactly will be your responsibility in this effort. Let us separately consider the roles of the classroom teacher and specialist. Doing so will make clear how each must collaborate with the other, and how each is crucial.

The Classroom Teacher

The questions you may be asking yourselves are "Why me?" "Why do I need to be concerned about teaching this subject?" "Will this not be the province of the physical education specialist?" "Will I not be too busy teaching an extremely large array of other subject matter?"

First consider the reality that you quite possibly will not be in a school in which a physical education specialist is available to provide daily or even frequent instruction to the children. Although there are variations throughout the States and in the different sized schools, the classroom teacher does the bulk of physical education; and the physical education specialists do virtually no instruction in health. The average elementary physical education instructor is responsible for something like 600 to 800 children. Furthermore, the number of physical education specialists has been decreasing in recent years because of the financial difficulties faced by schools. It would not seem unreasonable to expect schools to continue to face similar or even greater funding difficulties in the future. The states are demanding schools meet health and fitness standards at the same time schools generally lack funds to hire sufficient numbers of specialists. The most common situation is one in which you will have a physical education specialist about once or twice per week and in some schools there will be none at all. But even if your school is fortunate to have the most effective specialist on a fairly regular basis, he/she will unlikely be able to single-handedly produce the size of habit changes needed. Throughout this text I will be espousing the view that the lifestyle of children will not be significantly improved unless all teachers and administrators create a concerted front.

Secondly, there is no question that classroom teachers are being asked to teach more and more. More time needs to be devoted to the basics and yet many other critical subjects of concern are demanding attention. Is it fair for one more faction or interest group to be demanding a place in the curriculum? Yes it is entirely fair, not because physical education and health are inherently of greater importance than any other subject, but because full achievement in all other areas is contingent upon children being healthy. Children will not be as happy and they will not think and attend as well when inactive and unfit. This contention has been supported by curricular studies. In these studies, children typically have achieved better academic performance when schools have increased the curriculum time devoted to physical education. There is good justification to be encouraging school systems to put the fourth "R" back into education –Reading, wRiting, aRithmetic, and Recreation. It is developmentally indefensible to have children sitting for hours at school and at home, and that is what many young people are learning from our culture.

One other question you might have regarding your instructing of health and physical activity is this, "Even if I am convinced my children could benefit from instruction in this area, is it reasonable to expect that I can do it effectively if I have not had an athletic background and do not feel myself to be as physically fit as I should be?" You most certainly can! You do not need be a skilled athlete or the perfect template of fitness. Obviously, having a limited sports background will make it more difficult to teach some movement skills, but that does not mean there are not others you may be able to effectively instruct. As for health and fitness, if you believe in the importance of health and the active lifestyle, and particularly if you are making a sincere effort to realize their fulfillment, you have the essentials of being a powerful influence on the attitudes and behaviors of all those around you. There is no reason you should not be able to deliver a forceful message and one which will be credulously received by your students. I have had numerous beginning teachers come back to me and say that they initially feared teaching in this area because of perceived weakness in their motor and/or fitness abilities, but after attempting some instruction they were glad they had done so. They found the students liked and benefited from their efforts. As an added plus, some of the teachers felt as though working in an activity context enabled them to get to know and understand their students better.

If you have the will, the purpose of the rest of this book is to provide you with the way. In the following chapters you will be provided with the tools you will need. You will be introduced to guiding philosophies and goals, effective teaching methods and procedures, easy-to-use activity ideas, and answers to questions that are commonly voiced by classroom teachers as they begin to teach health and physical activity to children.

The Specialist

The current and looming health problems of your children have become so well recognized in recent years that society is demanding schools take serious action. As introduced in the Preface, in 2004 the Federal Government responded with passage of the Child Nutrition and Reauthorization Act. (Public Law 108-265: Section 204). The law requires every school district that participates in the federal school meal programs to establish a wellness policy. It states that a committee must set yearly wellness goals and assessment procedures. Besides ensuring that a healthy food environment is created, and that comprehensive nutrition instruction is occurring throughout the curriculum, the schools are responsible for pursuing various means of promoting regular physical activity. As introduced in the Preface, the schools are specifically charged with seeing to the following:

> 1. **Students are given opportunities for physical activity during the school day through physical education classes, daily recess periods for elementary school students, and the integration of physical activity into the academic curriculum.**
>
> 2. **Students are given opportunities for physical activity through a range of before and/or after-school programs including, but not limited to, intramurals, interscholastic athletics, and physical activity clubs.**
>
> 3. **Schools work with the community to create ways for students to walk, bike, rollerblade or skateboard safely to and from school.**
>
> 4. **Schools encourage parents and guardians to support their children's participation in physical activity, to be physically active role models, and to include physical activity in family events.**
>
> 5. **Schools provide training to enable teachers, and other school staff to promote enjoyable, lifelong physical activity among students.**

RECESS FOR ELEMENTARY SCHOOL STUDENTS
2006 National Association of Sport and Physical Education (NASPE) Position Paper

It is the position of NASPE that all elementary school children should be provided with at least one daily period of recess of at least 20 minutes in length.

Recess is an essential component of a comprehensive school physical activity program and of the total education experience for elementary school students. Various organizations including the U.S. Department of Health and Human Services and the United States Department of Education, Centers for Disease Control and Prevention, National Association for the Education of Young children, and American Association for the Child's Right to Play support school recess as an integral component of a child's physical, social, and academic development. Recess provides children with discretionary time to engage in physical activity that helps them develop healthy bodies and enjoyment of movement. It also allows children the opportunity to practice life skills such as cooperation, taking turns, following rules, sharing, communication, negotiation, problem solving, and conflict resolution. Furthermore, participation in physical activity may improve attention, focus, behavior, and learning in the classroom.

National recommendations state that school-aged children and youth should participate in at least 60 minutes per day of moderate to vigorous physical activity. Participation in a regularly scheduled recess period can make an important contribution toward meeting this recommendation. In addition, extended periods of inactivity (two or more hours) are discouraged for elementary-age children.

All children in elementary schools should engage in at least one daily period of recess for at least 20 minutes per period. Recess does not replace physical education classes. Physical education provides sequential instruction to enhance the development of motor skills, movement concepts, and physical fitness. Recess provides unstructured play opportunities that allow children to engage in physical activity.

Recess is not viewed as a reward but as a necessary education support component for all children. Therefore, students should not be denied recess so they can complete class work or as a means of punishment.

The mandates of PL 108-265 illustrate the broadened wellness role that is being expected of today's physical educators. Full and effective implementation of school/community-wide wellness practices such as those stated in PL 108-265 will not likely occur without the participation of physical education personnel. As the specialist, you must be a key player in activities such as: the school's wellness committees, the coordination of physical activity opportunities of everyone (students, faculty and staff) throughout the school day and beyond, and the establishment and maintenance of a healthy eating environment. In essence your role has changed from that of the traditional gym teacher to that of school/communitywide wellness director. As demanding as teaching physical education classes and coaching is, it is no longer sufficient. Teaching sports and movement activities in the gym and on the playing fields is only part of the new job description. Refer to the accompanying box, *Physical Education Needs Good People*. It summarizes the skills and interest you will need, and the rich rewards it will yield to you and society.

PHYSICAL EDUCATION NEEDS GOOD PEOPLE:
A PROFESSION FOR YOU?

The health of our society is at risk. Obesity rates, diabetes, high blood pressure, osteoporosis and other health problems have been significantly rising in recent years. This is occurring because both American adults and children are getting less physical activity, are not eating well, and often are not following other good health practices. There are many reasons for this: our workdays are longer and more sedentary; commuting is taking longer and we often don't have safe or convenient places to exercise; all kinds of labor saving devices surround us and rob us of activity; our rapid paced lives cause us to skip meals and rely more on high calorie fast and processed foods; and ever increasing media attractions bombard us with advertisements for unhealthy foods as we are enticed to sit more and more hours in front of TVs, videos and computers.

To reverse this trend elementary, middle, and high schools need to be encouraging and showing young people how to live healthfully in today's society. Just playing team games and sports in gym class will not be sufficient. Today's physical educators must also be introducing both individual sports and recreational activities. They need to be providing practical ways students can fit non-competitive, light-to-moderate paced activities into their daily routines. They need to help with goal setting and assessing the children's activity levels throughout the school day and beyond. They must teach young people how to eat better and show them how they can progressively begin to do so.

SKILLS AND INTERESTS YOU WILL NEED FOR THE JOB

Commitment to a wellness lifestyle
Living it is part of teaching it. You must be an excellent model of regular physical activity, good nutrition, and all other health practices (good hygiene, use of seat belts and helmets, avoidance of tobacco products and excessive sun exposure, appropriate use of drugs and alcohol, sound sleep and relaxation techniques for coping with stress, etc.).

Enjoy learning various kinds of physical skills
Many people maintain fitness through skill-based activities such as tennis, swimming, golf, basketball, aerobics, bicycling, hiking, and rock climbing. Although you do not have to be a great athlete you must be interested in, and able to provide, competent explanations and demonstrations of a variety of physical skills.

High energy level and interest in working with young people
You must be enthusiastic about working with a diverse population of children, particularly the lower skilled and unmotivated; it is they who are often at the greatest health risk. You will be on your feet and moving both throughout the school day and during after school programs and sports.

Team player within the school and community
You will not be able to accomplish the ambitious goal of changing the students' lifestyles by staying isolated in the gym. You will need to initiate interaction among the administration, teachers, staff, parents, and community leaders in order to develop a concerted school-wide health promotion effort. This will involve organizing and participating in extracurricular events/meetings.

Lifelong learner
You will establish the fundamentals of teaching health and physical education in your undergraduate degree program, but the person who dares to teach can never cease to learn. You must be the type of person who will want to remain active in professional organizations, attend conferences, read journals, and take classes.

> **BENEFITS YOU CAN EXPECT:**
>
> Teaching is a respected profession with good job security and health benefits. Although it is a time and energy-demanding job, it provides ample holiday opportunities throughout the year and during summer. Relocation potential is excellent in that teachers are needed from one end of the country to another and abroad. The possibilities exist for you to be able to work in rural areas, cities, suburbs, and with children of diverse ethnic and social backgrounds. Finally, the physical educator gets to share in the excitement of kids moving and learning. Nothing could be more important and rewarding than influencing kids' physical and social lives for the better. They will remember you for it and it will keep you young.

As with the classroom teacher, the purpose of the rest of this book will introduce you to some guiding philosophies and goals, effective teaching methods and procedures, and easy-to-use activity ideas that are appropriate for elementary aged students. Your other course work will have provided you with a sound foundation in the kinesiology sciences (anatomy, exercise physiology, motor learning, biomechanics, etc.) and in the pedagogy of movement skills (administration, adapted physical education, measurement and evaluation, etc.). This text will specifically show how that knowledge can be applied to teaching health and fitness in the schools.

Although the focus of this text is on teaching kindergarten through six-grade my own published research findings have determined that approximately 80 percent of health and fitness pre-service students are planning to teach in secondary schools. Along with coaching interests, their high school physical education experiences may have been the deciding factor in being predisposed towards the older grades. If such is the case with you, do not let it deter you from an honest perusal of this text and involvement in this course. Not only will it have relevancy for all of teaching, but contrary to expectations, circumstances may find you teaching in the elementary grades. The number of health and fitness job openings is expanding much more vigorously in elementary school as compared to secondary school. Also, you may come to learn that teaching at the younger levels has its unique rewards in terms of student enthusiasm and receptivity to lifestyle changes. I as an undergraduate student never thought of working at this level and yet here I am and have been for over 35 years.

CHAPTER COMPREHENSION CHECK

1. What is the approximate percent of children currently overweight or obese? (Preface)
2. Are both adults and children getting more or less exercise than 10 or 20 years ago? (Preface)

3. Have the nutrition practices of adults and children been improving, staying the same, or deteriorating (both with regards to nutritional value and calorie consumption)? (Preface) *Deteriorating*
4. What are the basic tenets of the *2004 Child Nutrition and WIC Reauthorization Act*? (Preface)
5. In what ways does exercise affect one's quality of life?
6. What is *exercise deficiency*?
7. What is *compressed morbidity* and how does exercise affect it?
8. Over the decades of aging through our 30s, 40s, 50s, 60s, approximately what percentage of our physical capabilities can we expect to lose?
9. What are the 3 leading causes of death and what is their relationship to lifestyle practices?
10. What approximate percentage of babies born in 2000 can expect to become diabetic unless lifestyles change a whole lot?
11. Approximately how much longer can someone expect to live as a result of following a good lifestyle compared to an unhealthy one? *15 yrs*
12. What is the approximate likelihood of an overweight/obese child becoming an overweight/obese adult? *80%*
13. Given a listing of the causes of death, which ones would be near the top, which ones near the bottom? What would be the approximate differential among them?
14. Approximately what percentage of the adult population could be classified as regular exercisers? what approximate percentage sedentary? *regular - 25   more than 25*
15. Approximately what percentage of youths quit sport by the age of 12? *50*
16. What are the reasons adults and children are getting less exercise today than 10 or 20 years ago?
17. Approximately what percent of children walk or bike to school? *10%*
18. Fat should make up approximately what percentage of one's diet? *20-30%*
19. Approximately what percentage of children get 5 fruits/vegetables in their diet each day? what percentage get 7 fruits/vegetables? *5-20%   7-5%*
20. What is the recommended grams of fiber to have in one's diet? What is the average consumed by children each day? *25 grams → 5 grams*
21. What is the recommended hours of sleep for children? What approximate percentage of children is getting it? *9 - 15% get it*
22. How often and how long should children be brushing their teeth? Approximately how often and how long are they doing so? *2 times, 2 to 3 mins → 1 min*
23. Relative to brushing, how important is flossing viewed? At what age should children be expected to begin flossing?
24. What are some basic sun-safety practices children should be following?
25. What is the approximate average starting age for smoking? How dangerous is the practice? *12.5 yrs   1x age*

- Is curriculum time allotted to Physical Education and Recess increasing, decreasing, or staying stable?
- What is meant by the broadened role of the physical education specialist?
- What is NASPE's stance regarding and amount and need for recess for elementary children? *At least one 20 mins*
- What approximate percentage of pre-service physical education teacher expect to teach at the high school level? What level shows the greatest increase in job openings?

[CHAPTER 2]

MODELS FOR PHYSICAL ACTIVITY AND NUTRITION

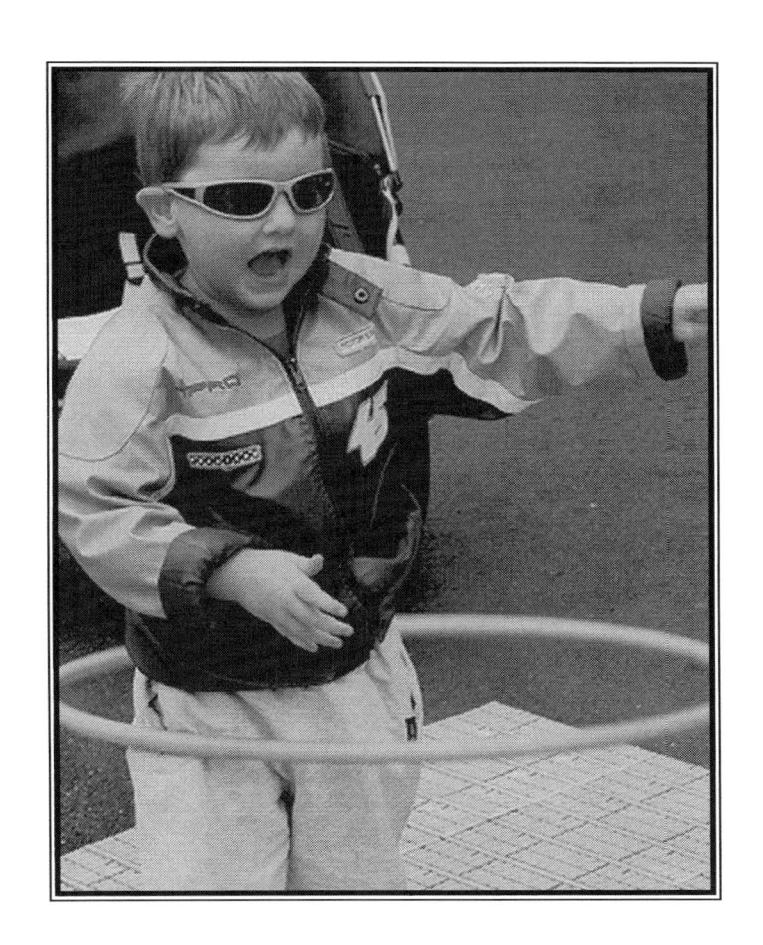

MODELS FOR PHYSICAL ACTIVITY

The Activity Pyramid

MODELS FOR NUTRITION

The Healthy Eating Pyramid
The Vegetarian Pyramid
Health Reasons
Environmental Reasons
Ethical Reasons

CHAPTER COMPREHENSION CHECK

> "*Not less than two hours a day should be devoted to exercise, and the weather shall be little regarded. I speak this from experience having made this arrangement of my life. If the body is feeble, the mind will not be strong.*"
> ~ Thomas Jefferson

> "*Health and good estate of body are above all gold, and a strong body above infinite wealth.*"
> ~ Ecclesiastics 30:15

Establishing physically active lifestyles and sound nutritional practices are central to healthful living. This chapter will review the major existing physical activity and nutrition models and will recommend those that might best be applied to the instruction of our children.

MODELS FOR PHYSICAL ACTIVITY

In recent American history three basic physical activity models have been developed. The first two, the *Exercise Prescription Model* and the *Lifestyle Activity Model*, were formulated for adult populations but used as guides for both adults and children. In this section brief histories of these two models will be given. Their strengths and weaknesses will be presented. It will become apparent that neither of them fully matches the physical and psychological needs of children. A separate section is then devoted to the *Activity Pyramid*. It is offered as a useful guide specifically designed to meet the needs of children and to lead them into valuing and adopting an active lifestyle.

Prior to the 1960s there had been relatively little research on the effects exercise had on the body. Myths were rampant. When I was in school in the 1950s and 1960s I was taught that strength training caused a loss in flexibility ("muscle boundness"), swimming resulted in a softening of muscles, running was not good for women's internal organs, and vigorous cardiovascular exercise risked over-stressing and damaging the heart. In consequence of these fears, and not knowing of the many physiological and psychological benefits exercise provided, the public generally left serious physical training to a rather small subset of mostly young male athletes. A seminal publication that began to change society's understanding and exercising practices was Kenneth Cooper's 1967 book entitled *Aerobics*. Cooper was a medical doctor who had been putting people through vigorous cardiovascular training programs, which have subsequently become known as the *Exercise Prescription Model*. The essence of the model has people engaged in three or four exercise bouts per week. Each bout usually is prescribed to last 20 to 40 minutes and the exercise is vigorous enough to raise and maintain heart rates in a target zone of something like 75 to 85 percent of maximum capability. Cooper found that when men and women followed this type of continuous-vigorous training for a number of weeks or months they experienced numerous health benefits. Short-term improvements were found in the forms of stronger stroke volume, lowered blood pressure, and decreased body fat. And tracking over a period of years began to show decreases in heart attacks, strokes, and diabetes.

Cooper's book and the work of other researchers had a profound influence on the exercise habits of Americans. The "fitness boom" of the 1970s and 1980's ensued with running events materializing in almost every community. Aerobic dance classes and videos became popular. The *Exercise Prescription Model* became commonly employed by instructors for all kinds of activities and all kinds and ages of participants. And it continues to this today to be widely followed. Step aerobics instructors have their students feeling for their pulses, elliptical and stair-climbing machines are fitted with heartbeat sensors, and school children have heart rate monitors strapped on to them in gym class.

The long-standing *Exercise Prescription Model* has bourn the test of time and research by proving itself to be an appropriate model for adults and individuals interested in high-level performance as well as accompanying health benefits. As more and more modern-day research has been done a wider and wider range of health benefits have been detected in those who follow the model's prescriptions. However, a major practical weakness of the model has been the failure of most of the population to adhere to it. Although a segment of American adults religiously abides by and benefits from faithfulness to its strictures, society at large has never done so. At least 80 percent of the population does not follow the model at all, or have done so only sporadically. Compliance with the model demands not only the motivation to work at a rather high energy level, but it requires good time management. In addition to the block of time needed for actually exercising, preparation and showering time must be factored in. In this busy adult world, these barriers have proven to be formidable to the majority of the population.

Although it could be generally expected that children do not face the same degree of time commitments as do adult, the inherent nature of children does not predispose most of them to enjoyment of steady-state continuous exercise. My experience with children has found them to be inveterate *interval trainers*. By that I mean that they naturally like to engage in spurts of activity. They are always ready to rush into vigorous excitement for short periods but soon tire and want to stop. They relish the thrill and drama of all kinds of games that call for burst of energy and stoppages. Because of this I do not believe we should view children as merely miniature adults. They are fundamentally different and expecting and forcing them to stay in a high steady state of exercise will not be inherently attractive to most of them. I fear that setting this as an exercise goal might actually be counterproductive and reduce their likelihood of developing an active lifestyle rather than advancing it.

In more recent years an alternative to the *Exercise Prescription Model* as been adopted by the federal government and various health organizations. It is known as the *Lifetime Activity Model.* Epidemiological research in the 1980s and 1990s was discovering that a person's total amount of moving was strongly related to his/her health profile. People who accumulated as much as an hour of physical activity each day, even though it might be of a light to moderate intensity, were significantly healthier than those who did not do so. The majority of adults do not get that much activity and only 36 percent of youths get 60 minutes of activity on all or most days of the week. As a result you likely have seen and heard many commercials and promotions advocating the goal of exercising for an hour each day, six or seven days a week. Walking, gardening, golfing, biking, are typical of the light to moderately paced activities that will count. Another salient feature of the *Lifetime Activity Model* is that the physical activity does not need to be concentrated into an exercise bout but can be dispersed throughout the day, maybe 15 minutes here, 10 minutes there, whatever is convenient and adds up to the minimum hour criterion. An obvious advantage of the *Lifetime Activity Model* is its feasibility in comparison to that of the *Exercise Prescription Model*. From a motivational perspective it should be far easier to select enjoyable light/moderate paced activities than those requiring target-zone heart rates. Also, the greater flexibility of breaking the activity up to fit one's schedule goes a long way toward solving the often real "don't have time" excuse. There would seem to be no reason all Americans, with a little time management, should not be able to adopt and maintain this agenda, a far better result than the 10 to 15 percent faithful adherence rate of the *Exercise Prescription Model.*

The weakness of the *Lifetime Activity Model* pertains to the degree of the health benefits that can be potentially conferred. While it is undeniably true that regular light/moderate exercise produces measurably better fitness than sedentary ways, more vigorous training of the body just as assuredly yields still healthier consequences. Some hardliners criticize the model as a backing off from intensities that are known to be most effective. They fear that lowering of standards leads to a lowering of effort and the belief that less is sufficient. While the absence of vigorous activity is a debatable shortcoming of the model in regards to adults, for children it seems especially problematic. Motor development experts uniformly advocate all levels of physical activity for children. Optimal bone and muscle growth is contingent upon strenuous activity. The vigorous activity does not need to be of the long-term continuous sort, but highly energetic play is what the young naturally love and thrive upon. Although the light to moderate activity of the *Lifestyle Activity Model* is to be appropriately encouraged in children, as it is in adults, that kind of activity alone is unlikely to fully satisfy either the physiological or psychological needs of children. A carefully reviewed, more comprehensive model designed for children would seem appropriate. The *Activity Pyramid* meets those specifications.

The Activity Pyramid

The *Activity Pyramid* was originally developed in the 1990s by Dr. Charles Corbin, a leading authority in children's physical education. *The Activity Pyramid* presented in figure 2.1 is an updated refinement sponsored by the *National Association of Sport and Physical Activity* (NASPE). It is a conceptual model designed specifically for the growth and health needs of children ages 5 through 12. Furthermore it does not view children as miniature adults but recognizes their unique psychological propensities. It describes four levels of physical activities. The general idea is to accumulate at least 60 or more minutes a day from the first three levels.

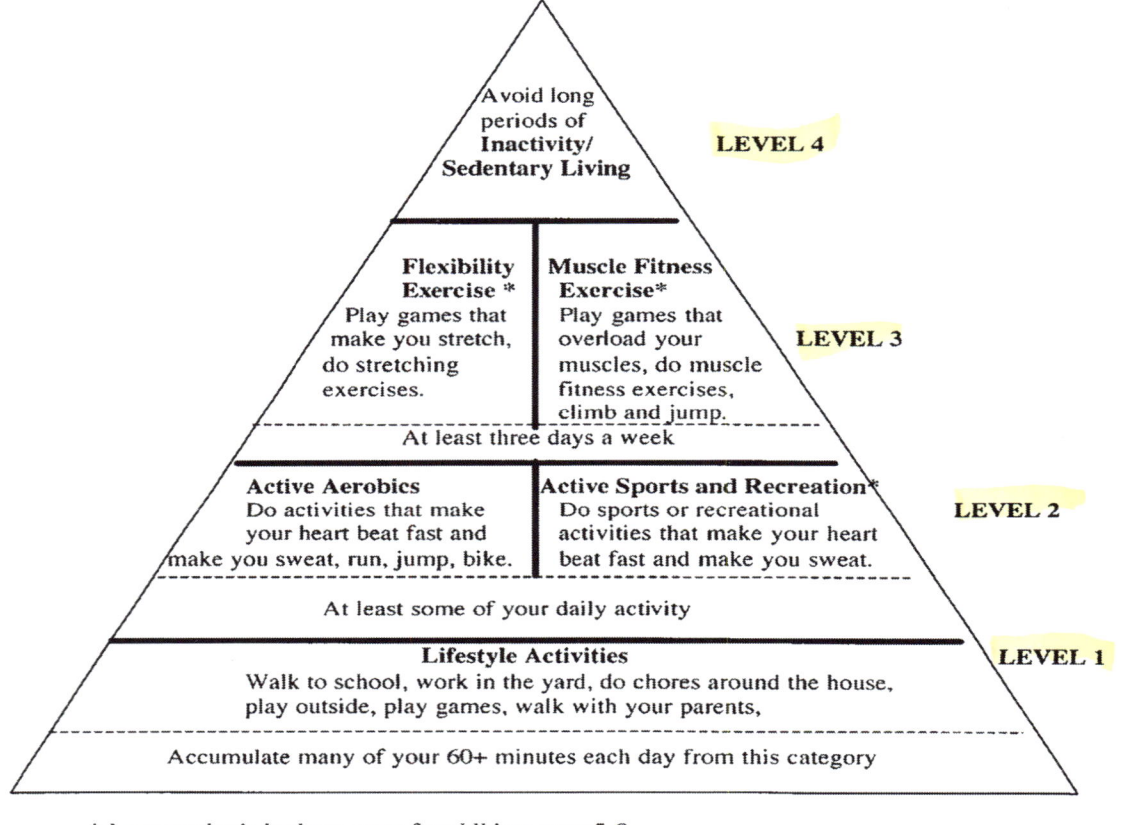

LEVEL 4 — Avoid long periods of Inactivity/Sedentary Living

LEVEL 3 — At least three days a week
- **Flexibility Exercise *** Play games that make you stretch, do stretching exercises.
- **Muscle Fitness Exercise*** Play games that overload your muscles, do muscle fitness exercises, climb and jump.

LEVEL 2 — At least some of your daily activity
- **Active Aerobics** Do activities that make your heart beat fast and make you sweat, run, jump, bike.
- **Active Sports and Recreation*** Do sports or recreational activities that make your heart beat fast and make you sweat.

LEVEL 1 — **Lifestyle Activities** Walk to school, work in the yard, do chores around the house, play outside, play games, walk with your parents. Accumulate many of your 60+ minutes each day from this category.

* Less emphasis in these areas for children ages 5-9.

Figure 2.1. The Activity Pyramid

At the base of the pyramid (level 1) lifestyle activities of a moderate intensity are emphasized. Such activities could be continuous or intermittent in nature and might include various games, loco-motor maneuvers, or dancing activities. A substantial portion of the accumulated minutes of daily activity should come from this tier, especially in younger children (ages 5 to 9).

The second tier (level 2) focuses on more vigorous activities (not necessarily continuous) that significantly raise heart rate and induce sweating. Fleeing and chasing activities, as well as sport activities involving large muscle groups (basketball, soccer) would fit into this tier. At least some of the daily activity should be performed at this level. Older children nearing adolescence (10 to 12 years of age) are more likely to choose aerobic or sport-based activities of a vigorous nature.

Exercises promoting flexibility and muscular fitness are stressed at level 3. The recommended frequency for this form of activity is a minimum of three times per week. In younger children such exercises might involve climbing, tumbling, and developmentally appropriate calisthenics. Older children can engage in stretching exercises and resistance exercises using resistive bands, light dumbbells, or body weight (calisthenics). More formal and regimented resistance training should be reserved for those who truly demonstrate an interest in the area and choose such a program

The fourth level of the pyramid addresses the final physical activity guideline in that children should limit extended periods of inactive pursuits.

THE PHYSICAL ACTIVITY PYRAMID GUIDELINES

Guideline 1: Children should accumulate at least 60 minutes, and up to several hours, of age-appropriate physical activity on all, or most days of the week: This daily accumulation should include moderate and vigorous physical activity with the majority of the time being spent in physical activity that is intermittent in nature.

Interpretation: Sixty minutes is the minimum amount of daily activity recommended for children. To attain optimal benefits, children need to accumulate more than 60 minutes per day. Physical activity minutes accumulated each day should include some moderate activity equal in intensity to brisk walking and some vigorous activity of greater intensity than brisk walking. Most physical activity accumulated throughout the day will come in intermittent activity bursts ranging from a few seconds to several minutes in length alternated with rest periods. Continuous vigorous physical activity of several minutes in length *should not* be expected for most children, nor should it be a condition for meeting the guidelines.

Guideline 2: Children should participate in several bouts of physical activity lasting 15 minutes or more each day.

Interpretation: Much of a child's daily activity will be in short bursts and accumulated throughout the waking hours. However, if optimal benefits are to accrue, as many as 50 percent of the accumulated minutes should be in bouts of 15 minutes or more. Examples of physical activity bouts are recess, physical education, play-periods, and sport's practices. Typically, most bouts of activity include both physical activity and inactivity for participants. For example, a child at recess may be active for 5 minutes and inactive for 10 minutes.

> *Guideline 3: Children should participate each day in a variety of age-appropriate physical activities designed to achieve optimal health, wellness, fitness, and performance benefits.*
>
> *Interpretation:* Three different levels of physical activity are described in the Physical Activity Pyramid. It is recommended that children select from all of the first three levels of activities in the pyramid each week.
>
> *Guideline 4: Extended periods (periods of two hours or more) of inactivity are discouraged for children, especially during daytime hours.*
>
> *Interpretation:* Research suggests that people (including children) who watch excessive amounts of television, play computer games, work on computers for extended periods of time, or engage in other low energy expenditure activities will likely fail to meet guidelines 1, 2 and 3. In general, extended periods (two hours or more in length) of sedentary behavior (in and out of school) are discouraged. Because many positive things can happen during times of relative inactivity (homework, studying, learning to read, write and think, and family time), some periods of relative inactivity may be necessary in a typical day. It is the accumulation of excessive inactivity (lack of activity accumulation) that is of concern. It is important that children be active when opportunities to be active are available such as before and after school, at appropriate times during school, and on weekends.

The specific guidelines of the *Activity Pyramid* are provided in the accompanying box. An important concluding implication to be drawn from the model is that sustained high-intensity exercise is not generally considered to be age appropriate for children. Most youths do not perceive continuous high-intensity exercise to be fun. When forced upon a child, this type of activity could have a negative effect on both current and future activity habits. Rather children should be encouraged to engage in unstructured active play and activities of an intermittent nature. Children might profitably be introduced to the concept that the heart rate changes with different levels and types of exercise, but the use of target heart-rate zones to monitor exercise intensity is not recommended for children age five to 12 unless the child is highly motivated and training for a sport.

MODELS FOR NUTRITION

In the 1960's when research unequivocally began to document the various health benefits of aerobic exercise, many of the authorities were claiming that here was a panacea for the rampant cardiovascular diseases the our nation. Dr. Kenneth Cooper, the author of the first aerobics book and considered the father of the aerobic movement, once believed that adherence to aerobic activities would actually have the benefit of allowing you to indulge all your dietary inclinations. Because activity would be burning those fats and calories you could eat about as much as you wanted, and whatever you wanted. It was just one of the joyous freedoms conferred by doing aerobics. Since those early days our knowledge of the benefits of physical activity has continued to expand but so has our appreciation of the critical role of sound dietary practices. To be truly healthy, physical activity and a sound diet must compliment each other. Americans, even if regularly active, will not be able to avoid cardiovascular diseases, diabetes, excessive body fat, cancers and other impairments if their nutritional practices continue as currently practiced.

You have heard many divergent views about what foods are good for you and which ones are bad. No doubt, friends and family have vowed, modeled and advised you as to the benefits of extremely different dietary practices. Each year new diet programs, supported by famous scientists and/or the testimonies of celebrities, are marketed in the popular media. The newspapers periodically have articles on some revolutionary nutritional data published in the likes of The New England Journal of Medicine or some other prestigious source. How then do we know what is correct and incorrect for our children and ourselves? It is necessary to say up front that nutrition is a complicated field and admit that there is much that researchers do not yet fully understand. As a consequence, we must realize that any model that is put forth will be necessarily subject to revisions as science progresses. Nevertheless there is a great deal that we have learned from thousands of nutritional studies done in the past couple of decades. In light of this current data I will be proposing the Harvard School of Public Health's Healthy Eating Pyramid (2008) or the closely related Vegetarian Pyramid as the most worthy nutritional goals. But prior to explaining each of these a brief history is needed to understand what has led me to select these models over that which is recommended by our federal government.

The federal government charges the United States Department of Agriculture (USDA) with the dual responsibilities of (1) providing the American public with nutritional guidance and (2) protecting the interests of American agricultural producers. Starting in the 1950s the USDA advised Americans about the four basic food groups: meat, milk and dairy, breads and cereals, and fruits and vegetables. Accordingly, if we ate from all four groups every day, especially the first two, we would be healthy. This advice reflected the nutritional knowledge of the day and it was pleasing to the powerful dairy and meat producers because of the larger market it created for its goods. Then, by the 1970s, medical research had began revealing the negative health effects of eating red meat and dairy produce, and scientists were lining up against its promotion. After lengthy debate throughout the eighties and early nineties the USDA Food Guide Pyramid was finally introduced to the public in 1992. This guide placed grains across the broad base of the pyramid as the food group we should seek out most. Fruits and vegetables took up a lot of space on the next level with meats and dairy as somewhat lesser players near the top, and sweets and fats taking up very little space at the pointed tip. Although this guide was a major improvement over the formerly unalloyed advocacy of greater dairy and meat consumption, it did not fully reflect the research concerns regarding the extent of their use. It was still encouraging a level of meat and dairy consumption (two to three 5 to 7 ounce servings per day) that simply was now known to be unhealthy. Clearly the continued unjustifiable encouragement of this level of consumption could be attributed to the influence of likes of *The National Cattleman's Association* and the *National Milk Producer' Federation.*

The next and latest in the saga of USDA guidelines occurred in 2005 with the release of *My Pyramid*. Its intent was to keep the pyramid approach but to provide more simplified nutritional advice. The picture of the newer pyramid provides little information in that it consists of a series of unlabeled multi-colored bars that run vertically down the pyramid. To understand the pyramid the public is directed to the web site www.mypyramid.gov. Once there, a click on its colored stripes takes you to the different food groups and for each group one or two descriptive phrases are given. For example, clicking on one column might get you VEGETABLES with the message "Vary your Veggies: eat more dark green vegetables; eat more orange vegetables; eat more dry beans and peas." Clicking on another column and up might pop MILK with the message "Get your calcium-rich food: go low-fat or fat-free; if you don't or can't consume milk, choose lactose-free products or other calcium sources." Clicking on yet another column and you might be given MEAT & BEANS with the message "Go lean on protein: choose low-fat or lean meats and poultry; bake it, boil it, or grill it; vary your choices with more fish, beans, peas, nuts, and seeds."

There are two main criticisms of *My Pyramid*. First, most health professionals feel that its messages are too vague and not readily assessable. They argue that the columns do not offer enough information to help people make informed food choices and to even get those messages requires a visit to the Internet. Millions of Americans do not have a computer and Internet, and those who do might not take the time to approach and explore the site. The second criticism comes from the food scientists and is the same as existed with the initial pyramid. The USDA *My Pyramid* persists in recommending meats and dairy products that are now not considered essential to good health, and may even be detrimental in the quantities prescribed.

The Healthy Eating Pyramid

In light of these concerns, the faculty in the Harvard School of Public Health was moved to develop the 2005 *Healthy Eating Pyramid* (Figure 2.2). Its goal was to create an easy to understand, trustworthy guide for choosing a healthy diet. As a result the guide is completely aligned with the latest research and unaffected by businesses and organizations with a stake in its messages. I am comfortable offering it as a better and more usable nutritional goal then that of the USDA. You will notice that the *Healthy Eating Pyramid* does not give specific advice about the numbers of cups or ounces to have each day of specific foods. That is because it is not meant to be a rigid road map, and the amounts can vary depending on your body size and physical activity. It is a simple, general, flexible guide to how you should eat.

Although the *Healthy Eating Pyramid* does seem to summarize the best dietary information available today, the Harvard developers appropriately do not see it as set in stone. They realize that nutrition researchers will undoubtedly turn up new information in the years ahead and the pyramid will need be reflective of that important new evidence. Also, they recognize that there exist other good, evidence-based vegetarian guides for healthy eating.

THE HEALTHY EATING PYRAMID

Department of Nutrition, Harvard School of Public Health

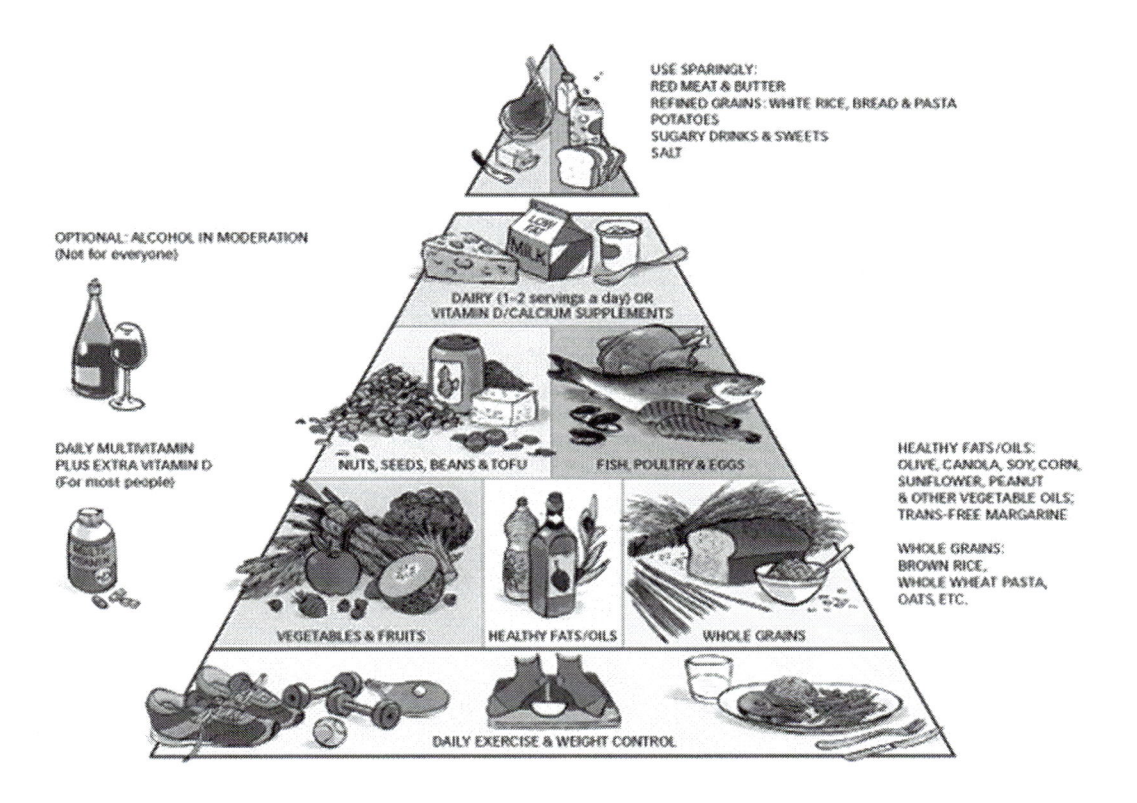

For more information about the Healthy Eating Pyramid:

WWW.THENUTRITIONSOURCE.ORG

Eat, Drink, and Be Healthy
by Walter C. Willett, M.D. and Patrick J. Skerrett (2005)
Free Press/Simon & Schuster Inc.

Copyright © 2008 Harvard University

Figure 2.2 The Healthy Eating Pyramid

There is just one basic guideline to remember: A healthy diet includes more foods from the base of the pyramid than from the higher levels of the pyramid. Within this guideline, however, there is plenty of flexibility for different styles of eating and different food choices. A vegetarian can follow the *Healthy Eating Pyramid* by emphasizing nuts, beans, and other plant sources of protein, and choosing non-dairy sources of calcium and vitamin D; someone who eats animal products can choose fish or chicken for protein, with occasional red meat.

Choosing a variety of fresh, whole foods from all the food groups below the "Use Sparingly" category will ensure that you get the nutrients you need. It will also dramatically lower your salt intake, since most of the salt in the U.S. diet lurks in processed food – canned soups, frozen dinners, deli meats, snack chips, and the like. Perhaps the only foods that are truly off-limits are foods that contain trans fat from partially hydrogenated oils.

The following Five Quick Tips capture the essence of the *Healthy Eating Pyramid*. In Chapter 4 we will be taking a more thorough look at the fundamentals we need know about good nutrition and in Chapter 5 we will address how we might practically help children begin to understand and adopt good nutrition practices.

> **1. Start with exercise:** A healthy diet is built on a base of regular exercise, which keeps calories in balance and weight in check.
>
> **2. Focus on food, not grams:** The *Healthy Eating Pyramid* doesn't worry about specific servings or grams of food, so neither should you. It's a simple, general guide to how you should eat when you eat.
>
> **3. Go with plants:** Eating a plant-based diet is healthiest. Choose plenty of vegetables, fruits, and healthy fats like olive and canola oil.
>
> **4. Cut way back on American staples:** Red meat, refined grains, potatoes, sugary drinks, and salty snacks are part of American culture, but they're also really unhealthy. Go for a plant-based diet rich in non-starchy vegetables, fruits, and whole grains. And if you eat meat, fish and poultry are the best choices.
>
> **5. Take a multivitamin, and maybe have a drink:** Taking a multivitamin can be a good nutrition insurance policy. Moderate drinking for many people can have real health benefits, but it's

not for everyone. Those who don't drink should not feel the need to start.

The Vegetarian Pyramid

The *Vegetarian Pyramid* presented in Figure 2.3 is really the same as the *Healthy Eating Pyramid* except instead of encouraging the minimization of meat consumption it entirely removes it. It is a flexible model in that it accommodates choice between the two fundamental levels of vegetarianism. The *lacto ovo vegetarian* is a person whose diet excludes meat, fish, and poultry but includes dairy products and eggs. The *vegan* is a person who eats no meat, fish, poultry, eggs, or dairy products. Notice that Figure 2.3 lists the dairy and eggs level as optional. Adherents to lacto-ovo vegetarianism would be including foods from the dairy and eggs level while the *vegan* would be more restrictive and not do so.

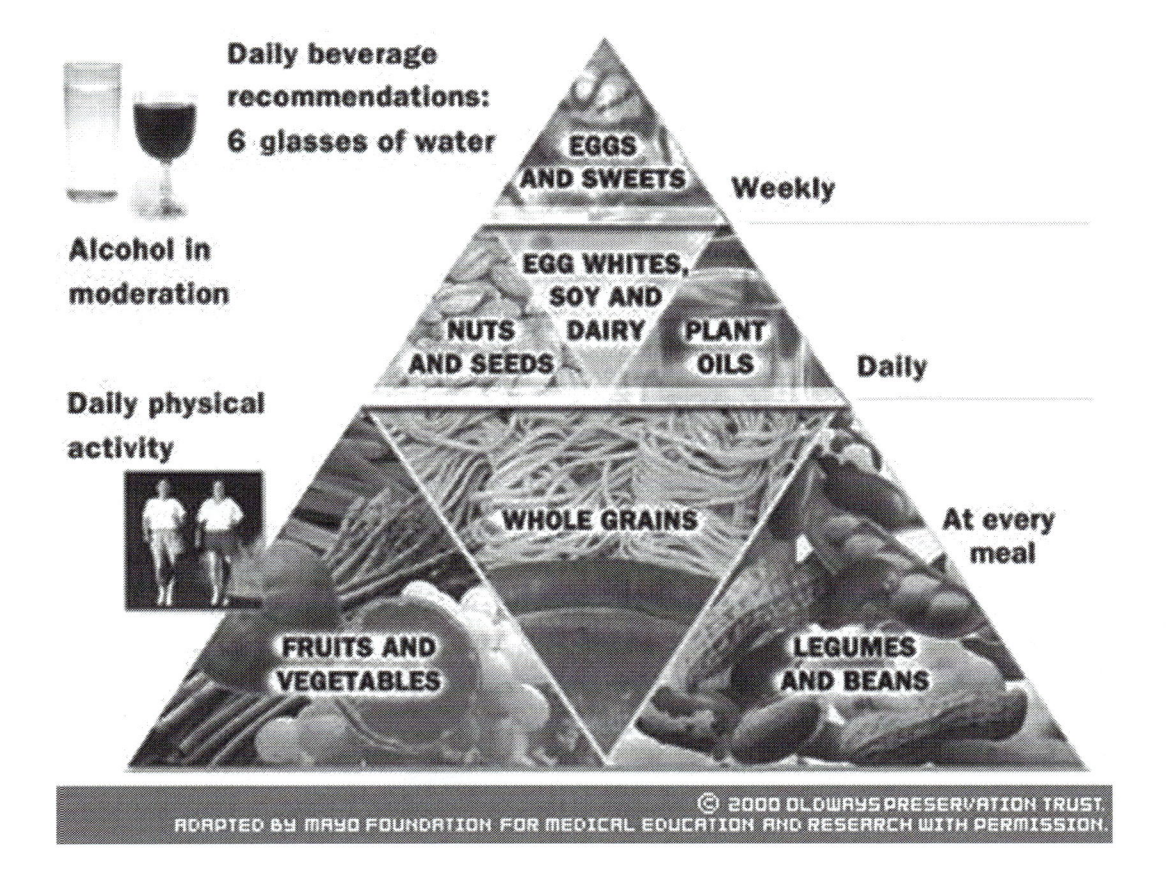

Figure 2.3 The Vegetarian Pyramid

Models for Physical Activity and Nutrition

Upon first thought the *Vegetarian Pyramid* might seem a radical eating model to be advocating. Most Americans probably view it rather suspiciously and it is estimated that less than three percent of the population excludes all meat from their diet and only one percent avoids both meat and meat products. Each year the average American eats 271 pounds of meat, 16 pounds of fish, 254 eggs, 180 pounds of milk, 32 pounds of cheese, 25 pounds of ice cream, 10 pounds of cream, and 8 pounds of yogurt. However, just because something is not commonly accepted or practiced does not mean that it might not be the best of all models to work toward. The major difference between the *Healthy Eating Pyramid* and the USDA *My Pyramid* was that the Harvard faculty determined that meat and dairy products were not a preferred or even necessary ingredient in a healthy diet. The same conclusion has been reached by the major health organizations. *The American Health Association*, *The National Academy of Sciences*, *The American Academy of Pediatrics*, and *The American Dietetic Association* all recognize the ability of plant-based diets to best meet our nutritional needs. They universally are stating that the less meat and dairy we consume the better off we will be. The three following sections summarize the health, environmental and ethical reasons in support of vegetarianism. I think you will see there to be an overwhelming array of cogent arguments rightfully deserving attention.

Health Reasons

Because it is sometimes difficult to separate the effects of vegetarian diets from other factors it is not possible to precisely quantify the lifespan of vegetarians vis' a vis' those who eat various amounts of meat. However, studies that look at correlation data generally discover that vegetarians do live longer, and the longer time spent on the vegetarian diet the greater was the decrease in mortality risk. Clearly they have fewer heart attacks and strokes. If a person eating *The Standard American Diet (SAD)* cut his/her consumption of animal products in half the occurrence of heart attack would be lowered by 45 percent. And that drops to nearly 90 percent with a move to *veganism*.

Vegetarians have lower blood pressure and cholesterol levels. Two percent of vegetarians have high blood pressure compared to 26 percent of non-vegetarians of the same age and social circumstances. The average person on the *SAD* has a total cholesterol level of 193. The average *lacto-ovo vegetarian* is significantly better at 181 and *vegan* comes in at 158. This 158 number is lower than the cholesterol profile of the average Boston marathoner. To qualify for the Boston Marathon a runner must be very fit and regular in their exercise habits. While regular exercise is known to lower cholesterol levels it is instructive to see that diet, namely a vegetarian diet, seems to have a more pronounced influence on cholesterol than even especially high amounts of vigorous exercise.

Vegetarians are less likely to be overweight or obese. Two-thirds of American adults are now classified as overweight or obese; fifteen percent of vegetarians are overweight or obese. Vegetarians have a far lower incidence of type II Diabetes and significantly lower levels of breast and colon cancer. Men are almost 4 times less likely to get prostate cancer. Vegetarians have fewer kidney stones and less kidney disease than non-vegetarians.

In recent years worrisome amounts of toxic metals, pesticides, hormones, antibiotics and disease organisms have been discovered in human bodies. While various environmental sources could be contributing to these rises, the eating of animals is thought to be the primary factor. *Bioamplification* is the concept that each step up the food chain produces a higher concentration of toxic chemicals than in the one below it. Today's factory-farm animals (beef, milk cows, pigs, chickens) are persistently stressed and fed and injected with large doses of antibiotics and hormones. Their diets are unnatural and the remains of other animals are commonly mixed with their feed. These practices result in high contamination and pathogen levels which can be passed on to humans that dine on them. Some disease outbreaks in humans have been attributed to this process and other long-term consequences will have to uneasily await the future.

Finally, there is the issue of vegetarianism and athletic performance. A long-held pervasive perception is that ingestion of meat is the *sine qua non* of developing strong bones and large powerful muscles. The evidence is otherwise. Vegetarians have a measurably lower incidence of osteoporosis. In fact, generous consumption of meat has been found to decrease the density and strength of bones. The countries with the highest intakes of dairy products and animal protein also have the highest rates of hip fracture. The reasons for the increase in osteoporosis will be explained in Chapter 4 as will the discoveries that balanced, plant-based diets are fully capable of providing the protein needed to develop muscle for everyday health, extreme physical performance and even body-building. For now, look at Figure 2.4. It consists of an impressive list of undeniably strong boned muscular vegetarians who have achieved remarkable feats of strength and endurance.

Figure 2.4. Vegetarian Athletic Exemplars

Athlete (Country)	Athlete Achievement
Surya Bonaly (France)	Olympic figure skater
Andreas Cahling (Sweden)	Champion body builder and Olympic gold medalist in ski jump
Chris Campbell (USA)	Olympic wrestler
Desmond Howard (USA)	Professional football player and Heisman trophy winner
Peter Hussing (Germany)	European super-heavyweight amateur boxing champion

Billie Jean King (USA)	Champion tennis player
Carl Lewis (USA)	Olympic runner
Ingra Manecke (Germany)	Champion discus thrower
Bill Manetti (USA)	Power-lifting champion
Edwin Moses (USA)	Olympic gold medalist and world record holder in track
Martina Navratilova (USA)	Champion tennis player
Paavo Nurmi (Finland)	Long-distance runner, Olympic gold medalist (20 world records)
Bill Pearl (USA)	Weight lifter and four-time Mr. Universe
Dave Scott (USA)	Six-time winner of the Ironman triathlon
Scott Jurek (USA)	Badwater Ultra-long-distance champion (vegan – winning by two hours)

Environmental Reasons

Although health concerns are the focus of this discipline, I am sure that all teachers recognize their encompassing duty to instill children with an appreciation of the earth that supports them. In fact, federal law states that care for the environment is to be integrated into academic instruction throughout the curriculum. We understand that students need be receiving an integrated cross-disciplinary message of what citizens of the 21st century must do to care for the environment and live sustainably in it. We have all heard the statistics on a wide variety of environmental problems ranging from soil erosion, fresh water depletion, air pollution, forest fires, desertification and decline in bio-diversity. Virtually everyone now knows that the scientific community has established solid evidence for man-made climate changes which are exacerbating these problems and producing yet others. The predictions are indeed dire and it is urgently necessary that we employ every means of conservation possible as the industrial world moves from fossil fuels to the more environmentally friendly energy sources of wind, wave, solar, geo-thermo and nuclear. We need to be taking the small, easy conservation steps such as turning off lights and appliances, recycling products, driving less and generally living more materialistically simple lifestyles. Furthermore we need to be taking the bigger steps that yield more substantive impacts. These switches involve moving to efficient appliances, vehicles, homes and vegetarianism.

You may not have thought it but yes, vegetarianism belongs on the list of major steps that can be taken to address the environmental problems facing us. An unbiased assessment would actually place it at the top of the list as having the greatest potential ramifications. Here is why. As environmental science has advanced, it has become apparent that the human population's appetite for animal flesh is a driving force behind virtually every major category of environmental damage now threatening the human future – deforestation, erosion, fresh water scarcity, air and water pollution, climate change, biodiversity loss and the spread of disease. It has been calculated that the energy demands and CO_2 emissions required to raise, transports and process livestock in the United States generates more CO_2 emissions than the entire transportation industry (that includes cars, trucks buses, trains and airplanes). The average American switching to a vegetarian diet would save more energy then if he/she switched from the typical car to a fuel-efficient hybrid. Land, energy and water resources for livestock agriculture range anywhere from 10 to 1000 times greater than those necessary to produce an equivalent amount of plant food. About 40 percent of all land area in the United States is used for grazing livestock. Two-thirds of all the grain we grow goes to feed livestock. The amount of land resources needed to raise animals for their meat is exponentially greater than the amount needed to grow enough plant matter to feed the same number of people directly. A steer has to eat 7 pounds of grain or soybeans to produce 1 pound of beef. Over half the water used in the U.S. goes toward irrigating land to grow food for livestock. It takes about 25 gallons of water to grow 1 pound of wheat, but it takes about 390 gallons of water to produce 1 pound of beef. The aquifers that lie deep below the earth's surface hold the kind of water that we need to irrigate our land and to drink. Those giant pools of fresh water are dwindling rapidly because we are sucking up great quantities of the stuff to irrigate the vast amount of land needed to graze the animals from which we get a relatively small amount of food – a very inefficient use of a very precious resource. And livestock agriculture does not merely use these resources, it depletes them. According to a Congressional study, 1.4 billion tons of waste is generated by animals on mega farms in more than 40 states. That is more than 130 times the amount of waste that the entire American population produces in a year. None of this waste is treated as is human waste. Not only does this pollution kill fish and aquatic life, it also seeps into our drinking water.

> We (in 2010) have killed off 90 percent of the big fish that were in the world's oceans just sixty years ago.

The world's population has increased from 2.5 billion in 1950 to 6.5 billion today, and that rate of increase continues. If numbers in the billions are too hard to grasp, translate that into the fact that the earth's population is increasing by a million people every four days. Global analyses confirm that the earth's environment is being stressed in order to feed today's population. That stress on the environment will be greatly magnified as the population increases. Albert Einstein said "Nothing will benefit human health and increase the chances for survival of life on earth as much as the evolution of a vegetarian diet." Adopting a vegetarian lifestyle might be duty we must assume if in fact we are to be stewards of a sustainable earth. The world's population is forecasted to grow to 9 or 10 billion by the end of the century. There is no question that that number of people cannot continue eating meat and dairy products as we are doing now.

Ethical Reasons

As powerful and individually sufficient as both the health and environmental reasons might be, surveys reveal that ethics is the foremost determinant for practicing vegetarians. Specifically, most vegetarians have concluded that they cannot morally support the inherent cruelty they see in today's factory farms. Cattle, chickens and pigs do not live in idyllic pastures and barnyards anymore. It is inescapably true that the vast majority is raised under methods that are systematically abusive. For them, discomfort is the norm, pain is routine, growth is abnormal, and diet is unnatural. Disease is widespread and stress is almost constant. The plight these animals experience from birth to death cannot be chronicled here, but review a few representative examples. Ninety-nine percent of chickens sold in American come from factory-farms where they typically live their entire lives crowded in 8.5" X 11" spaces. Egg-laying hens are stacked in small cages and their beaks are seared off because in frustration they would injure or kill those about them. Ninety percent of pigs, animals more intelligent than dogs, never get to go outside or root around in pasture. They live in cement confinement without any straw, and have no alternative but to lie in their excrement, something no free pig would ever do. Veal calves are the babies of dairy cows, removed from their mothers when they are only one day old. Each calf is placed alone in a tiny, dark stall just a bit longer than a standard bathtub. Chained at the neck, a calf in such a stall cannot even turn around its entire life.

Some could conclude that the solution to this repellent situation lies in reform of factory farming methods rather than vegetarianism. Although many improvements should be demanded and made, there is a realistic limit to making these farms and slaughterhouses more merciful. In a global, high-tech economy of six and a half billion consumers, perhaps nine or ten billion by the year 2100, livestock animals simply cannot be raised under humane conditions. The average American now eats more than 200 pounds of red meat, poultry, and fish per year (more than a half-pound each day). That is an increase of 23 pounds over 1970. American's slaughterhouses kill around 10 billion birds and mammals each year to meet that demand – that is 40 million in less than two days! That sort of demand is not going to be met by local independent farmers with chickens strutting about the yard and a few cows lazily grazing in a lush green pasture.

Because of this reality we are faced with a rather stark dilemma. We can ignore the problem by not thinking about the dark aspects of the factory farms and slaughterhouses; we can belittle it by telling ourselves that animals are here for our use and that it is okay to exploit them because of their more limited cognitive capacities and self-awareness; and we can rationalize that our individual choice to not eat meat would have no measurable effect upon the totality of the industry. On the other hand, we can decide not to ignore the ugly reality of factory farming and resolve ourselves to action. We could attenuate the problem by becoming *semi-vegetarians* by cutting back on meat and dairy consumption, or completely remove our contribution to it by becoming vegetarians and vegans. Mahatma Ghandi said, "The greatness of a nation and its moral progress can be judged by the way it treats its animals." And the vegetarian philosopher Peter Singer asks us to weigh the following question. "If, within our own species, we don't regard differences in intelligence, reasoning ability, or self-awareness as grounds for permitting us to exploit the being with lower capacities for our own ends, how can we point to the same characteristics to justify exploiting members of other species?" These are basic ethical, philosophical questions we must ask ourselves, and as educators, pose and discuss with the young inquiring minds of our students.

CHAPTER COMPREHENSION CHECK

1. When and by whom was the *Exercise Prescription Model* developed? *Ken Cooper 1967*
2. What are the specifics of the *Exercise Prescription Model*? *3 to 4 times a week, 20-40 mins target*
3. How well has the *Exercise Prescription Model* been adhered to? *Very well*
4. What is meant by thinking of children as *interval trainers* and what implication does that have for applying the *Exercise Prescription Model* to them?
5. What are the specifics of the *Lifetime Activity Model*? *60 minutes 6 to 7 times broken up*
6. Approximately what percentage of children currently adhere to the *Lifetime Activity Model*? *36*
7. Why is the *Lifetime Activity Model* considered a more feasible model than the *Exercise Prescription Model*? *flexible in breaking up activities*
8. What is considered a major weakness of the *Lifetime Activity Model*? *lowers standards of intensity*
9. What are the specifics of *The Activity Pyramid* (all 4 levels)? *page 30*
10. How does *The Activity Pyramid* view involving children in steady-state aerobics and weightlifting activities? *3 days a week*
11. What are the two charges of the *United States Department of Agriculture (USDA)*? *pg 33*
12. What were the specifics of the 1992 *USDA Food Guide Pyramid*?
13. In what ways is the new USDA 2005 *My Pyramid* different from the 1992 *Food Guide Pyramid*?
14. What are the two main criticisms of the 2005 *My Pyramid*?
15. What are the specifics of the Harvard School of Public Health 2005 *Healthy Eating Pyramid* (all 4 levels)? *pg 35*
16. What does the *Healthy Eating Pyramid* say about the eating of meat and meat products, about the eating of trans fats from partially hydrogenated oils? *use sparingly*

Models for Physical Activity and Nutrition

17. What does the *Healthy Eating Pyramid* say about the taking of a multivitamins and drinking alcohol?
18. What is the difference between the *Healthy Eating Pyramid* and the *Vegetarian Pyramid*?
19. What are the definitions of the *lacto ovo vegetarian* and the *vegan* diets?
20. Approximately what percentage of the population is vegetarian?
21. Approximately how many pounds of meat, and how many eggs does the average American eat?
22. What is the stance of the major health organizations (AHA, NAS, AAP, ADA) regarding the eating of meat and meat products?
23. Approximately how much would the incidence of heart attack decrease with a move from *The Standard American Diet (SAD)* to consumption of one half as much meat? with a move to a vegan diet?
24. What are the approximate cholesterol levels of those on the *SAD*, *lacto-ovo vegetarian* and *vegan* diets?
25. Who likely would have the lowest cholesterol level, the Boston Marathon runner or the vegan?
26. What is *Bioamplification* and why is the problem increasing?
27. Who likely would have a problem with osteoporosis, the vegetarians or those on the SAD diet?
28. Which aspects of the environment are compromised by a meat-eating diet?
29. Which step would conserve more energy, moving from a typical car to a fuel-efficient hybrid, or moving from a *SAD* to a vegetarian diet?

Is it environmentally sustainable if the world's current population (6.5 billion people) adopted a *SAD* diet? What if the population grows to 9 or 10 billion by century's end, as forecasted?

30. What is the major reason people choose vegetarianism?
31. What are the major ethical arguments for vegetarianism?

[CHAPTER 3]

EXERCISE PHYSIOLOGY: WHAT YOU NEED TO KNOW

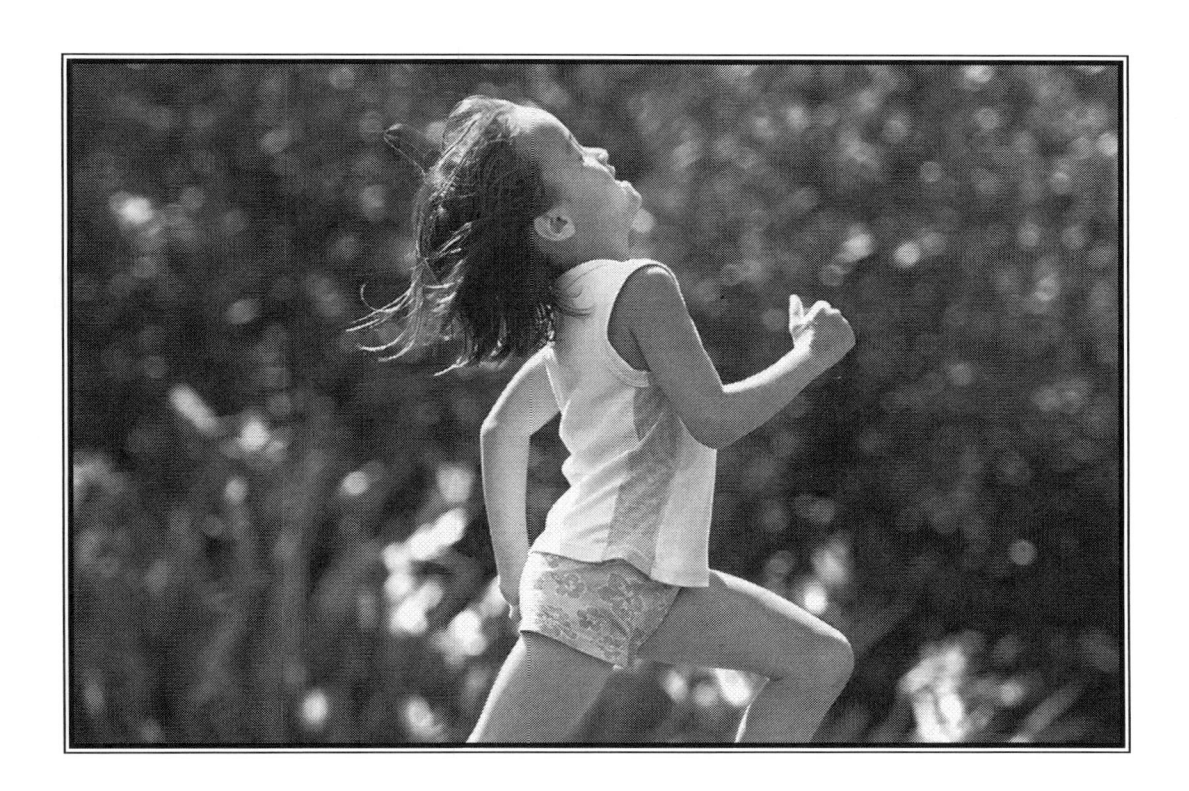

WHAT IS PHYSICAL FITNESS

Component of Cardio-Respiratory Fitness
Component of Dynamic Flexibility Fitness
Component of Muscular Fitness
Component of Body Composition Fitness

HOW TO DEVELOP AND MAINTAIN THE COMPONENTS OF FITNESS

(F)requency (I)ntensity (T)ime Principle
F.I.T. Principle Applied to Improving Cardio-Respiratory Fitness (Aerobic)
F.I.T. Principle Applied to Improving Cardio-Respiratory Fitness (Anaerobic)
F.I.T Principle Applied to Improving Dynamic Flexibility Fitness
F.I.T. Principle Applied to Improving Muscular Fitness
F.I.T. Principle Applied to Reducing Body Composition Fitness
Qualification of the F.I.T. Principle
Overuse Principle
Reversibility Principle
Readiness/Trainability Principle
Warm-up and Cool-down Principle

CHAPTER COMPREHENSION CHECK

> *"Everyone agrees with the educational catchphrase 'A child's mind is a terrible thing to waste.' But what about the hearts, lungs and legs of those same young bodies?"*
> ~ Tom Weir

> *"Science teaching (for children) should begin, not with the mythical body in rest or uniform motion, but with the human body."*
> ~ J.B.S. Haldane

In the previous chapter the *Activity Pyramid* was offered as a useful model for achieving a physically healthy lifestyle. As specified in the base of the pyramid, adherents to the model would generally be accumulating an hour or more of light to moderate activity each day. This kind of activity would play a key role in burning calories and hence preventing the accumulation of excess body fat. These low-intensity activities would also yield modest improvements in muscular strength, flexibility and cardiovascular function. The second and third tiers of the pyramid prescribed more vigorous sports and exercises that would promote higher levels of muscular strength and endurance, flexibility, and both aerobic and anaerobic cardiovascular fitness.

In this chapter we will take a closer look at: (1) what is physical fitness and the components of which it is comprised; and (2), what kinds of physical activities develop and maintain each component. The intent will be to avoid complexity while introducing the basic physiological concepts we need to know in order to take care of our bodies. These are the concepts we must also begin teaching the children if they too are ultimately going to assume self-responsibility for their fitness.

WHAT IS PHYSICAL FITNESS?

Physical fitness can be divided into two levels. The *health fitness level* would represent minimal fitness for which everyone should strive throughout his or her life span. Those in possession of it would have sufficient physical fitness to carry out daily activities without pain or significant restrictions. They could shop, climb stairs, mow and trim the yard, garden a small plot, clean the car or house, and even hurry after the bus without undue risk of injury or sore muscles. They would not feel run down and exhausted by the end of the day. They could live physically comfortable, independent lives, free of the degenerative *hypokinetic diseases* associated with an inactive lifestyle (cardiorespiratory diseases, type II diabetes, excessive body fat, lower back pain, etc.).

The *performance fitness* level would permit us to go beyond everyday tasks. We would be capable of expanding movement horizons to include recreational/sports activities. These activities could vary from long neighborhood walks and golfing to climbing mountains and competing in "ironman" length triathlons. Performance fitness would enable us to safely enjoy these challenges and reach the fullest physical potential for which we might strive. This level would yield a higher level of protection against hypokinetic diseases and might also afford greater psychological benefits such as better self-concept, body image, and anxiety reduction. Various philosophers have argued that it is the civic duty of everyone to strive for what would be considered performance fitness. According to Socrates, "No citizen has any right to be an amateur in the matter of physical training. It is part of his profession as a citizen to keep himself in good condition, ready to serve his state at a moment's notice… What a disgrace it is for a man to grow old without ever seeing the beauty and the strength of which his body is capable!" The American poet/philosopher Walt Whitman admonishes every man and woman to join those with sweet and determined bodies, "Allon! After the great Companions, and to belong to them!"

Regardless of which of the two levels of fitness sought, physical fitness must be recognized as being made up of a number of components. To have health fitness we must possess a minimal degree of certain components of fitness; other components and higher levels of those components may be needed for performance fitness. Each of the major components of physical fitness is described below.

Component of Cardio-Respiratory Fitness

The cardio-respiratory system can be divided into two basic components of fitness: aerobic and anaerobic. In simplified terms, the word *aerobic* is referring to "with oxygen." When we exercise we breath faster and deeper to take in more oxygen, and the heart beats faster and more forcefully to transport that oxygen from the lungs to the needful working muscles. It is obvious that we want a strong, efficient aerobic system in order to perform vigorous sports and activities, which last for a period of time. In fact, a good aerobic foundation is considered essential for all sports/recreational activities and health fitness. A sound aerobic capacity is an indispensable underlying energy system if we are going to comfortably complete everyday tasks. Furthermore, the leading causes of death and disability are a result of a deteriorated aerobic system. Narrowed and hardened arteries restrict oxygen flow to virtually all body organs and are associated with numerous impairments as diverse as strokes, heart attacks, decreased mental alertness, sexual disfunction, and loss of skin suppleness. An efficient aerobic system can play a role in reducing chronic high blood pressure and its concomitant health problems. There are good arguments for saying that aerobic capacity is the most critical component of health fitness. The two foundation levels of the Activity Pyramid are there primarily because of their contribution to aerobic fitness.

Anaerobic refers to "without oxygen." When the body is called upon to exert a large amount of energy in a short period of time the cardio-respiratory system does not have the capability of providing adequate oxygen to the muscles: kayaking in a particularly swift patch of water, swimming a fifty-meter race, or sprinting to hit a number of tennis shots in quick succession would be examples. The body has a short-term means of accomplishing such tasks by producing energy through chemical reactions that do not require oxygen. However, these reactions can only be maintained to up around 90 seconds before an "oxygen debt" is incurred, byproduct lactic acid builds up in the blood, and activity falters and stops. Although a good functioning anaerobic system is not important in more moderately paced sports/recreational activities, the above examples attest to its importance in others. Anaerobic fitness is not considered to be nearly as important to health fitness as we saw aerobic fitness to be. Unlike aerobic diseases, we do not have to worry about degenerative disabilities as a result of anaerobic problems and it is rare to be faced with anaerobic tasks in our normal daily routines. Nevertheless, it is well to recognize that even in our humdrum existence there arise emergencies when we may wish to vigorously push a car out of a snowdrift or sprint some place when others or we are in danger. The Activity Pyramid does not specifically dictate anaerobic experiences although many of the second level recreational and sports experiences have anaerobic aspects to them.

Component of Dynamic Flexibility Fitness

Dynamic flexibility can be thought of as the capacity to move joints through a full range of motion. The major factor limiting the normal range of movement in a joint, other than the bone structure of the joint itself, is the tightness of the tendons, ligaments, and other muscular connective tissues involved. Everyone requires at least a moderate range of motion to carryout normal daily activities. Successful performance of sports and recreational activities call for higher degrees of movement that are activity specific. For example, dancers and gymnasts obviously require great flexibility in most every body part, golfers need good trunk rotation, swimmers need good shoulder and ankle flexibility, and football kickers need an extreme suppleness in the hip.

Flexibility can also be a factor in posture, chronic joint pain, and personal safety. For example, some postural problems such as rounded shoulders might be traced to over tightness in the chest; chronic neck and lower back pains are sometimes attributed to tight extensor connective tissues in these regions. Elderly people naturally become more restricted and might evince a shorter stride length when walking or have difficulty turning their heads to monitor traffic while driving. Larger losses in flexibility accompanying more sedentary aging can pose many other safety problems and restrict even self-care tasks.

The third tier of the Activity Pyramid specifies that activities/exercises promoting a full range of movement should be done at least 2 or 3 times per week.

Component of Muscular Fitness

The muscular system can be divided into two basic components of fitness: *muscular strength* and *muscular endurance*. These components are not completely unrelated to one another in the sense that developing one will have some developmental effect on the other.

Muscular strength is determined by how much force someone is capable of producing. Bench-pressing as much weight as possible would be a test of the strength of the chest and arm extensor muscles. Squeezing a hand gauge with maximal force would be a measurement of hand contraction strength. Muscular strength may come into play in weight lifting, wrestling, rock climbing. A child may not have enough strength to swing a bat or shoot a basketball with proper technique. As for general health, muscular strength is only minimally important. Moving the refrigerator and loosening the bolts to change a tire are a couple of examples of when strength is required around the house and garage. My elderly mother has difficulty twisting off jar lids.

When a resistance must be repeatedly moved we are relying on the component of *muscular endurance.* This ability is needed in virtually all sports-recreational activities. Running distances demands that our legs continually thrust the body upwards and forward. When swimming, the arms must pull through the water again and again. As do the majority of sports/recreational activities, hiking, paddling, biking, and swinging rackets all require sustained, repetitive movement. When muscular endurance wanes, skilled performance is impaired. Muscular endurance affects our daily health in more ways than just walking about; it plays a crucial part in posture. For instance, while standing, abdominal muscles must maintain a degree of tautness to keep the hips from rotating too far forward and letting the abdomen protrude. Likewise, having strong thigh muscles (quadriceps) sometimes are helpful in preventing knee pain. The Activity Pyramid calls for muscular fitness exercises (strength/endurance) to be done 2 to 3 times each week.

Component of Body Composition Fitness

Body composition is considered another component of fitness. Here we are referring to the body's percentage of body fat relative to lean mass. The lean mass is primarily made up of bone, muscle and connective tissue. Fat is chiefly necessary for protection of internal organs, brain function and transmission of neural messages, insulation to preserve body heat, and as a reservoir of energy supplies. For most all sports-recreational activities it is good to have a relatively lower percentage of body fat because any more than is necessary results in extra weight that must be moved. The extra weight will reduce the speed with which we can move and it also places greater stress on the cardio-respiratory system. Furthermore it will result in greater forces being placed on joints thus increasing the chances of muscle and joint injuries. A couple of sports where a somewhat higher percentage of fat may be beneficial would be distance swimming in cold water, because of the need for insulation, and football linemen, where the greater weight of the individual would make it more difficult for an opposing player to apply enough force to move him out of the way.

With regards to health, it is very important that children or adults do not accumulate more fat than necessary. We saw in Chapter 1 that the percentage of effected American has been rapidly increasing. Excess body fat makes all daily activities more fatiguing and is associated with cardiovascular diseases, type II diabetes, arthritis, some kinds of cancer, and low back pain. Excess body fat is also the most readily observable of fitness components and is generally viewed negatively. Because many people hold an unfavorable view of being overfat it can have restricting social and psychological implications. Of course, all of the activities of the Activity Pyramid contribute to the burning of calories and hence to fighting excessive fat accumulation. A primary purpose of the pyramid is to ensure that people have a good quantity of movement, at least an hour a day of lifestyle activities in addition to aerobic and muscular fitness activities.

Having a healthy body composition is not always about burning calories and reducing body fat. While too little body fat is not nearly as common a health problem as is having too much, it can have serious, even life threatening, consequences for those effected. Because of the prevalent negative views that society has toward fat, some adults and children do acquire anorexic, bulimic, and excessive exercise behaviors. The message needs to be one of moderation. The role of the Activity Pyramid is to promote adequate activity with some room for rest and recovery. The role of the various food pyramids is to moderate excessive fat and sugar consumption, not eliminate it.

HOW TO DEVELOP AND MAINTAIN THE COMPONENTS OF FITNESS

We now know that physical fitness is multifarious. To be physically healthy we must achieve, and maintain throughout our lives, a healthy level of functioning in a variety of components of fitness: aerobic, muscular strength/endurance, dynamic flexibility and body composition. For the fuller athletic life, higher degrees of functioning in those components may be necessary. Additionally, well-developed muscular strength/endurance and anaerobic cardio-respiratory capacities will be required in some sports and recreational activities. We shall now direct our attention to some physiological principles relating to the development and maintenance of each of the components of fitness that we have been discussing. An effort has been made to keep this coverage focused on the bare essentials. The principles should be easy to comprehend and remember, and yet be a sufficient guide for leading a healthy life of physical activity and exercise. Not only do you the teacher need to understand these principles, to some level you must be able to communicate them to the children. Students in the upper elementary grades need to be beginning to take some degree of responsibility for their own physical fitness. That will not be possible without them having some basic appreciation of the relationship between the components of physical fitness and different kinds of physical activities and exercises.

The (F)requency (I)ntensity (T)ime Principle

F.I.T. is an acronym for Frequency, Intensity, and Time. Frequency refers to how often someone needs to exercise, intensity refers to how hard or vigorous that exercise needs to be, and time relates to how long the exercise must persist. Figure 3.1 contains a listing of the generally recommended training guidelines for developing each of the components of fitness. Justification for the guidelines is derived from research studies showing that significant improvements can be clearly verified when people follow them over a period of weeks, months, and years. The gradual progressive stresses of these magnitudes, when placed on the body as a result of these guidelines, will result in adaptation in the cardio-respiratory, musculoskeletal, and body composition regulatory systems.

Figure 3.1. F.I.T. Training Guidelines for Developing the Components of Fitness

	Frequency	Intensity	Time
Cardio-respir. (Aerobic)	3-7/week	60-95% max HR	20 mins. +
Cardio-respir. (Anaerobic)	2/week	near max HR	sport specific multiple bout
Dynamic flexibility	2-7/week	repeated dynamic movement through the full range of the joint	
Muscular Strength/	2-3/week	near exhaustion	12 reps Endurance
Body Composition	daily	low to moderate	1 hour plus

F.I.T. Principle Applied to Developing the Cardio-Respiratory Fitness (Aerobic)

The recommended guidelines for achieving a more efficient oxygen delivery system is to exercise with an intensity sufficient to elevate the heart rate into a target training zone, maintain it in that zone for a time of 20 minutes or more, and repeat such an exercise routine at a frequency of 3 to 7 times per week. The *target heart rate zone* is usually defined as having the person exercise at an intensity, which will elevate the heart rate to between 60 and 95 percent of maximum heart rate. *Maximum heart rate* is simply how many beats per minute a person's heart will achieve when that person exercises as strenuously as possible. *Maximum heart rate* varies from individual to individual but a rough way of approximating it is to use this simple formula: *maximum heart rate = 220 minus and person's age.* Using this formula it would be determined that a 20 year old would have a maximal rate of 200. A 40-year old would be able to achieve a maximum rate of about 180. You can see that as people age their hearts gradually loose some capacity to beat rapidly. Now to determine the target zone for the 20 year olds we would multiply their maximum 200 by 60 percent (.60) and 95 percent (.95) and come up with a range between 120 and 195 beat per minute. The zone for the 40-year old would be 108 to 171.

Although I believe it is good to teach both children and adults how to monitor their exercise heart rates and determine whether or not they are exercising in their prescribed training zones, the calculations involved in using the *F.I.T. Principle* might be more complex than what is always necessary. Also, calculating one's zone from the 220 minus age method is only a rough estimate and can have an error of as much as 17 beats for some individuals. A much simpler way of determining appropriate aerobic training intensities is to use the *1-10 Perceived Exertion Scale* shown in Figure 3.2.

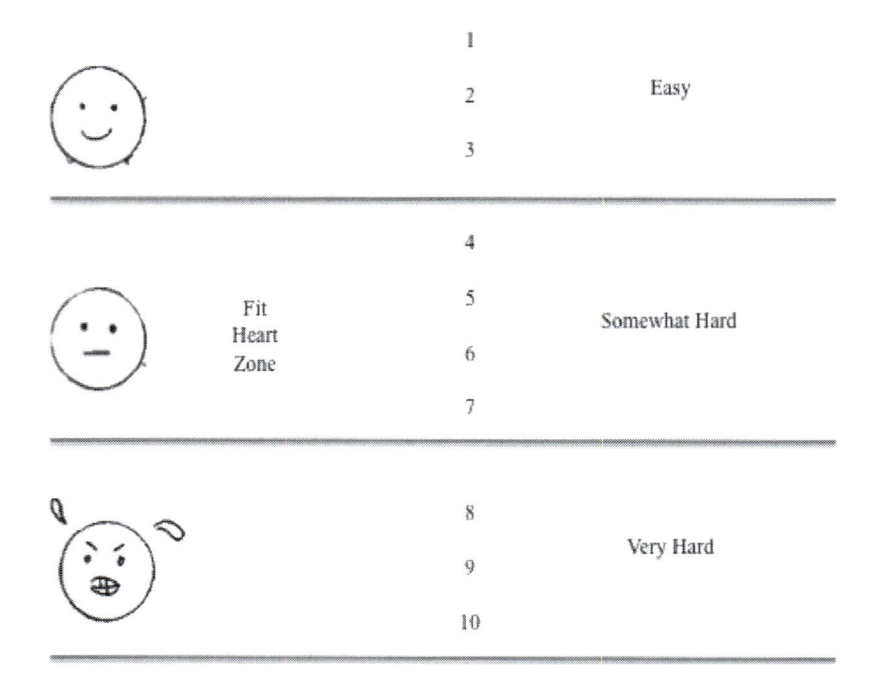

	1	
😊	2	Easy
	3	
	4	
	5	
😐 Fit Heart Zone	6	Somewhat Hard
	7	
	8	
😠	9	Very Hard
	10	

Figure 3.2. Perceived Exertion Scale
This simple 1-10 scale allows people a quick and easy way to estimate the intensity of their aerobic activities. Here the children are told that if they are feeling they are exercising somewhat hard (4,5,6,7) they are in a good heart training zone, if they are below it they might want to go just a little faster. If they are above it, be careful because they might not be able to keep it up. Your chart might also place greater emphasis on facial diagrams rather than verbal descriptors.

F.I.T. Principle Applied to Improving Cardio-Respiratory Fitness (Anaerobic)

As you may recall, anaerobic processes occur when exercise is very vigorous and the cardio-respiratory system cannot supply adequate oxygen to the muscles. Preparing the body to function under anaerobic conditions dictates that training intensity needs to be very close to maximum. The most common activity is to have the performers do sprints; other examples would be near all out execution of certain drills or calisthenics. The T of the *F.I.T. Principle* is usually determined by the specific activity for which you are preparing. If the softball player might face 30 seconds or less of sustained effort in the game as he/she rushes about the bases, then that is considered the best length of time to make the training bouts. But of course, that does not mean that the whole anaerobic workout ends after just one 30-second bout. The concept of repeated bouts or sets is used to promote greater physiological training effects. The softball players might be required to sprint or go near full speed on a drill for 30 seconds, allowed to recover by walking it off for about a minute (twice as long as the exercise phase), then go again and again, doing a series of repeats (maybe 10 or more). This type of training is called *interval training*. See Figure 3.3 regarding specific suggested interval training lengths for some common sports.

Figure 3.3. Interval Training Guidelines for Common Sports

Sport	Interval Training Recommendations
Softball and Football	Short intervals of 30 - 60 sec.
Basketball, Wrestling, Tennis	Medium intervals of 1-2 min.
Soccer, Lacrosse, Middle-distance Swimming	Long intervals of 2-10 min.

Because anaerobic interval training is difficult and stressful on the body, the F.I.T. Frequency guideline is to keep the workouts for young adults to twice a week. While aerobic training is thought best to do year round, four to six weeks of good anaerobic training has been found to be sufficient to achieve anaerobic peaking. Thus, interval training is often begun in the weeks of pre-season and then periodically during the season. If the performers are regularly performing anaerobicly as a result of game play then it may not be necessary. But if there are breaks in the schedules and players are not getting full game time, it may be needed. With regards to prepubescent children, many authorities caution us against an over emphasis on anaerobic training due to its demanding physiological and psychological nature. Perhaps significant moderation of the F.I.T. standards would be appropriate. Having the youngsters do a bout or two on an occasional basis might be sufficient to give them an idea of the potential importance of anaerobic fitness for future performance. Just making sure that everyone has an opportunity to regularly participate to vigorous games is probably the best solutions. Kids naturally love games calling for many burst of energy followed by short rest periods. I think of children as innate interval trainers. Later in the chapter under the heading of readiness, I will have more to say about children and anaerobic training.

F.I.T. Principle Applied to Improving Dynamic Flexibility Fitness

Before defining the *F.I.T Principle's* specific recommendations for developing dynamic flexibility, it should be made clear that in recent years a revolution has occurred in the realm of stretching and flexibility exercises. For many decades the ubiquitously approved advice and practice has been to stretch statically. *Static stretching* is where a person slowly and gradually moves to the limit of the joint and then holds that position or only very gradually extends it. Examples would be reaching towards the toes and holding that position in order to stretch the hamstring muscle in the back of the leg, or holding your hands in an extended clasped position behind the back so as to stretch the chest muscles. The belief was that static stretching was the best way to warm-up prior to physical activity. It would both improve subsequent sports performance and reduce the incidence of injuries. Furthermore, it was often recommend as a stand-alone practice, especially effective when done as a post-activity cool-down. Doing so was thought to reduce muscle soreness and because the connective tissue would be warm and supple after exercise, greater range could be achieved. It was thought that that greater static flexibility in turn would them lead to more efficient everyday movement and better future sports performances.

Today's exercise physiologists and top-level trainers and coaches no longer support the efficacy or advisability of static stretching either before or after exercise, or as a separate training technique. Static stretching before exercise was thought to reduce injuries and improve performance. Research data has failed to confirm either. No significant difference in injury rates has been found nor have improvements in performance occurred. In fact, performance has been documented to be poorer following this kind of stretching. Yes, you read that correctly. Static stretching has been shown to decrease strength by up to 9 percent for as long as 60 minutes. Specific activities requiring strength and muscular power, such as sprinting and jumping, have suffered measurable decreases in speed and height respectively. Distance runners with tighter hamstrings and calve muscles have been found to be more efficient runners.

Static stretching following exercise, or as an isolated practice, was believed to reduce muscle soreness and improve flexibility that would contribute to better performances in the future. Here again the current research has failed to verify either of these claims. In controlled studies estimates of subsequent muscle stiffness and soreness have been the same whether or not static stretching was done after participation. As for improving flexibility we need to understand this important and perhaps unintuitive concept: *static stretching improves static flexibility, but it does not improve dynamic flexibility (the ability to move joints through a range of motion).* In other words, the flexibility results have been determined to be specific to the type of stretching performed. For example, within a 4 to 6 week static stretching program a 5 to 20 percent increase in the ability to hold a stretched position can occur. However, that increase in static flexibility would not translate into a greater ability to dynamically move that joint through a full range of motion. And it is precisely that ability to dynamically move through a full range of motion that is the essence of good performance, whether it is everyday activities or sports skills. There are relatively few lifetime activities and sports where achieving a high degree of static flexibility is advantageous. Even instructors of athletes in sports such as dance and gymnastics, which demand extreme suppleness, are judging there to be little or no need for *static stretching*. Instead, the emphasis is on training dynamically.

Dynamic stretching uses movement speed, momentum and active muscular effort to bring about stretch. Unlike *static stretching* the end position is not held and the movements tend to be more sports specific. Arm circles, exaggerating a kicking action and walking lunges are examples of *dynamic stretches*. You may have seen track athletes executing these kind of hopping and skipping actions prior to their events. *Dynamic stretching* prior to an athletic event has been shown to improve performance and reduce muscle tightness that is associated with musculotendinous tears. Performance improvements have been especially evident in movements requiring strength and power. Figure 3.4 offers a sampling of common *dynamic stretches*. If those descriptions do not give you a clear image of what these kinds of exercises look like I suggest you "google" *dynamic stretching*; you will readily see various videos clips. As seen in Figure 3.1 the F.I.T. Principle designates no set number of repetitions for dynamic exercises. But regardless of the exact repeats of the movement, the (I) demands building up so as to move through the greatest possible range. (F)quency-wise at least two exercise bouts per week is considered the minimum needed to derive gains. Doing so more often, even every day, should be more effective and would not be harmful unless some noticeable muscle strain is noticeable.

Exercise Physiology: What You Need To Know

Figure 3.4. Common Dynamic Stretches

Dynamic warm-up exercises are designed to elevate core body temperature and maximize active ranges of motion. They typically include low, moderate, and high-intensity hops, skips, jumps, lunges, and various other exercises for the upper and lower body.

1. *Low Jacks*: While moving feet apart and together, lift arms from hips to shoulder level. Progress to high jacks by lifting arms from shoulder level to overhead.
2. *High-Knee March*: While marching in place, lift right knee towards left elbow then return to starting position and repeat on opposite side. Drive with a high knee lift and bring opposite elbow towards knee. Progress to a high-knee walking march by performing this drill while marching forward.
3. *Standing Flutter*: Stand with both arms extended above head and feet at shoulder width. Extend left arm and right leg backwards a few inches while maintaining an erect body position. Return to starting position and perform with opposite limbs. Keep arms and legs extended during the movement. Progress to a continuous and repetitive flutter performed with full extension of all limbs.
4. *Standing Toe Touches*: Stand with both arms extended in front of the body. Lift one extended leg towards the extended arms and then return to starting position. Alternate movement with other leg and repeat. Progress to a walking standing toe touch by performing this drill while moving forward.
5. *Stepping Trunk Turns*: With hands clasped behind head, march in place and turn hips to the right 90 degrees then the left 90 degrees while upper body remains forward. Progress to trunk rotations by placing both hands behind your head and then hop forward as you turn your hips to the right then the left. Focus on trunk rotation and an erect body position during both movements.
6. *Crunches*: Begin by lying on ground with knees bent at 90 degrees, feet flat on the ground, and arms crossed on chest. Crunch upward, aiming the elbows toward the thighs. Progress to crunch punches by increasing the velocity of the crunch action while pushing both arms from a chest-crossed position to an extended arm position above the knee. Emphasize a slow controlled return to starting position for safety and proper technique.
7. *Marching Lateral Shuffle*: From a standing side-stance with feet at hip width, hop and land with feet at shoulder width and body lowered to a semi-squat position. While maintaining this position, move laterally by taking a lead step followed by a short secondary step. Progress to a quick lateral shuffle by increasing the speed of the lateral movement.

8. *High-Knee Skips*: Rapidly skip forward while focusing on knee lift, arm action, and reduced ground time. To progress to kick away, jog forward while kicking heels backward with extended leg. Emphasize proper form by allowing the knee to bend at the end of the kick away to assist the return of the foot to the ground quickly.
9. *Partial Push-ups*: From a standard push-up position, lower body until elbows are at 90 degrees, then return to the starting position. Progress to push-up and lift one hand a few inches off the floor after returning to the starting position. Maintain a three-point base of support for a few seconds, then return hand to starting position and repeat on opposite side.
10. *Run and Go*: From a standing position, lean forward as you run to the five-yard mark and then sprint through the 10-yard mark. Focus on arm action, knee height, and accelerating as fast as possible. Progress to run and stop leaning forward as you sprint through the five-yard mark and then stop at the 10-yard mark. Focus on decelerating by lowering your body, bending your knees, and increasing foot contacts (i.e., chop feet several times).

F.I.T. Principle Applied to Improving Muscular Fitness

As you will recall, there are two basic types of muscular fitness: strength and endurance. Normally, different F.I.T. guidelines are set when adults are training for *muscular strength* as opposed to *muscular endurance*. The difference lies in the number of repetitions the resistance is to be moved. When working on strength, the recommendation has been to have a resistance great enough so that it can only be moved 6 to 12 times. This appears to be the optimal range to increase muscle size and its ability to complete one repetition with a heavier weight (which is the definition of *muscular strength*). For developing *muscular endurance* the guideline calls for a lesser load, one that the exerciser can move 13 or more times before the muscle becomes fatigued. Such training prepares the muscle for being able to continue functioning over a longer period of time (which is the definition of *muscular endurance*). If a student did 25 curl-ups and was nearly incapable of doing any more, this would be an example of a *muscular endurance* exercise done according to F.I.T. prescription. But also, if a runner's legs were beginning to become heavy and wobbly after a mile run, this too would be evidence of a good *muscular endurance* workout for his/her specific sport.

When dealing with elementary aged children it is unnecessary to make separate time or repetition guidelines between muscular strength and muscular endurance training. Children 5-12 years of age have been found to develop both better strength and muscular endurance when doing 13 repetitions or more. This working with more moderate loads also has the advantage of decreasing the possibility of injury. While there is no evidence that resistance training is physiologically harmful to children, having them straining to move very heavy weights does not seem prudent because their lifting techniques might be poor and they might not always appreciate the amount of caution required.

In the past there has been a concern that heavy resistance training could damage the soft growth plates of children's bones. No evidence has been found to support this thesis. In fact, children's bones, like those of adults, respond to the stress by becoming denser and less susceptible to breakage. It is never recommended to have children straining to see how much they can bench-press on one attempt, or how heavy an object they many be able to pick up. Such efforts even pose a health risk to adults who are physiologically mature and trained, and who are well-versed in proper mechanical techniques.

Before leaving the issue of repetitions a word should be said about exercise bouts or sets. Recall that when training the anaerobic system our Figure 3.1 guidelines specified doing multiple bouts. Traditionally the same idea of multiple bouts has been recommended for strength training. It has been a long accepted practice that doing around 3 sets of exercises was best for strength gains. Notice that our Figure 3.1 guidelines do not require repeated sets for the development of muscular strength and endurance. The reason for this deviation is that some recent research has not shown repeated sets to result in significantly greater increases in strength when compared to single set procedures. According to many exercise physiologists, doing the extra work of repeated bouts might produce some small extra strength gains, but the key ingredient in stimulating muscle growth seems to be if the muscle has had to contract at, or very near, maximal force.

As outlined in Figure 3.1, the I of the *F.I.T. Principle* demands a fairly high intensity level or "near exhaustion." This means that you do not have to go until you cannot move that muscle any more, but on the other hand, you should be approaching that threshold. Only as you draw near that threshold will measurably significant muscle fiber adaptations be stimulated. Remember, any level of activity will develop some strength, but maximal gains occur with maximal effort and muscle overload.

The F guidelines are for 2 to 3 bouts per week. The reason for this is that when you exert the body to near exhaustion levels it is important for the body to have a day or two of recovery time (remember how highly stressful anaerobic training was also recommended only twice per week). Some serious weight trainers who lift everyday do so by varying the muscles they work. They might train their upper body muscles one day and the following do exercises for the lower body.

The drawings in Figure 3.5 illustrate a few basic muscular strength/endurance exercises. They are designed to exercise the major muscle groups of the body. You will note there is a balance between the exercises. For example, some of the exercises use *extensor muscles* that increase the angle of a joint, they push and extend away from the body (push-ups, back extensions overhand press, calf raises, or raising up from a forward lunge or squatting position). Other exercises employ *flexor muscles* that decrease the angle of a joint, they draw and curl towards the body (rowing, curl-ups, pull-ups). A balanced muscular strength/endurance program will train the muscles that make counter movements. The muscles are known as *antagonistic muscles* when one functions to flex a joint and the other serves to extend it in the opposite direction. More and more schools are acquiring weight-training pieces of equipment and even weight machines. In my diagrams I have tried to show that when such equipment is not available calisthenics can be done and makeshift weights can be improvised. Plastic drink containers that are about a quart in size, when filled with water, can make a reasonable resistance.

Figure 3.5. Muscular Strength/Endurance Exercises
Upright Rowing: the muscles of the back (trapezius) and front of the arms (biceps) flex the weights up toward the body.
Push Ups: The antagonistic muscles of the chest (pectoralis) and back of the upper arms (triceps) extend the body's weight away from the floor.

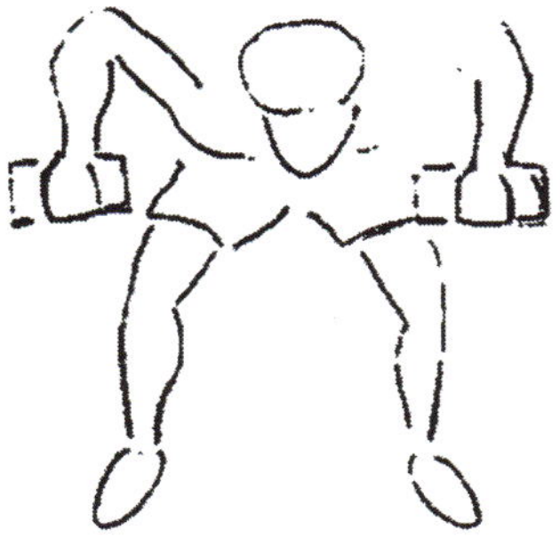

Upright Rowing 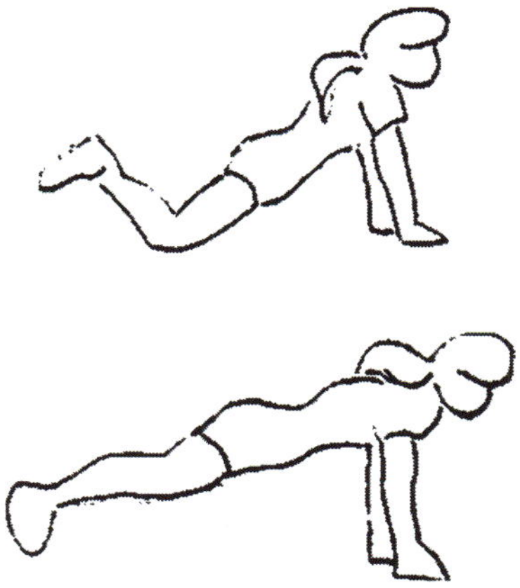   *Push-Ups*

Exercise Physiology: What You Need To Know

Overhead Press   *Pull-Ups*

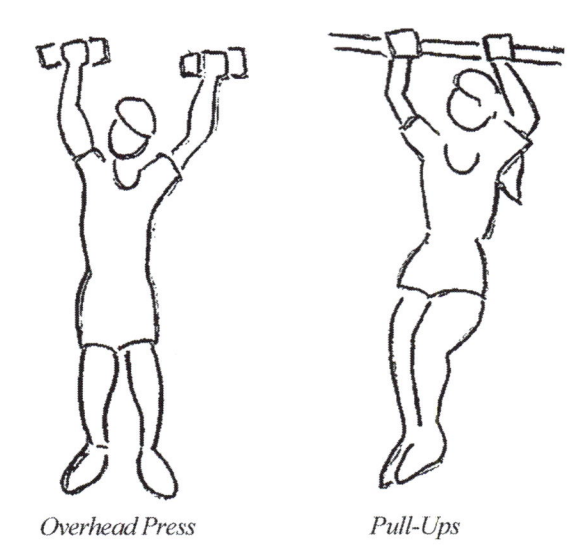

Overhead Press: the muscles of the shoulders (deltoids) and back of the arms (triceps) extend the weights up away from the body.

Pull-Ups: the antagonistic muscles of the back (trapezoids) and front of the arms (biceps) flex the body up towards the bar.

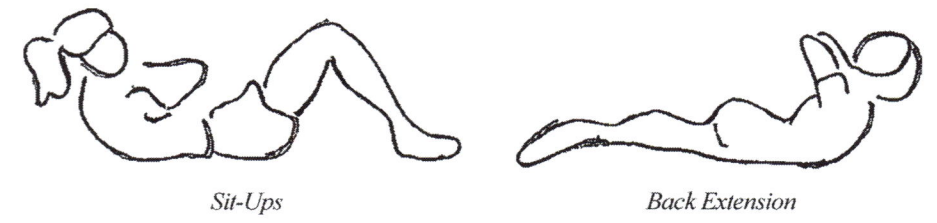

Sit-Ups   *Back Extension*

Sit-Ups: the muscles of the stomach (abdominals) flex the waist as the performer comes up.

Back Extension: the antagonistic muscles of the lower back (erector spinae) contract to extend the waist and raise the upper body upwards.

To this point in our discussion of muscular fitness we have been talking only of moving resistance through the range of motion. This type of training through a movement range is called *isotonic training* and is the most common means of training. There is another type of muscular strength training known as *isometric training*. Here we are referring to training without movement. Examples would be a student forcefully pushing his/her hands together or pushing mightily again a wall or against the offsetting force of another student. This kind of *isometric training* can be as effective as *isotonic.* A couple of major drawbacks of it is that the student might not as readily witness muscular gains as would be seen in accomplishing a greater number of pull-ups or being able to move a resistance a greater number of times. Also, the muscular strength gains made in *isometric* exercises seem to be quite specific to the joint positions used in training. Therefore, either the exercises need to be executed at a number of joint positions or significant strength gains at other joint angles can be expected to be small. Perhaps a good place you could utilize *isometric* exercises is in the classroom. As an activity break to get the blood flowing you could design a few exercises in which the students push and pull against himself or herself or against a partner

F.I.T. Principle Applied to Reducing Body Fat

For the reduction of body fat, the F.I.T. guidelines call for an hour of daily, low to moderate exercise. To understand the rationale for these guidelines some fundamental knowledge of calorie burning is useful. To begin with, we shall assume our body composition is at a stable level and we are not going to alter our caloric input by making any dietary changes. To lose one pound of body fat a person must do an extra 3,500 calories worth of exercise. Remember that relationship, *Three thousand five hundred calories must be burned to lose one pound of body fat.* Next, realize that if a 150-pound individual walked a mile on level terrain, he/she would burn approximately 100 calories above the normal resting metabolism rate. This figure would not vary much from individual to individual because, barring disabilities, most everyone walks with comparable efficiency. The only factor, which would pronouncedly affect this caloric figure, would be the weight of the person. A 300-pound person would burn about twice as much and a 75-pound child might burn half as much. If you are impressed with the above figures as I am, you are probably thinking, "Wow, a lot of walking must be done just to lose one single pound of fat!" The 150-pounder must walk 35 miles, the 300-pounder 17.5 miles, and the 75-pounder nearly 70 miles.

Now consider the caloric burning when our three people have run a mile. Because of the greater work inefficiencies in running compared to walking, our people would consume more calories during the activity: the 150 pound person would burn approximately 120 calories, the 300 pound person 240 calories, and the 75 pound person 60 calories. However, the net caloric effect of vigorous activities like running is not quite so simple. When people engage in vigorous activity their metabolisms get revved up and remain elevated for a period of time following the cessation of movement. You probably have noticed how your rate heart is somewhat higher and your cheeks and skin glow with the stronger flow of coursing blood. The more intense the exercise has been, the more this effect occurs. The metabolism can be thought of as a revolving wheel, the faster you get it going the longer it will continue to go after the applied forces have been terminated. Researchers have labeled this post-exercise calorie burning, due to a stimulated metabolism, *residual calorie burning*. Before we become overly excited about the benefits of residual calorie burning, we need to recognize that its contribution to total calorie expenditure is probable rather limited. The metabolism seems to be only significantly elevated following sustained high intensity exercise and even then it quickly returns to baseline levels within an hour or two. While it is difficult to calculate precise figures, and investigators are not yet in full agreement, most estimate that only around 20 to 40 residual calories will be burned up following robust aerobic efforts. If we return to our three runners once again we might come up with a best guess of their calorie usage by allotting each a mid-range figure of 30 residual calories. Doing so would see our 150 pounder consuming 150 calories as a result of the mile run (120 during + 30 residually); our 300 pounder 270 calories (240 during + 30 residually); our 75 pounder 90 calories (60 during + 30 residually).

So what are the implications we might draw from the above information? Firstly, as we already noted, a great deal of walking miles must be covered to lose just one pound of body fat (35 miles for the 150-pound person, 17.5 for the 300-pound person, and 70 for the 75-pound person). This is a sad fact of life that we need to understand, *the amount of weight you lose through exercise is grossly exaggerated.* You probably have to walk a mile to burn up the calories consumed in a bite-size Snickers (95 calories). This is indeed a sad fact of life if we are hoping to exercise so as to lose excess body fat. Our distant ancestors who were scrambling to find enough food to eat certainly would not view it as a sad fact. When considered in that light the efficiency of the body deserves to be appreciated.

Secondly, it is apparent that exercising more strenuously, given the same distance is covered, does not radically increase the total number of calories used. More will be burned during and following exercise but still, the 150-pound person might have to run at least 30 miles, the 300-pound person 13 miles, and the 75-pound person 39 miles. An initial despairing reaction you might have to the above data could be to conclude, "Why bother! Exercise, even vigorous exercise, seems so ineffectual in fat loss. Why put out such a great amount of effort for so small a return?" Although such a response is understandable, there is a more optimistic counterpoint to be made. Granted, exercise, either light paced or vigorous, will not produce large reductions in body fat in the short run, but let us look at the situation with a more long-term eye. What happens when we adhere to the *F.I.T. Principle* for body fat reduction over a period of time? Say our 150-pounder did an hour of walking or a comparable light-paced activity. We already know that an hour of steady walking would net about 3 miles or 300 calories. Now if this were done 7 days throughout the week, as the guidelines suggest, we would be talking about 2,100 calories. The weight scales would not yet show rewarding evidence of a pound of fat loss, but the needle would be wavering in that direction. Next assume that we have habituated this week's walking regimen and have continued it faithfully for the next 52 weeks. Now we are talking about real calories and fat loss, 109,200 calories and over 31 pounds. The moral of this story is clear. A lifelong active lifestyle will make a difference. Application of the *F.I.T. Principle* can be an effective, long-term approach to fat loss. People normally gain unwanted body fat over many months and years in a creeping fashion and we need to go about reducing in the same manner.

Perhaps a concluding point is warranted pertaining to the *F.I.T.* recommendation of light and moderate activity vis' a vis' vigorous activity. It should not be construed to mean that vigorous activity could not be effectively used as an avenue for weight loss. A better interpretation is that it is not a necessity. Light to moderate activity is suggested because, given equal amounts of total work, nearly as many calories are expended in light as in vigorous movements, and because data show that more people enjoy lighter paced activities and tend to better persevere at them for extended periods of time. But realize that participation in vigorous activities has its advantages. Those who become accustomed to and can enjoy more robust activities will be effectively burning calories and will also be deriving additional benefits. Training at more vigorous aerobic heart rate zones can give rise to greater psychological gains and to physiological gains in the cardio-respiratory and muscular fitness systems. Another benefit of higher paced activities is that more calories are burned in a shorter period of time and hence, for the same caloric loss, less time needs to be devoted to exercise; a 3 mile jog can be completed in probably half the time of a walk. This can be an important factor when we consider that lack of time is by far the most common reason given for not exercising. Figure 3.6 quantifies how, when time of exercise is held constant, modestly increasing the vigorousness of activity will significantly up the number of calories burned.

Figure 3.6. Calories Burned Per Hour

	\multicolumn{6}{c}{**Weight (pounds)**}
	95	125	155	185	215	245
Slow walking	86	114	140	168	196	222
Walking, moderate pace	172	228	280	336	392	555
Hiking	258	342	420	504	588	666
Jogging	430	570	700	840	980	1,110
Running	480	770	945	1,134	1,323	1,499
Heavy housework	194	256	315	378	441	500
Sweeping	108	142	175	210	245	278
Scrubbing	237	313	385	462	539	611
Tennis	301	399	490	588	686	777
Golf (carrying clubs)	237	313	385	462	539	611
Golf (in a cart)	151	200	245	294	343	389
Swimming (light laps)	344	456	560	672	784	888
Swimming (hard laps)	430	570	700	840	980	1,110

Qualification of the F.I.T. Principle

In concluding our discussion of the F.I.T. Principle as it relates to each of the components of fitness, a qualifying point is worth making. While the F.I.T. Principle provides a good training guideline and has scientific support, we need recognize that failure to fully comply with these guidelines does not mean some fitness improvements will not take place. Any amount of exercise, even though far below the F.I.T. guidelines, is good for us. Would no aerobic benefits be achieved if a person's target heart rate zone was 120 to 160 and he/she exercised at 119 beats per minute? Of course not. The body does not operate in an all or nothing manner. In fact, research documents that people who regularly engage in activities such as walking and gardening derive important cardiorespiratory benefits. Those people are not exercising at 60-95 percent of their maximum but at more like 20 for 30 percent. Likewise, should we expect no gain in abdominal muscle strength if the sit-ups were terminated before a near maximal effort was reached? No, the gains would be greatly lessened but some strength and muscular endurance improvements would take place. Choosing any level of movement is going to yield greater dynamic flexibility compared to doing nothing at all.

Perhaps we should think of exercise as having a dose effect. That simply means that small amounts of exercise and low intensities will produce small benefits, be they improvements in fitness components, protection from hypokinetic diseases, or many diverse psychological aspects of our lives. Larger doses of exercise will produce larger benefits. Figure 3.7 depicts a linear dose effect relationship established between a disability (strokes) and different levels of exercise. Such linear relationships are not always found when exercise levels are increased to quite high levels. For example, one study showed that for every additional mile run per week – up to 50 miles a week for men and 40 for women, the subjects had better blood pressure, better blood cholesterol, and less estimated risk of heart disease. Beyond 50 and 40 miles no further improvements were found. Another study found that subjects who were moderately fit had half the risk of early death as those who were not fit. Those who had attained high fitness fared even better, but not to quite the same degree – their premature death rate were 10 percent to 15 percent lower than the moderately fit group. And sometimes, when exercising to very extreme levels, a point of diminishing returns may be passed and health could be negatively impacted. That topic of overuse will be addressed in the next section.

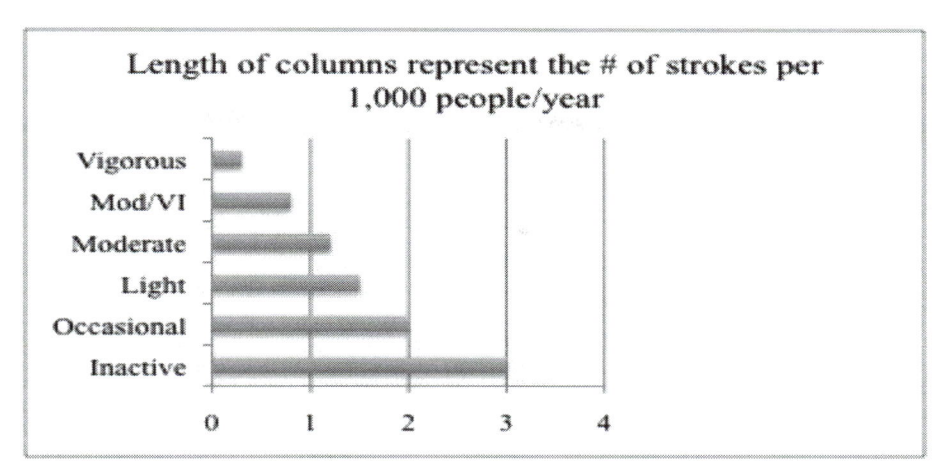

Figure 3.7. Dose Effect of Exercise as it Relates to Incidence of Stroke
Subjects studied were men aged 40 through 50 years old.

    Perhaps the most balanced stance to take relative to the F.I.T. Principle is to see it not as unbendable requirements but a useful guideline. I believe that teachers should make students aware of the F.I.T. Principle and the consequences of complying with differing degrees. Very little activity is bad, some regular activity is good, more regular activity is better. We should then let them know that they are responsible for the level of activity they choose to follow. I do not think it fruitful in the long run for us to be martinets and demand strict compliance. Such an approach may be discouraging to many whose exercise histories are many fathoms below these prescribed levels. Some of these people may never become comfortable with vigorous activities. And yet, if given an encouraging okay, they will be able to find light and moderate activities that can be a joy and benefit to their welfare.

    Having given my imprimatur to backing off of the F.I.T. Principle so as to stay in one's comfort zone, a cautionary word is in order. People must be aware that authorities view the guidelines as rather minimal standards that need to be followed if a fully healthy life is to be attained. If a person does 30 minutes of light activity each day he/she will indeed be much healthier than the person who chooses to be sedentary. However, this modest level of activity will not produce a well-trained cardio-respiratory and muscular fitness system. Nor will it likely be sufficient to enable the maintenance of an ideal or even good ratio of body fat. Our genetic inheritance is a product of physiological beings that survived by almost constant and unrelenting physical exertion, supported by an unreliable and worst than plain diet. Is it therefore unreasonable to expect that we need provide ourselves with at least an hour a day of moderate/vigorous activity to partially compensate for hour after hour of sitting, and plate after plate of succulent foods? Considered in this light, is one or more hours, out of 16 waking hours, really so exorbitant and unnatural? Is a person an obsessive health nut for vigorously exercising an hour everyday, or is he/she a bigger nut for not doing so?

Overuse Principle

The *Overuse Principle* is the simple statement that more is not always better. We need remind ourselves that most health behaviors, if advocated and taken to the extreme, can actually be harmful to wellbeing. Attempting to reduce fat intake down to near zero is not a good idea; being obsessively worried about sun exposure, germs, or other environmental hazards can also become needlessly debilitating. There is often wisdom in moderation and virtue in the mean.

With regards to exercise, it is important to remember that more is not always better. Generally speaking, unless there is a specific physiological problem, exercising at intensity levels well beyond the *F.I.T.* guidelines does not need to be dangerous for adults. Joy and peak physical fitness benefits can be safely found even in long arduous training sessions, running Marathons, climbing mountains, and competitively lifting heavy weights. However, it should be obvious that the stresses on the body may be too great if workloads are not slowly and progressively increased; and it is always essential to listen to warning limits of the body. When coaches and athletes operate according to the motto of "no pain, no gain," they are dangerously pushing the very upper limits of training intensity and injuries are not an uncommon consequence. If we are running and dancing with painful knees, and throwing with sore arms, we must know that our muscles and joints are saying that excessive trauma is occurring; the body is not successfully adapting to the strain and is in danger of breakdown. Overtraining without adequate recovery times can also effect more than limbs. Chronic fatigue and weakening of the body's immune system to colds and other stresses may occur. It is a good habit to regularly check one's resting heart rate. An unusual elevation may be a sign of overtraining or infection.

Prepubescent children are more susceptible to overuse. They may become hyperenthused about activities and they may poorly monitor warning signs. Additionally, their physiological defense systems are immature and less capable of coping with large forces and prolonged poundings. We have already made the point that children should not be seeing how much weight they can lift. When they do resistance training they should have a weight that can be safely controlled for at least a number of repetitions (13 or more). As for determining how far it is safe to have a child walking or running the following *Children's Walk/Run Formula* is useful: *miles to walk/run = age divided by three*. This means a nine-year-old should be able to buildup to 3 miles but be careful about much exceeding that. As with any such standard, still pay attention to individual differences. Children with disabilities, excessive body fat, etc., may need an individualize standard.

The American Academy of Pediatrics has identified a number of concerns centered on distance running, including potential long-term adverse effects that may not be seen for many years after a running program has started. Two main areas of concern are psychological consequences and physical consequences.

Psychological problems can result when adults set unrealistic goals for distance running by children. A child who participates in distance running primarily for adult approval may tire of it after a time and quit, or may push on unadvisedly while chafing under the pressure. In either case, psychological damage may be done and the child discouraged, either immediately or in the long run, from participating in future activity. Elementary school children should be given opportunities to run for the sheer joy of it, without fear of adult assessment. Children's sense of accomplishment, satisfaction, and appreciation – by parents, teachers, and peers – simply for participating will foster their involvement in running and other physical activities throughout childhood and in later life.

For school-age children, participation in distance running training and competitions also poses physical dangers. A position taken by the International Athletics Association states, "The danger certainly exists that with over-intensive training, separation of the growth plates may occur in the pelvic region, the knee, or the ankle. While this could heal with rest, nevertheless definitive information is lacking whether in years to come harmful effects may result." In view of this concern, it is the opinion of the committee that training and competition for long-distance track and road-running events should not be encouraged in young children. It is suggested that up to the age of 12, children not run more than 800 meters (one-half mile) in competition.

AEROBIC TRAINING FOR OVERWEIGHT CHILDREN

Being overweight reduces children's ability to perform physical tasks. Overweight children must expend more energy compared to normal-weight youngsters to accomplish the same task, and they perform at a higher percentage of their aerobic capacity. This gives overweight children less reserve capacity and causes them to perceive activities as requiring more effort, which indeed they do.

Despite these differences, some physical educators and classroom teachers require their entire class to participate in the same aerobic activity. Most commonly, teachers instruct their students to run a certain distance. When their increased exertion causes overweight students to perceive the task as too demanding, these teachers perceive the "overweight kids don't like to run." Indeed, many overweight children don't like to run because they cannot keep up with their peers. Thus, their needs for both peer acceptance and physical competency go unmet. Furthermore, running may not even be a physically appropriate activity for them because it can place too much stress on their joints. For all these reasons, it is inappropriate and counterproductive to require overweight children to run – or to perform other types of aerobic activities – to the same standards as normal-weight children.

To avoid this problem, rather than basing your performance expectations on distance, speed, or number of repetitions, base them on *time*. A principle to keep in mind is that the intensity of the activity is secondary to the amount of time a student is involved in it. In weight control, for example, long bouts of moderate activity are more effective than short bouts of intense exercise. Allow students to adjust the intensity of a physical activity to fit their individual needs. They know better than anyone else what

> they are capable of performing. When you base your expectations on time, you will not fault overweight runners for covering less distance than lean runners during a stipulated time period, or for performing fewer repetitions of an assigned exercise. Instead, you will reward all children for doing their best.

Reversibility Principle of Training

The Reversibility Principle simply means that physiological adaptations will not long be maintained following the cessation of training. It is a sad tale but true, you cannot store fitness. This is probably the most violated of all exercise principles. We all have at one time or other engaged in activities that have resulted in improvements to some component or components of fitness. Maybe we worked at a job that required heavy lifting and we noticed a significant increase in the strength and endurance of our arms. Maybe we played regular racquetball one term and could tell that both aerobic and anaerobic fitness had advanced. When we terminated these activities, and were not doing others that taxed those particular components of fitness, it was not long before those gains were lost. It is easy for researchers to document the reversibility process, it is not easy to say exactly how rapidly it occurs. The level of fitness that had been achieved, the component of fitness involved, the person's age, and innate individual differences can affect the rate of loss. A rough estimate might be something like a 10 percent decline of capability each week until the return to baseline. Although the exact rate of loss is not always clear, it is clear that no significant chronic effects should be expected. If an adult attributes his/her well-developed shoulder muscles to a youthful swim team experience, he/she is not correct. Either he/she is continuing to do some exercise which is maintaining it, or he/she naturally has a larger than normal baseline level for big shoulders.

    The moral of the *Reversibility Principle* is that if a certain level of fitness is acquired or possessed, and we wish to maintain it, then we must habituate ourselves to lifelong continuance of comparable activity. Children need to understand that gains made in school or during a sports season will be quickly lost if they become inactive over holidays or the summer months. Riding bicycle in the summer will not produce aerobic fitness throughout the winter months. Physical fitness is a dynamic process, a way of life.

Readiness/Trainability Principle

We have been saying that the various fitness components will respond to progressive training loads. However, this *readiness* to adapt to the stresses of exercise depends upon maturity. Before puberty, children do not fully possess the physiological mechanisms that will enable them to acquire the degree of fitness gains that can be garnered by post-pubescent children and adults. They are not nearly as *trainable* or amenable to exercise effects. A recent meta-analysis of 28 studies found that exercise programs had little, if any, increase in aerobic power in pre-pubescent children. When we see pre-pubescent children make improvements in fitness activities we must attribute most of that to their simply learning how to do those skills better; they are demonstrating more effective neuromuscular changes in technique, pacing themselves better, and/or benefiting from more self-confident motivation. Particularly little gains should be expected in the components of fitness requiring high intensity efforts: strength and anaerobic fitness. For those components, *muscle hypertrophy* (increased muscle diameter size) is a major factor for improvements and young children do not yet have all the hormones to simulate this growth.

What is the implication of low *trainability* in young children? To my mind, it means the improvement of elementary children's physical fitness levels should not be a priority goal. Any efforts here will be of limited avail, particularly with regards strength and anaerobic fitness. However, it does not mean that young people should not be learning the importance of exercise and should not be formulating the exercise habit.

Warm-up and Cool-Down Principle

Warm-up activities can be most any light or moderate paced activities or exercises that you do at the beginning of the lesson. Warm-ups should precede any strenuous activity because it increases respiration and blood flow and helps to guard against muscle, tendon, and ligament strains. As said earlier, newer research has suggested that *static stretching* is not a good activity for this purpose. Gradually going from walking to jogging to running is effective. Finally, progressing through dynamic flexibility exercises specific to the task is always called for.

Slower paced activities have long been advocated as a cool-down. The thought has been that if someone suddenly stopped moving following vigorous effort the pumping action of muscles would stop. That in turn would result in many bad things happening. Metabolic waste products such as lactic acid that built up in the muscles during exercise would not be removed as well and the result would be greater muscle soreness and slower recovery from fatigue. It was also thought that heart arrhythmia, that is more common immediately following strenuous efforts, might be lessened with a more gradual tapering of movement.

Upon close inspection of the research literature there is little evidence that these things actually happen. Differences in muscle soreness and recovery time from fatigue have not been documented between those who immediately sat down following exercises and those who did cool-down procedures. Nor is there evidence of differences in abnormal heart behaviors.

My conclusion is that each of us should do whatever feels best. If you like to move about that is fine, if you like to collapse, that too is all right. With your classes I still do advise ending with slower paced activities. It gives everyone a chance to cool off a little and to settle down. I always like to have a discussion at the end of class to summarize what was learned. By having a slower activity and a reflection time you will find that you have better behaved students in the hallways and back in the classroom. Vigorous exercise can promote more attentive and calm behaviors in the classroom but the transition should not be expected to be instantaneous.

CHAPTER COMPREHENSION CHECK

1. What are the *hypokinetic diseases*?
2. What is the difference between *health fitness* and *performance fitness*?
3. What are the components of physical fitness?
4. What are the two components of cardio-respiratory fitness? How is each defined?
5. Which component of fitness is considered most important to your health? What disabilities are associated with a lack of it?
6. How is *dynamic flexibility* defined?
7. What is the difference between *muscular strength* and *muscular endurance*?
8. How is *body composition* defined?
9. What are the main functions of body fat?
10. What are the main problems associated with having excessive body fat?
11. The *F.I.T. Principle* stands for what?
12. What are the specific *F.I.T. Guidelines* for developing each of the components of fitness?
13. How can maximum heart and target heart rate zones be determined?
14. What is the purpose of *the Perceived Exertion Scale*?
15. What is the difference between *dynamic* and *static flexibility* and how is each trained?
16. What has current research found regarding static stretching and athletic performance, injuries and muscle soreness?
17. What approximate percent reduction in strength has been found as a result of prior static stretching? For how long has the reduction occurred?
18. What is the relationship between *static* and *dynamic flexibility*?
19. Does a distinction between muscular strength and muscular endurance need to be made when training elementary children?
20. What is the minimal number of repetition suggested for developing muscular fitness in children?
21. Is there evidence that heavy resistance training could damage the soft growth plates of children's bones?
22. What is meant by *antagonistic* muscles? What are a few major muscles groups that are antagonistic to each other?
23. What is the difference between *isotonic* training and *isometric* training?
24. What does the number 3,500 represent in terms of calories?

| **Health** AND *Fitness* An Elementary Teacher's Guide

25. Approximately how many calories would a 150-pound person burn up by walking one mile? By running a mile?
26. What is meant by *residual calorie burning*? When does residual calorie burning occur most and how powerful of an influence does it produce?
27. What is the *dose effect* and how does it relate to exercise? Running beyond 50 miles per week for men and 40 miles per week for women was found to have what effect on the incidence of heart disease?
28. What is the *Overuse Principle*?
29. What is the *Children's Walk/Run Formula*?
30. What is the American Academy of Pediatrics psychological and physiological concerns about children and long-distance running?
31. The International Athletics Association has set a maximum distance for competitive running events for children 12 and under. What is it?
32. It is recommended that aerobic expectations for overweight children should be based upon which: distance, speed, or time? Why?
33. What is the *Reversibility Principle*?
34. What are the principles *of readiness* and *trainability*?
35. What is *muscle hypertrophy* and how susceptible are pre-pubescent children to it?
36. What are the guidelines for effective *warm-up* and *cool-down* activities?

Exercise Physiology: What You Need To Know

[CHAPTER 4]

NUTRITION: WHAT YOU NEED TO KNOW

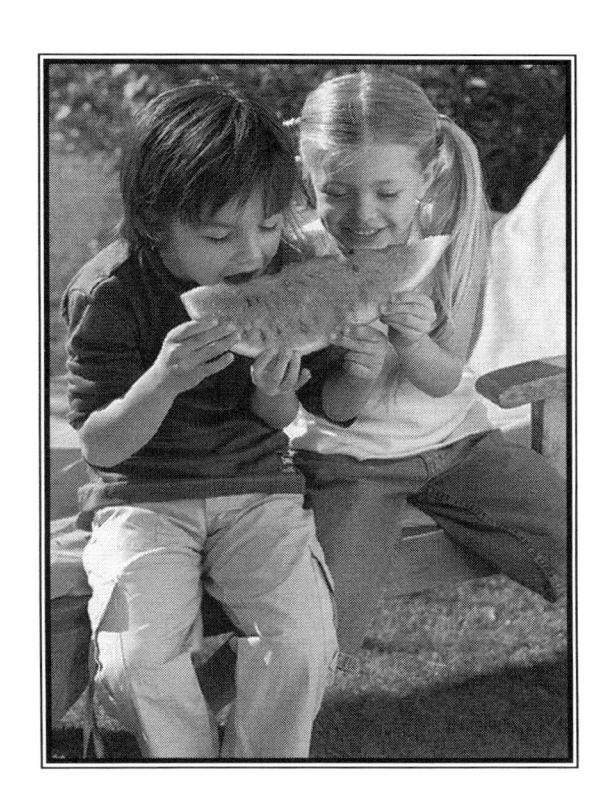

CARBOHYDRATES

FATS AND CHOLESTEROL

Unsaturated Fat
Saturated Fat
Trans-Fat

PROTEINS

FIBER

WATER AND BEVERAGES

Soda
Juice and Fruit Drinks
Tea and Coffee

VITAMINS

MINERALS

Calcium
Salt

OMEGA-3 FATTY ACIDS

CALORIC BALANCE

Anorexia

CHAPTER COMPREHENSION CHECK

> *"How can one play and think and find truth when stuffed with jelly doughnuts?"*
> ~ Anonymous

> *"We never repent having eaten too little."*
> ~ Thomas Jefferson

Chapter 1 made clear that poor nutrition, along with insufficient physical activity, warrants being classified as a leading health concern. Remember the estimates that unless lifestyles significantly change, 90 percent of the American population will become overweight or obese at some stage in their lives. If they do not gain excess body fat during childhood or young adulthood it is almost certain they will do so in their later decades. That means that virtually all Americans who maintain the Standard American Diet (SAD) will sooner or later experience some of the many unpleasant and deadly health problems that accompany excess body fat (i.e. psycho/social challenges, mobility limitations, high blood pressure, diabetes, arthritis, cancer). And even if those poor nutrition practices do not lead to weight gain many other health impairments will be the nearly inevitable consequence. Foremost of these would be the many variants of cardiovascular disease. It is well established that diets high in cholesterol and saturated fats lead to poor blood flow and hence progressively degrade the function of every part of the body (i.e. the brain, heart, other internal organs, limbs).

The body of evidence supporting a diet rich in whole grains, vegetables, and fruit, moderate in protein and in total fat, low in saturated and trans fats, abundant in vitamins and minerals and fiber is, quite simply, overwhelming. It is based on literally thousands, tens of thousands, and perhaps even hundreds of thousands of scientific studies. Chapter 2 explained why The Harvard Healthy Eating Pyramid and the kindred Vegetarian Pyramid best reflect this research and can serve as easy to follow working models. The strength of these models lies in simply directing us to what foods we should be eating and what foods we should be reducing, and they can be followed without being overly concerned about counting numbers of servings and grams.

This chapter covers the basic concepts that must be understood in order to eat in accordance with the models' recommendations. There is a section allotted to each of the fundamental aspects of nutrition: carbohydrates, fats and cholesterol, proteins, fiber, water and beverages, vitamins, minerals, omega-3 fatty acids, and caloric balance. The intent has been to be thorough without becoming too technical. These are the fundamentals you need to know in order to eat healthily. What is more, they are the concepts you will need to be introducing to your students if they are ultimately going to develop sound self-responsible eating behaviors. Now with the table set, let's get down to the food and drink.

CARBOHYDRATES

Carbohydrates (should be 55 to 60 percent of total calorie intake): Choose good carbs, not no carbs. Whole grains are your best bet.

In some circles carbohydrates have gained a bad name. A number of fad diets make blanket pronouncements on the dangers of carbohydrates. They say that promotion of carbohydrates by the USDA Pyramid has been the cause of the dramatic increase in obesity over the past couple of decades. After all, carbohydrates is what we feed pigs to fatten them up. This is wrong. Carbohydrates are essential and are a significant part of good diets. They provide the body with the fuel it needs for physical activity and for proper organ function, and they are an important part of a healthy diet. But some kinds of carbohydrates are far better than others. Complex carbohydrates are what we want and simple carbohydrates are what we want to minimize. Complex carbohydrates are slowly digested and provide sustained energy for the muscles. They promote good health by delivering vitamins, minerals, fiber, and a host of important phytonutrients (natural substances found in foods of plant origin which play a potentially beneficial role in the prevention and treatment of diseases).

Good sources of complex carbohydrates are vegetables, fruits, legumes, brown rice, whole grain pastas, whole grain cereals, and whole grain breads. Be careful when selecting whole grain products. Companies often make foods sound like they are whole grain when they are not. The package might say something like "nutritious wheat bread" or "wholesome multi-grain cereal" and not be in the least whole grained. You need to read the labels. True whole-grain products list as the main ingredient whole wheat, whole oats, whole rye, or some other whole grain cereal. Also, this shopping process is now much easier with the addition of the newly required *Whole Grain Stamp*. Look for this golden label. It will be found on all truly whole grain products.

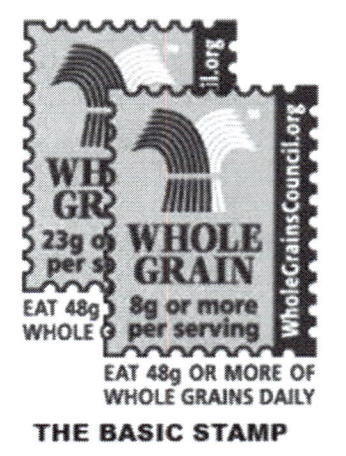

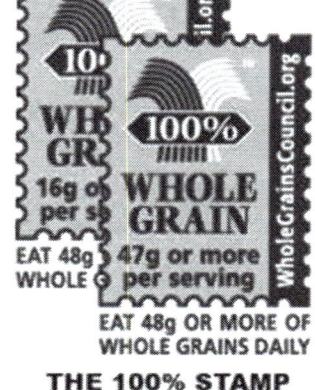

THE BASIC STAMP   THE 100% STAMP

If a product bares *The 100% Stamp*, then all its grain ingredients are whole grains. If a product bears *The Basic Stamp*, it contains at least 8 grams of whole grains, but may also contain some refined grain.

Simple carbohydrates are classified as *hyperglycemic (hyper* – meaning excessive, *glyc* – sweet, *emic* – of the blood) foods. That means that when they are eaten they are quickly digested and an abrupt rise in blood sugar occurs. This is why diabetics carry some type of candy or other sweets with them. It gives them an immediate fix when they detect the symptoms that their sugar level has become depleted. Although that is effective first aid for them, it is not something beneficial for the non-diabetic person to be frequently doing to their bodies. Simple carbohydrates cause quick rises that are soon followed by a rebounding drop in blood sugar. The result is that they do not provide a stable energy supply. The advertisement for a Snickers pick-me-up to get you through the afternoon is in reality counter-productive. More importantly, the long-term consequences of eating lots of hyperglycemic foods have been determined to contribute to weight gain, interfere with weight loss, and promote diabetes and heart disease. The calories they provide are considered "empty" in that they are not good for providing sustained energy and they are lacking in fiber, minerals and vitamins.

Typical sources of simple carbohydrates are white bread, white rice, potatoes, pastries, sugared sodas, and other highly processed foods. This might give you pause the next time you think of heading to a regularly frequented fast food restaurant for a hamburger, soft-drink, and fries. The hamburger bun is white bread, the potato in the fries is highly *hyperglycemic*, and the soda is totally so. Do not expect such a meal to effectively fuel any ensuing activity/sports plans, nor are you doing your body any long-term favors.

Up to this point I indeed have been uncompromisingly severe on all things *hyperglycemic*. In closing let me be somewhat equitable and defend them against one prevalent criticism. Although researchers have confirmed a link between consumption of simple sugars and the various deleterious health consequences identified above, there is one commonly thought consequent for which they are not guilty. It is a myth that giving students sugary treats will result in the dreaded "sugar highs." There is no physiological reason sugar ingestion should lead to hyperactivity, and well-controlled investigations have not documented any effect of this kind. The restiveness following parties and snacks is attributed to the relaxing of rules and greater exuberance that generally accompany breaks.

FATS AND CHOLESTEROL

Fats and Cholesterol (should be 20 to 30% of calorie intake): Choose healthy fats, limit saturated fat and cholesterol, and avoid trans fat.

As with carbohydrates, fats have a bad reputation in the minds of many. Over the years different diets have recommended deducing fats drastically. Proponents saw fat consumption to be the leading cause of obesity and cardiovascular disease. Obesity was linked to fat ingestion because high fat foods pack a much greater calorie wallop than do carbohydrates and proteins. Each gram of fat delivers 9 calories whereas a gram of carbohydrate or protein carries only 4 calories. Fatty diets were linked to cardiovascular disease because earlier epidemiological studies found strong correlations between the two. Populations that ate large amounts of fats were shown to experience greater incidence of heart disease.

Today's research shows that fats are not uniformly demons and that some fats are an integral part of healthy diets. In light of this more complete understanding, all three of the food pyramids (*USDA's My Pyramid, Harvard Healthy Eating Pyramid, Vegetarian Pyramid*) advocate the inclusion of a moderate amount of fat and differentiate among the types of fats that support or diminish health. The recommendation is for the total fat in one's diet accounting for between 20 to 30 percent of total daily calories. This range means that those "fat phobic" people who have eliminated almost all fat from their diets would be wise to assess if they are getting enough of the health contributing fats. On the other hand, this recommendation for moderation in fat consumption means that most Americans need to be reducing the quantity of fat they are eating, and by a sizeable amount for many of them. The typical American is deriving over 35 percent of his/her calories from fats and that figure has been continuing to creep upwards ever since the 1970s. Current figures show 80 percent of adults are above the 30 percent upper limit. High fat consumption is even more prevalent in the young; 82 percent of children aged 6 to 11 are above the 30 percent; 86 percent of adolescent boys and 82 percent of the girls are above the 30 percent. And overriding the common problem of too much total fat is the kinds of fats that are predominant. Approximately one half of total fat calories are currently coming from the deleterious types. Let us separately look at four major types and how a better ratio of good fats can be achieved.

Unsaturated Fats

Unsaturated Fats (should be 20 to 25 percent of total calorie intake)

Unsaturated fats, both monounsaturated and polyunsaturated, are a types of fats that are liquid at ordinary temperatures. Being liquid at body temperatures allows them to be digested quickly and not to linger in the stomach. They are thought of as the "good" fats that should account for at least two-thirds of total fat intake. They perform essential roles such as cell construction, energy supply, absorption and transport of vitamins/nutrients, hormone production, and maintenance of healthy hair and skin. Furthermore, contrary to past thought, they play a significant part in reducing arthrosclerosis by dissolving other unhealthy fats and cholesterol in the blood stream.

Health AND *Fitness* An Elementary Teacher's Guide

The vast majority of plant-based foods are low in total fat and generally the fat that is there is of the unsaturated kind. Unless fats are added to them in processing and cooking, the amount of fat in vegetables, fruits, legumes, grains, cereals and breads is a small percentage of total calories. There are a few plant-based exceptions. Coconut and palm oil are both high in saturated fats (the "bad" fat). Thus when choosing cooking oils, or looking at the oils added to processed foods and baked goods, it is better to select alternatives to palm and coconut. The way I remember which to avoid is to think of palm and coconut as the *Tropical Oils*, and to visualize a palm tree with coconuts hanging on it. One other vegetable oil that is high in the "bad" saturated fats is cocoa butter. It is found in chocolate – but don't despair. Guilt-free enjoyment of all things chocolate might still be possible. The saturated fats in chocolate seem to be of a special kind that does not raise cholesterol levels in the blood. The conclusion is that while light-milk chocolate should be limited, purer dark chocolates actually provide some health benefits. Although the dark chocolate is preferred, remember that all fat in-take is calorie rich and hence quantity needs to be guarded.

THE NUT CASE

Nuts have long had a bad rap for being high in fat and calories, prompting many to relegate nuts to their lists of forbidden foods. Nuts are delicious, crunchy foods that are packed with vitamins, minerals, and antioxidants. And that fat we were so wary of? Turns out it's good for our hearts. The Food and Drug Administration (FDA) states that eating 1.5 ounces (about a handful) of nuts a day may reduce the risk of heart disease. That is because most of the fat in nuts is monounsaturated and polyunsaturated, which have been shown to lower levels of LDL (so-called "Bad" cholesterol). However, not just any nut will do. The FDA includes six nuts in its qualified health claim. Those six winners are walnuts, almonds, peanuts, pistachios, pecans and hazelnuts. Those missing the cut include Brazils, macadamias, and cashews. These nuts have relatively high levels of saturated fat, which over time can clog arteries and lead to heart disease. It's also a good idea to steer clear of prepackaged nut mixes, which are often coated in oils and salt.

Saturated Fats

Saturated Fats (should be less than 10 percent of total calorie intake)
Saturated fats are a type of fat that solidifies at ordinary temperatures. Being less liquid at body temperatures results in slower digestion and a longer stay in the stomach. Although a moderate amount of dietary fat is needed, for the reasons already given (cell construction, energy supply, absorption and transport of vitamins/nutrients), saturated fats are known as the "bad" fats. They have earned this moniker because they are perhaps the main dietary cause of high blood cholesterol. As a consequence

of this effect on cholesterol they are associated with an increased risk for several medical conditions, such as obesity, heart disease, high blood pressure, insulin resistance, gallbladder disease, and certain cancers (for example, breast, colon, and prostate cancers). The Standard American Diet (SAD) typically sees 15 percent of more of total calories coming from saturated fats. Medical researchers would be pleased to see the figure significantly reduced. Seven to 10 percent is a commonly cited target.

Although we have learned that there are a few plant sources of saturated fat (coca, coconut, palm), saturated fats normally derive from animal products. In fact, approximately two-thirds of the fat in dairy products is saturated fat. Specific products particularly high in saturated fats include beef, beef fat, veal, lamb, pork, lard, poultry fat, butter, cream, milk, cheeses and other dairy products made from whole and 2 percent milk. All of these foods also contain dietary cholesterol. Saturated fat is more highly concentrated in red meat than in chicken. Fish is an animal exception because in contains a lower percentage of saturate fat and important amounts of Omega-3 fatty acids that work to lower cholesterol. Most shellfish is naturally low in total fat and saturated fat, and moderate in cholesterol content. Specific recommendations regarding different kinds of fish and shellfish will be discussed in the Omega-3 section.

It follows that the most efficacious way to lowered saturated fat consumption is to reduce or eliminate animal products. That is exactly what the Harvard Healthy Eating Pyramid and Vegetarian Pyramid advocate. Doing so is far easier than in the past. Many plant-based substitutes are much more flavorful, reasonably priced, and widely marketed. Soy and rice milk has become a happy substitution for many people. These milk substitutes have no saturated fat or cholesterol and yet provide the same proportion of protein as cow's milk. They are also typically enriched with calcium. There exist a wide range of meat substitutes that are rich in protein but minus the saturated fat. Smart-ground soy products can be used in toppings, stews and casseroles (i.e. spaghetti and taco sauce, soups and chilies, "Sloppy Joe" sandwiches and meat loafs). A diverse array of "veggie" meat substitutes exist in the forms of burgers, sausages, hot-dogs, and chicken strips. Egg-beater substitutes are made from egg whites and hence contain no saturated fat or cholesterol.

Selecting lower-fat animal products is another means of reducing saturated fats and calories. Chicken contains less saturated fat than does red meat. Choosing leaner cuts of meat and removing the skin from chicken helps. The white meat of chicken is a better selection than the dark pieces. Moving from whole milk to low-fat versions makes a much greater reduction in fat and calories than is realized by public. The 2 percent and 1 percent labels on milks and cheeses are deceiving because they represent how much of the weight comes from fat. Milk-fat is much less dense than the other milk components, that is why cream floats to the top. The relevant reality is that 8 ounces of whole milk contains 150 kcal – 55 percent of which is fat. The same amount of 2 percent milk has 120 kcal - 34 percent fat. One percent drops to 100 kcal - 22 percent fat. Non-fat milk (80 kcal – 0 percent fat) is at almost one-half the calories of whole milk but provides just as much protein and calcium. The medical organizations recommend the adoption of low fat milk and cheese for everyone aged two and beyond.

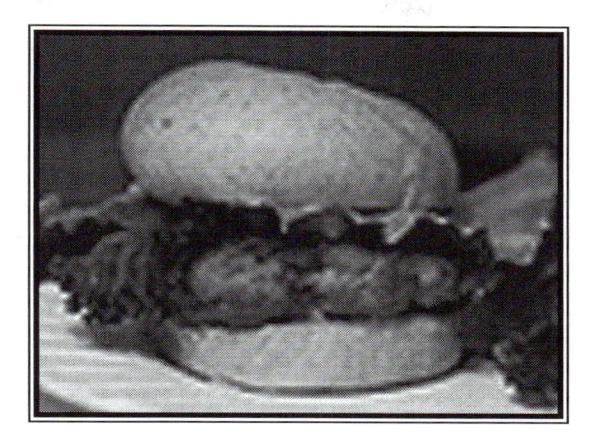

A large federal study of more than 500,000 middle-age and elderly Americans (age 50 to 71) found that those who consumed the equivalent of about a *small* hamburger every day were more than 30 percent likely to die during the 10 years they were followed, mostly from heart disease and cancers. Sausage, cold cuts and other processed meats also increased the risk. This, in the above photo, is not a *small* hamburger.

Trans-Fats

Trans-Fats (should be less than 1 percent of total calorie intake)
    Trans fats (or trans fatty acids) are almost entirely created in an industrial process that adds hydrogen to liquid vegetable oils to make them more solid. Another name for trans fats is "partially hydrogenated oils." Food manufactures and businesses like using trans fats in their foods because they are easy to use, inexpensive to produce, and last a long time. Trans fats give foods a desirable taste and texture. Many restaurants and fast-food outlets use trans fats to deep-fry foods because oils with trans fats can be used many times in commercial fryers.
    In recent years trans fats have been determined to be extremely bad for our bodies, even worse than animal fats. They raise both bad (LDL) cholesterol levels and lower good (HDL) cholesterol levels. Eating trans fats increases your risk of developing heart disease and stroke. It is also associated with a higher risk of developing type-2 diabetes. The American Heart Association recommends limiting the amount of *trans fats* to less than 1 percent of total daily calories. That means if you need 2,000 calories a day, no more than 20 of those calories should come from trans fats. That is less than 2 grams a day. Given the amount of naturally occurring trans fats you probably eat every day, this leaves virtually no room at all of industrially manufactured trans fats. Small amounts of trans fats occur naturally in some meat and dairy products, including

beef, lamb and butterfat. It is not clear whether or not these naturally occurring trans fats have the same bad effects on cholesterol as trans fats that have been industrially manufactured.

Some food producers and restaurants have moved away from the use of *trans fats* because of pressure from medical and consumer groups. However, it is still prevalent in many foods. It is especially common in fried foods like French fries and doughnuts, and baked goods including pastries, pie-crusts, biscuits, pizza dough, cookies, crackers, and stick margarines and shortenings. You can determine the amount of *trans fats* in a particular packaged food by looking at the Nutrition Facts label. You can also spot *trans fats* by reading ingredient lists and looking for the ingredients referred to as "partially hydrogenated" oils.

Finally, when discussing *trans fats* two products warrant individual attention. The first is peanut butter. It is a common product that can make a nice addition to a healthy diet. It is a good source of protein and the vegetable oil in peanuts is largely of the health promoting unsaturated sort. However, "hydrogenated fats" are added to most brands of peanut butter to keep the peanut oil in suspension and prevent it from separating and settling at the top of the jar. The cardiovascular system pays a high price for this convenience of not needing to stop and stir. The choice between hydrogenated and non-hydrogenated brands should be a no-brainer.

To use butter or margarine is another consequential health decision. Butter is rich in saturated fat, cholesterol and calories. One tablespoon has 100 calories (7.4 grams of saturated fat and 30 grams of cholesterol). It obviously needs to be used sparingly. But is margarine a better substitution? It depends. Most margarine is made from vegetable fat (low in saturated fat) and provides no dietary cholesterol. They thus are by far the wise alternative. The problem is that hydrogenated oils have been added to some margarines. The medical advice is to stay away from them, even butter would be preferable. Your best bet is read labels and to look for margarines in tubs or liquid form. The more liquid the margarine the less hydrogenated it is and the less *trans fats* it contains.

Supermarket shelves are loaded with products claiming zero grams trans fat per serving. But that "zero" on the label is not necessarily really zero. In fact, it can mean almost as much as half a gram of trans fat per serving. What consumers do not know is that many companies are taking advantage of the FDA trans fat labeling rules. According to FDA guidelines, products only need to have less than 0.5g trans fat per serving to claim zero grams trans fat. But even that is still too much. Just one of these so-called "zero grams trans fat" servings at each meal could add up to almost 1.5g trans fat per day over breakfast, lunch and dinner – and that is not including snacks. That is almost 75 percent of the American Heart Association's recommended daily limit of 2g. Consider the trans fat content of the following buttery spread brands that list zero trans fats: Country Crock (.436g), Blue Bonnet (3.92g), Land of Lakes (4.68g), I Can't Believe Its Not Butter Spread (.340g), and Smart Balance (.071g). Clearly the latter is the best choice.

CHOLESTEROL

Cholesterol: You make enough, consume as little as possible.

Cholesterol is a waxy substance produced in the liver and carried in the blood stream. It plays many useful functions such as building cell membranes and sex hormones. The liver easily produces enough to fully fulfill this role and the optimal dietary amount is zero. The health result of imbibing extra cholesterol is uniformly bad. It results in waxy plaque deposits forming in our arteries. This restricts blood flow and although no short-term symptoms might be noticed it leads to the serious cardiovascular impairments that are the primary cause of disability and death in America. We are not talking about just strokes and heart attacks. Weakened blood flow also degrades every limb and organ of the body, from tip of the toes to highest functions of the brain, and everything in between.

Because of the dire health consequences it is recommended that everyone know his or her total cholesterol level and have it checked every 5 or 10 years. The test entails a simple analysis of a small blood sample. Many people are unaware that they have dangerously high cholesterol because of their genetic predisposition, others do not realize how their food choices have caused it to be elevated and to change over time. A desirable total cholesterol is one that is positioned between 140 to 200 mg/dl. Readings from 200 to 239 are classified as borderline high. Two-hundred-forty and above is dangerously high. Thirty-eight percent of the population is in this category. That puts them at twice the risk of coronary heart disease as someone below 200.

A more thorough blood analysis is capable of separating cholesterol into two categories. That segment which is known as low-density lipoprotein (LDL), or "bad" cholesterol, is the true culprit responsible for the clogging. High-density lipoprotein (HLD) or "good" cholesterol actually plays an alternate part by counteracting the plaque build-up. Testing for the ratio of low to high lipoprotein gives a more precise picture of the degree of danger. This testing procedure is usually done as a follow-up to the more general total cholesterol count. It necessitates a fasting period of 9 -12 hours without food, liquids or pills.

As is the case in humans, animals naturally produce cholesterol in the liver. That means that all our dietary intake of cholesterol come from animals and their products. You can verify this by looking at the Nutritive Values Appendix in the back of the book, and checking the cholesterol column on the far right hand side. You will see that all types of meat contain high levels of cholesterol. Even though chicken and fish contain less saturated fat than red meat, they contain just as much cholesterol. The products of animals are likewise as high in cholesterol and many cases much more concentrated. Have a look at butter, cheese, whole milk and eggs. Notice that foods of plant origin contain zero grams.

It logically follows that if we wish to minimize our cholesterol levels, and our good health says we surely do, the course of action is to reduce the amount of meat products in our diets. Remember the numbers in Chapter 2 on the dramatically divergent average cholesterol levels of non-vegetarians vis-à-vis vegetarians: *Standard American Diet (SAD)* 193, vegetarian 181, vegan 153. If someone on the *SAD* cut the quantity of animal products in half, his/her chance of having a heart attack would be cut by 45 percent. If he/she went further and became a vegan, incidence of that occurring would fall by 90 percent. It needs to be realized that what we eat throughout the day has an immediate and pronounced effect on and amount of cholesterol floating about and sticking to our artery walls. Every 100 milligrams of cholesterol in a person's daily diet adds roughly five points to the total cholesterol level in the blood. For example, 100 milligrams of cholesterol are found in four ounces of trim beef or four ounces of chicken breast without the skin. Four ounces is not very much (remember we can equate three ounces of meat to a serving the size of a deck of playing cards). And of course these numbers precipitously jump if we are eating fatter cuts and the skin of chicken. The situation it much the same, or worse, with the products of animals. Three cups of whole milk will get you just about the same 100 milligrams and five points added to your cholesterol level. A cup of whole milk Ricotta cheese yields well over 100 milligrams as does half an egg. Given these facts it is easy to see that the *SAD* is resulting in chronically high cholesterol levels. The average American is far from eating four ounces of lean meat, four ounces of skinless chicken breast, a cup of cheese or half of an egg. The more accurate picture is that of regular selection of Extra-Cheese Pizzas, Egg-McMuffins, Woppers, Hot Wings, Grande Beef Tacos, etc.

GOOD EGG – BAD EGG?

It is understandable that you might be confused. Eggs are very high in cholesterol, and a diet high in cholesterol contributes to elevated blood cholesterol levels. On the other hand, the extent to which dietary cholesterol raises blood cholesterol levels is not clear. Many scientists believe that saturated fats and trans fats have a greater impact than does dietary cholesterol in raising blood cholesterol. Adding to the confusion, the *American Health Association* recently acknowledged that as long as you limit dietary cholesterol from other sources, it may be possible to include a daily egg in a healthy diet – a statement that was heavily reported in the media.

Here are the facts: One large egg has about 213 milligrams (mg) of cholesterol – all of which is found in the yolk. If you are healthy, it is recommended that you limit your dietary cholesterol intake to less than 300 mg a day. If you have cardiovascular disease, diabetes or high LDL (or "bad") cholesterol, you should limit your dietary cholesterol intake to less than 200 mg a day. Therefore, if you eat an egg on a given day, it is important to limit or avoid other sources of cholesterol for the rest of that day. If you like eggs but do not want the extra cholesterol, use egg whites. Egg whites contain no cholesterol. You may also use cholesterol-free egg substituted, which are made with egg whites.

To this point we have thought of cholesterol levels to be wholly a product of your hereditary make up and the amount of cholesterol acquired from the consumption of meat and animal products. It is not as simple as that. Two other significant factors are involved. The most important of these two is the influence other types of non-cholesterol foods have on lowering or raising the LDL blood levels. Some researchers believe that the impact of these other foods is even greater than the quantity of high cholesterol foods eaten. Foods high in fiber, unsaturated fats, and Omaga-3 fatty acids work effectively to remove the LDL "bad" cholesterol from the blood. Foods with these qualifications are those same complex carbohydrates advocated in the previous section: vegetables, fruits, legumes, brown rice, whole grain cereals and breads. Some specific complex carbohydrates that have been found to be particularly good at lowering cholesterol are oatmeal, kidney beans, apples, pears, bananas, barley, flaxseed and prunes. The other foods that lower cholesterol and LDL levels are those that are high in unsaturated fats and Omaga-3 fatty acid. The foods that have a major counter effect of worsening our cholesterol profiles are those with large amounts of saturated and trans fats. The specific foods processing unsaturated fats, saturated fats and trans fats were discuss earlier in this section and the Nutrition Values Appendix is helpful with columns for each. Foods with Omaga-3 fatty acids will be introduced in a later section along with a discussion of them.

The other factor that affects the total cholesterol count and the ratio of HDL and LDL is the amount of exercise one gets. Some people think that as long as they are exercising regularly, and are not over-weight, they will not have a problem with cholesterol and related cardiovascular problems. They rely upon it to control their cholesterol and free them up to not worry about the quality of their diets. The facts are that exercise definitely helps but not to the degree it can be solely relied upon. Any level of activity is known to help but those of a more vigorous nature produce the most benefit. For exercise to measurably lower cholesterol levels a relatively high volume is required. Adhering to a vigorous program can reduce total cholesterol by 10 to 20 percent. For example, participating in 1,500 kcal or more a week for 12 to 16 weeks produces these degrees of reductions. Fifteen hundred calories expended during exercise is equivalent to three to four hours per week for the average unfit person performing moderate-intensity walking, swimming, walk-jogging or cycling.

So what should be the lessons for us to draw regarding exercise and cholesterol? One would be that you can not run it away. The other is that a regular long-term program makes an undeniably useful contribution. Recall how marathon runners have lower cholesterol levels than the general population, but not as low as those lacto-ovo vegetarians and vegans. And remember too that if one persists in long-term exercise it tends to result in weight loss and that in turn lowers cholesterol.

PROTEIN

Protein: (should account for between 8-20 percent of calorie intake)
Pay attention to the protein package. Beans, nuts, seeds, fruits and vegetables and whole grains are your best bets. They provide the right amount of proteins along with other healthy things like fiber, vitamins and minerals.

The Food and Nutrition Board of the National Research Council states that you need 8-10 percent of your calories from protein. Other Health or organizations recommend the somewhat higher level of 15 to 20 percent. The average American diet provides much more than that, usually one to two times the recommended levels. We should be worrying much less about not getting enough protein, and a lot more about getting too much. Protein, unlike fats and carbohydrates, cannot be stored in the body and various health risks are incurred when the recommended levels are exceeded. When people eat too much protein, they take in more nitrogen than they need. This places a strain on the kidneys which must expel the extra nitrogen through urine. Diets rich in animal protein cause people to excrete more calcium than normal through their kidneys and thus increase the risk of both kidney stones and osteoporosis. Countries with lower-protein diets have lower rates of osteoporosis and hip fractures. Also, although fat is the dietary substance most often singled out for increasing cancer risk, some types of cancers are related to elevated protein intake.

Meat and animal products are rich sources of protein that contain all nine essential amino acids that cannot be synthesized in the body. However, because of the saturated fat, cholesterol and lack of fiber that accompanies the animal protein, plant protein sources are considered the better alternative. While individual plants might not offer all nine essential amino acids, a varied daily diet of beans, lentils, grains, and vegetables contains the entire compliment of complementary proteins. It was once thought that various plant foods had to be eaten together, at the same meal, to get their full protein value. Current research has determined that not to be the case. The American Dietetic Association states that protein needs can easily be met by consuming a variety of plant protein throughout the day.

As long as sufficient calories are being consumed to meet daily energy needs it is nearly impossible to be protein deficient. A diet rich in beans, nuts, seeds, vegetables and whole grains is abundantly capable of providing the 8 to 20 percent recommended levels. To confirm this point, look at the protein percentages found in this sampling of common plant based foods. You may be surprised at the quantity they contain: spinach 49%, broccoli 45%, mushroom 39%, tomato 20% pumpkin 15%, corn 15%, potato 11%, lentils 29%, pinto beans 26%, chickpeas 23%, peanuts 18%, sunflower seeds 17%, wheat 17%, oatmeal-cooked 15%, cashews 12 %, rice-brown 8%. You can refer to the Nutritional Values Appendix in the back of the book to see the grams of protein distributed across the plant spectrum.

Before leaving the subject of proteins, two frequently asked questions should be answered. The first is whether or not an active lifestyle demands a greater intake of protein. For a long time it was thought that athletes needed much more protein than other people in order to repair and build muscle mass. Many of today's researchers question whether physical activity level affects the body's need for protein at all. Others feel that increased physical activity levels require some increase. Both the American and the Canadian Dietetic Associations recommend that "highly active" athletes aim for nearly double the amount recommended for non-athletes. However, that recommendation is for the athlete who is engaging in more than 20 hours of vigorous weekly activity. Much smaller increases are advocated for more moderate amounts of exercise. Surprisingly the extra protein is not needed so much for muscle development as might be thought. Instead, it is needed to compensate for the protein that athletes burn up as fuel. Some athletes need a tremendous number of calories to meet their energy needs, and if they do not have enough fuel from carbohydrates and fats, their bodies turn to protein for energy. Regardless of exactly how much protein athletes may need it is certain that flooding the body with protein powders, egg white shakes, and big steaks does not build muscle. Any surplus calories from these powders, eggs and meats will just be converted into body fat.

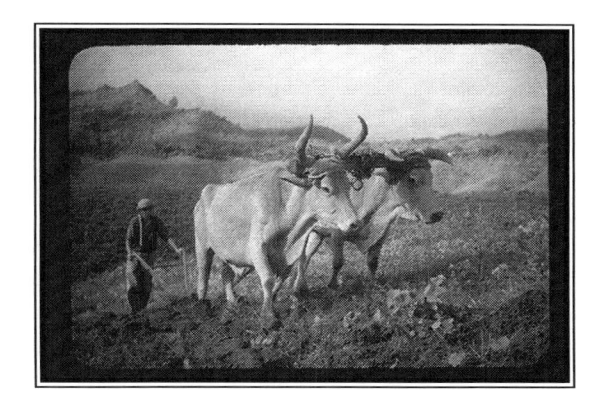

"One farmer says to me, 'You cannot live on vegetable food solely, for it furnishes nothing to make the bones with;' and so he religiously devotes a part of his day to supplying himself with the raw material of bones; walking all the while he talks behind his oxen, which, with vegetable-made bones, jerk him and his lumbering plow along in spite of ever obstacle." – Henry David Thoreau

The other common question relates to the advisability of adopting a high protein diet (Atkins, Zone, Protein Power, Sugar Busters and Stillman diets). As you probably expect, the answer is a definite no. These diets are especially popular because they are effective in producing a quick drop in weight. However, the quick drop in weight can be attributed to not just a drop in calories, but due to the dehydrating effect produced by minimizing or eliminating carbohydrates. The long-term effectiveness of these diets is questionable. And, of course, the really bad news is that they blatantly violate almost every tenant known essential for good health. Stressing meat and animal products and discouraging complex carbohydrates is essentially turning the research-supported pyramids on their heads. Inverting them this way means copious amounts of saturated fat and cholesterol and a dearth of the fiber, minerals and vitamins that are found in fruits and vegetables.

BIOAMPLIFICATION:
Another Health Reason for Choosing Plant Protein Over Animal Protein

When farm animals eat their feed, or fish eat plankton or smaller fish, they store and concentrate the toxic chemicals in their bodies. They in essence become piggy banks for toxic chemicals, storing them all their lives in their muscle and fat tissue. When we eat them, we break into the bank and receive a large load of toxic chemicals. Then, if we follow a diet that regularly includes animal products, we become toxic chemical piggy banks ourselves. When we eat meat, fish, dairy, and eggs, we are consuming a more concentrated source of chemicals, so the levels of toxic chemicals that accumulate in our bodies are even higher than in the animals we eat. This process is known a bioamplification and is a well-understood bio-chemical phenomenon. Levels of pesticides and industrial toxic chemicals, such as PCBs and dioxin, are often 100 times higher in animals than they are in greens and grains. The levels of pesticides and other toxic chemicals from the environment have been shown to be much lower in the bodies of vegetarians than in non-vegetarians. Many scientists consider this one of the reasons that vegetarians have lower rates of certain cancers.

FIBER

Fiber: Choose a fiber-filled diet, rich in whole grains, vegetables, and fruits.

Dietary fiber includes all parts of plant foods that our body cannot digest or absorb. It passes through our digestive systems supplying no calories and performs a number of valuable health functions. High-fiber foods require more chewing time and that in turn gives the body an opportunity to register when we are no longer hungry; overeating is less likely and more successful weight control results. Fiber in the digestive track has the effect of slowing absorption of sugars. This moderation of ups and downs in blood sugar levels is important in maintaining daily energy levels. This in turn plays a critical role in preventing and controlling diabetes. Fiber plays a significant part in lowering total blood cholesterol and hence is a component in fighting heart disease.

Finally, as is well known, fiber relieves constipation by softening stool and producing bulk. Hemorrhoids are a common difficulty when fiber intake is deficient.

The general recommendation is for adult women to shoot for over 20 grams of fiber a day; men should shoot for over 30 grams. Significantly higher intakes up to 50 grams per day would be better still. The only reason the number of grams is greater for men than for women is that they are typically larger and hence are consuming more total calories. The lesson to draw is that all men, women and children should be getting the majority of calories from complex carbohydrates because that is where the fiber is. Currently that is decidedly not happening. The average intake among American adults is approximately a meager 12 grams per day.

This gross disparity between fiber requirements and actual consumption should not be surprising. The great sources of fiber are whole fruits and vegetables, whole grain breads and breakfast cereals, and all manner of beans. These are the foods occupying the foundations of all three of the food pyramids and they are the very things of which our diets lack. When meat and animal products make up a major part of the *Standard American Diet (SAD)*, it necessarily displaces the amount of plant-based foods. Remember, all these animal products provide absolute zero grams of fiber. Compounding the problem is the prevalent practice of removing the fiber from the plant foods that are regularly eaten. Refined or processed foods – such as fruit juice, white bread and rice, pasta, and non-whole-grain cereals – are far lower in fiber content. The grain-refining process removes the outer fibrous coat (bran) from the grain. Similarly, removing the skin from fruits and vegetables decreases their fiber content. Those carbohydrates in restaurant hot dog/hamburger buns, taco/burrito shells, and rice/egg noodles have been denuded of much of their original fiber. And most of the supermarket offerings of cereals, breads, bagels, crackers, pastas, and desserts are much the same.

As we have stated elsewhere, the food environment that surrounds us is indeed toxic and we must take the time to read and understand labels. Be seeking "whole" grain foods and do not be misled by "wheat," "healthy," "nutritious," and other such empty claims.

WATER AND BEVERAGES

Water and Beverages: Drink water regularly. Stay away from pops and fruit drinks. Even juice is not the best.

Water is the body's principal chemical component, making up around 60 to 70 percent of body weight. Every system in your body depends on water. Water flushes toxins out of vital organs, carries nutrients to your cells and provides a moist environment for ear, nose and throat tissues. Every day you lose water through your breath, perspiration, urine and bowel movements. For your body to function properly, you must replenish its supply by regularly consuming water or beverages and foods that contain water. Even mild dehydration can drain your energy and make you tired.

There is no simple answer to how much water should be drunk each day. Studies have produced varying recommendations over the years. However, the 8 X 8 rule (eight 8-ounce glasses of water a day) is pretty well accepted. Some would be advocating higher levels if the person was physically large, exercised regularly, and lived in a warm climate that promotes perspiration. Others might downgrade the need for drinking water based upon the types of foods normally eaten. A diet high in fruits and vegetables provides more total fluids than one high in fat, meat, and dairy foods. Fruits and vegetables are 80 to 95% water. Obviously it is also possible to be getting water through other liquids: soda, juice, coffee, tea, alcoholic drinks, and milk. However, even though these beverages can be effective in increasing body fluids, they are not recommended as regular substitutions for water.

It is best to spread the intake of water throughout the day and evening. Drinking water with or just after meals is not encouraged because it can dilute digestive juices and reduce food digestion and nutrient assimilation. Some people like to drink a glass or two in the evening to help flush out their systems overnight, even though this may result in getting up during the night to urinate. Will increasing water intake result in many more trips to the restroom? Yes. But after a few weeks bladders tend to adjust and urination happens less frequently and in larger amounts. A practical guide as to whether or not a person is adequately hydrated is to monitor urine color; it should be a pale straw color and not a darker yellow.

Finally, a few words about water and exercising vigorously in hot weather. Those who exercise in hot environments are naturally at greater risk to becoming dehydrated. The recommendation is for them to drink a few gulps of water every 15 to 30 minutes. Water is the best choice for exercise sessions or athletic events that last up to 90 minutes. After that, there is a benefit to getting some carbohydrates in addition to the water to help boost blood sugar and prolong the period of time before muscles tire out.

Although rather rare, it is now known that there can be danger in drinking too much water. *Hyponatremia* is a condition that arises with excess fluid consumption and causes a dilution of sodium in the blood. Some marathoners have experienced *hyponatremia* because their fear of becoming dehydrated actually caused them to over compensate and drink much water. In recognition of this problem race literature has been changed from "drink as much as you can tolerate" to "drink as needed, but do not exceed 800 ml per hour." Eight hundred milliliters is equivalent to 3.2 cups.

Health AND *Fitness*   An Elementary Teacher's Guide

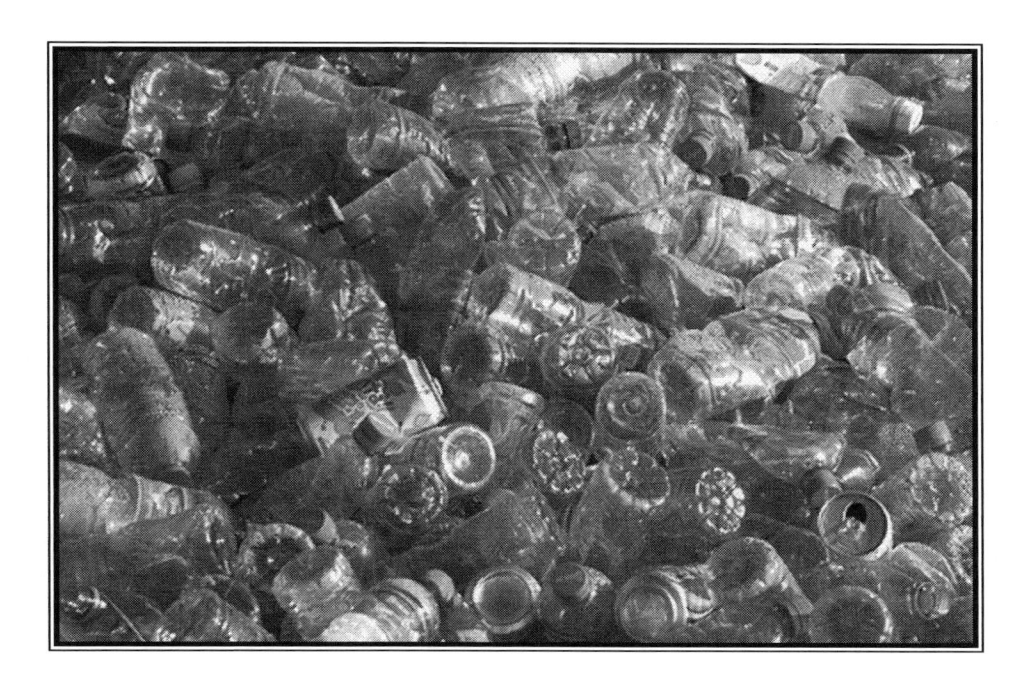

A CASE AGAINST BOTTLED WATER

You feel good when reaching for the bottled water instead of a soft drink –and rightly so. After all, who needs the empty calories and artificial sweeteners? But perhaps it would be in your interest, and the interest of the world, to forego the bottled water as well.

Cost
These distressed economic times accent the need for individuals and the world to conserve their finances. Consider this: global consumption of bottled water reached 41 billion gallons in 2004, up 57 percent from just five years earlier. That works out to between $50 and $100 billion with the market expanding at the startling annual rate of 7 percent, and of course the United States is the world's leading consumer. The average American is consuming 145 twenty-ounce bottles a year. Whether you purchase those bottles at $1 or $2.50 it is easy to calculate that we are talking about real money. That water is costing approximately 1000 times more than tap water. Does the expense of today's gasoline seem high? Realize that you are choosing to pay twice as much for the water.

Health
Municipal water falls under the purview of the *Environmental Protection Agency (EPA)*, and is regularly inspected for bacteria and toxic chemicals. Bottled water is regulated by the *Food and Drug Administration (FDA)*, which has weaker regulations than the *EPA* regulations for tap water. Furthermore, about 70 percent of bottled water never crosses state lines for sale, making it exempt from *FDA* oversight. When the *National Resources Defense Council (NRDC)* tested more than 1,000 bottles including 103

bottled water brands, they found contamination exceeding allowable limits in at least one sample from about one-third of the brands, including arsenic, synthetic organics, and bacteria.

In addition to the evidence that impure water is frequently put into the bottles, there is concern about the leaching of harmful chemicals from the bottles themselves. Research results have been equivocal thus far. But further testing remains to be done on bottles that have undergone ageing and temperature changes. It is known that these factors significantly increase leaching processes. Bottled water commonly undergoes significant storage periods and temperature changes during transportation over long distances.

Energy and Global Climate Change
Just saying NO to bottled water is a simple way to reduce our carbon footprint. Every year about 1.5 million tons of plastic goes into manufacturing water bottles for the global market, using processes that release toxics such as nickel, ethylbenzene, ethylene oxide and benzene. *The Pacific Institute* estimates that production of bottled water for U.S. consumption in 2006 required the equivalent of more than 17 million barrels of oil. This released over 2.5 million tons of carbon dioxide, a major global warming gas. Additionally, these figures do not factor in the sizeable energy and emissions costs of transporting the water. The water is first transported to the bottling plant, then the filled bottles are shipped to warehouses, stores, homes, and finally to landfills or recycling centers. By contrast, municipal water requires only a little energy to pump the water through pipes to our homes.

According to *The Pacific Institute*, the total amount of energy embedded in the use of bottled water is the equivalent of filling a plastic bottle one quarter full of oil. It also takes three liters of water to produce one liter of bottled water. Would it not seem rather profligate to dump that portion water down the drain prior to filling and drinking a glass of tap water?

Garbage
Bottled water currently accounts for 1.5 million tons of yearly waste, and each year the tonnage increases. Over 80 percent of plastic bottles are simply thrown away. In the U.S., more than 30 billion of them end up as garbage or litter each year. That is over 80 million bottles every day! The bottles take up to 1,000 years to decompose. Not only do they litter our cities, highways and parks, but they ultimately reach the ocean. The Central Pacific Garbage Patch eventually accumulates all the plastic that is washed to or dumped into the ocean. This vortex of undecaying waste is rapidly expanding. It now covers over 10 million square miles (about the size of Africa) and extends 30 meters below the surface. Tortoises, albatross, and other species are starving and dying as their stomachs fill with indigestible plastic pieces.

Conclusion
In light of the above reasons, purchasing bottled water is decidedly unnecessary and unsustainable. The environmental cost would remain large even if every bottle were diligently recycled. Recycling helps but does not negate the major amount of energy expended in reprocessing and transportation to and from various sites.

Soda

Drinking soda in place of water has become common and is easy to criticize. The average American is drinking 56 gallons per person per year. That is nearly 600 12-ounce cans. The typical 12-ounce soda has 150 calories and the equivalent of 8-10 teaspoons of sugar, mostly in the form of high-fructose corn syrup. The USDA recommends consuming no more than 8 teaspoons (32 grams) of added sugar (sugar that is added at the table or to processed foods and drinks) a day for those who follow a healthy 2,000-calorie-per-day diet. It usually works out to a 6 teaspoon limit for women and a 9 teaspoon limit for men. Children are consuming 30 pounds of sugar from soda a year.

The role of soda in America's bulging waistline has been hotly debated, but a new analysis says that it has been an increasing source of calories for children and adults, a trend that likely has led to weight gain and obesity. It has been found that drinking soda has no affect on hunger and the amount of food eaten. Drinking one soda a day can lead to a one-year weight gain of 15 pounds. Soda is also associated with increases in diabetes, fractures and cavities.

Some concerns have been expressed about diet and zero calories soda drinks. The fear has been that artificial sweeteners might increase the desire for more sugary foods or have other long-term deleterious health consequences. No research has of yet supported these claims. For now, they seem like a good alternative to sugary sodas, but maybe not as safely healthy as water.

Juice and Fruits Drinks

Selecting 100 percent fruit juice is thought to be better than drinking soda but not as good as eating the whole fruit. It is superior to soda in that it offers the nutritious vitamins and minerals present in the fruit or mixture of fruits from which it is extracted. It is inferior to whole fruit in that contains little or none of the vitally important fiber and a concentrated abundance of the fruit's sugars. For example, an orange has two times as much fiber and half as much sugar as a 12-ounce glass of orange juice. Because of the high caloric content of juice it is recommended the people who are looking to maintain or lose weight should be drinking no more than 8-ounces a day.

Innumerable popular fruit drinks are on the market. The percentage of juice in them can be misleadingly small. A fruit "cocktail" drink, for example, might contain as little as 5 percent juice with the other 95 percent water, added flavorings, and sweeteners. The obvious recommendation regarding these drinks is to minimize them as much as possible. They provide little in the way of vitamins while promoting weight gain, cavities and diabetes.

Tea and Coffee

Is tea and coffee good for us or not? Likely you have heard a variety of views pro and con. Although some of the research findings have been equivocal and much more investigation is needed, both drinks seem to qualify as part of a healthy diet. Light to moderate levels of daily use (1 to 2 cups and 3 to 4 cups respectively) has consistently been shown to increase alertness and improve both cognitive and physical performance on a variety of tasks. Some studies have found moderate coffee use to reduce risks of colon cancer, liver cancer, cirrhosis of the liver, Parkinson's disease and diabetes. Other studies have shown moderate tea drinking to lessen the incidence of diabetes, cancer, cardiovascular disease, and bone and joint problems.

Both coffee and tea contain significant amounts of caffeine. Coffee normally has about twice as much as does tea. A long-held common perception has been that caffeinated drinks are not effective in hydrating the body and actually contribute to dehydration. Studies have unequivocally shown otherwise. Both tea and coffee can help to hydrate the body. But caffeine certainly has a downside for some individuals, particularly when consumed in immoderate amounts. The caffeine that is responsible for stimulating better cognitive and physical performance can also cause wakefulness, jitteriness, elevated pulse, anxiety and higher blood pressure. Caffeine definitely is addictive and withdrawal symptoms include headache and lassitude.

Finally, a plain cup of tea or coffee contains zero fat and only a couple of calories. But as with most things we consume, what is added to it in the preparation process can change the landscape. One tablespoon of whipping cream adds more than 50 calories and 5 grams of fat to a cup of coffee, and 1 tablespoon of sugar adds nearly 50 calories. One tablespoon of fat-free milk, on the other hand, adds only 5 calories.

VITAMINS

Vitamins: A daily multivitamin is a great nutrition insurance policy.

Trying to follow all the studies on vitamins and health can make your head swirl. So many vitamins are important to different aspects of our health in so many complex and diverse ways. However, for the scope and purpose of this book, it is not necessary for us to cover the multitude of essential vitamins and their functions/symptoms. The important thing we need to grasp is that "no vitamin deficiencies occur when a balanced diet is followed." Hardliners take this summary fact as unassailable justification for redoubling efforts to eat better and get what is needed from whole foods. They fear that moving into the business of advocating supplements will lead to some people becoming less vigilant about eating well. They will rationalize that eating a balanced diet is not quite as critical because they have taken a pill to compensate. Although this argument is well taken, most nutritionists are aligning themselves with a more pragmatic approach and recommending a daily multiple vitamin and mineral supplement for everyone. They are cognizant of how severely imbalanced and erratic the Standard American Diet (SAD) is. Until society begins regularly eating quantities of fruits, vegetables and whole grains, they will continue to be at risk and would unquestionably benefit from appropriate supplements. Taking a one-a-day multivitamin and mineral supplement should be thought of as insurance for those who are conscientiously eating well, and absolutely essential for those not yet doing so. It is also essential for people over 50 to supplement their diet because the capacity to process vitamins is reduced as aging occurs.

The expense is not great for a basic multivitamin. And in light of today's knowledge it is probably wise to say no to any mega doses and "super" supplements. Future research might confirm that extra benefits can be gained from larger doses of certain vitamins, but at this stage such benefits are in dispute and there is more evidence that large amounts of vitamins can have unhealthy consequences.

Finally, a word should be said about vitamin B12. Because B12 is an essential vitamin that is only found in animal products, many have voiced this as an argument against vegetarianism. It is true that a strict vegan diet, which is completely based on plant matter, does not provide any B12. However, in practice there is little difficulty and vegans have rarely been found to suffer any symptoms. Firstly, many commonly available foods are fortified with B12. For example, soy milk, rice milk, and many breakfast cereals are fortified with it. And it is a regular ingredient in multi-vitamin tablets. Secondly, only a miniscule amount of B12 is required. The body hoards and recycles that which it receives. Very little is excreted and most people have at least a three-year supply stored in their livers and other tissues. Some people can go without it as long as 20 years.

MINERALS

Calcium and Milk: Calcium is important. But milk isn't the only, or even best, source. And leave more of the salt in the salt mine.

Calcium, the most abundant mineral in the human body, has several important functions. More than 99 percent of total body calcium is stored in the bones and teeth where it supports their structure. The remaining 1 percent is located throughout the body in blood, muscle, and the fluid between cells. The major concern about not getting enough calcium is osteoporosis. Getting enough calcium from childhood through adulthood helps build bones up and then helps slow the loss of bone as we age. Some other functions associated with calcium are lowering of blood pressure, reducing colon cancer, and aiding weight management. It is believed that the majority of Americans, especially girls and women, are not meeting the recommended intake for calcium. The deficiency estimate for girls ages 6-11 is 58 percent. Those estimates increase to 87 percent for adolescent girls and 78 percent for women over 20.

A common perception is that dairy products such as milk, cheese, ice cream and yogurt are the best means of get adequate calcium. These animal products do provide significant amounts of calcium but they are far from being the only source and they also have more than one downside. First of all, a diet replete with plant-based foods has no difficulty in achieving desirable intake standards. Specific foods that are naturally rich in calcium are beans (black and navy), dark leafy vegetables, cabbage, soymilk, cornmeal, wheat-flower, almonds, and sesame seeds. Ounce for ounce broccoli has more calcium than milk and the absorption rate of the calcium is almost double. There is much more calcium in 4 ounces of tofu or ¾ cup of greens than in one cup of cow's milk. Also, there are various regularly eaten products that are fortified with calcium. Breakfast cereals, juices and fruit drinks are good examples.

One of the reasons plant sources of calcium are preferable is that they contain healthy amounts of fiber and little or no saturated fats and cholesterol. That is decidedly not the case with cow's milk and cheeses. Selecting low-fat versions of these would helpfully lower the amount of saturated fats but they still would have some cholesterol and provide none of the fiber that would be found in soymilk.

The other problem with relying upon animal products as a calcium source has to do with absorption rate. Animal products are very high in protein. Excessive protein has the effect of countering calcium absorption and results in more of it being excreted in the urine. Some studies have determined that doubling the animal protein in the diet increases calcium loss by 50 percent. As a consequence, counter-intuitive as it may seem, demographic data finds osteoporosis rates are lower in countries where people consume fewer animal products. And vegetarians, even vegans, have been found to have bone densities as great or greater than the general population.

In consequence, the recommendation is to limit milk and dairy foods to no more than 1 to 2 servings per day. More will not necessarily do bones any good. Consuming less is fine as long as the diet contains the fruits, vegetables and complex carbohydrates prescribed by the *Harvard Healthy Eating* or *Vegetarian Pyramid*.

In closing the discussion of calcium it is worth stating that sodas, caffeinated drinks and exercise affect bone density. The phosphorus in soft drinks causes the body to lose calcium, as does the caffeine found in such things as cola drinks, other soft drinks, coffee, and tea. More than moderate intake of these drinks is thus discouraged. And no matter what level of calcium is ingested, regular weight-bearing exercises is needed to fully store calcium in the bones. Walking, running, step aerobics and resistance training are examples of exercises that cause your bones and muscles to work against gravity while they bear your weight

Salt

Sodium chloride is the primary electrolyte that regulates the extra-cellular fluid in the body. It is essential for hydration because it pumps water into the cells. The standard guideline is to have a daily intake of between 500 to 2,300 milligrams (2,300 milligrams is equivalent to one teaspoon of salt). The only people who might not be getting sufficient salt would be endurance athletes exercising in hot weather and who have been closely following a low salt diet of fresh fruits and vegetables. Most Americans take in 3,000 to 5,000 milligrams per day, about twice the recommended level. The major health problems with doing so are heightened blood pressure and calcium loss. High blood pressure, hypertension, is the serious "silent killer" that puts individuals at far greater risk of heart disease, stroke and kidney problems. The incidence of high blood pressure has been steadily increasing. In less than 10 years the number of suffers has doubled and physicians fear a growing epidemic in young people. The consequences of calcium deficiency upon osteoporosis have been previously discussed.

Excessive salt intake is so ubiquitous among Americans because large amounts are added to almost every processed food. Seventy-five to 80 percent of daily salt consumption comes from processed foods and we are eating a lot of processed foods! You might expect the sodium content to be high in snack food like pretzels and potato chips, and they are. Just one ounce of potato chips has 183 milligrams. But consider these representative examples of processed foods for which you probably have not given thought to salt: one teaspoons of soy sauce = 304 mg, one ounce of American cheese = 304, one cup of caned chicken soups = 850 mg). I like to pack an 11.5-ounce can of V8 juice in my lunch each day because I have come to like it and it contains a good variety vegetable juices and fiber. Nevertheless I must understand that it contains 690 mg of salt. That constitutes 29 percent of the upper cutoff allotment. The point I am making is that large quantities are added to almost every processed food unless it is a specifically marketed low sodium version. And the high salt situation is much the same or worse for the meals bought at fast food and family restaurants. They typically lace their offerings with copious salt because it is an inexpensive spice and they know most people's taste buds have become accustomed to it.

So what is a person to do? The best solution is the same old story, eat more fresh fruits, vegetables and whole grains, and rely less of processed foods. Beyond that, reading labels is needed to make wise selections, and learn to gradually decrease the amount of salt used in the course of preparing meals. Various spices help compensate for lower levels of salt and with time taste preferences do adjust downwards.

OMEGA-3 FATTY ACIDS

Omega-3 fatty acids are polyunsaturated fatty acids that are essential nutrients for health. Many food scientists believe that raising their levels could be as important as lowering cholesterol. Among other things, omeg-3 fats protect against heart disease and are vital in building cell membranes in the brain.

Since our bodies cannot make omega-3 fats we should aim to get at least one rich source of omega-3 fatty acids in your diet every day. Even though the amount needed is quite small, the typical American diet seldom includes the good sources of omega-3s, and certainly does not contain them on a daily basis. Look at this list of rich sources of omega-3s and you will see that they are not foods on the radar screen of most Americans: fish, tofu, soybean oil, canola oil, flaxseed, walnuts and various green vegetables (i.e. Brussels sprouts, spinach, and salad greens).

Introducing these foods into the SAD will undeniably require major changes for most people. However, it should not be as unrealistic as it might first seem. The required quantities of these sources are remarkably small: 3-ounces of fish, a tablespoon of vegetable oil, a handful of walnuts, a salad with lunch or dinner, etc. Also, supplements, although an imperfect replacement, can be an easy and helpful backup. For safety, a daily 500 mg fish oil supplement is recommended. Vegans can find supplements derived from algae, the fishes' omega-3 source.

Doctor's normally advise eating fish at least twice a week for the omega-3 benefits. Fish classified as "fatty fish" are best (mackerel, lake trout, herring, sardines, albacore tuna and salmon). The heart-healthy benefits of fish are best maintained when baked or grilled. High heat can destroy omega-3 molecules. Also, wild fish tends to have higher levels of omega-3s then do those that are farm-raised. This is because of the greater amounts of algae in their diets. Of course, vegetarians, and people who do not regularly purchase fish, can still meet their omega-3 requirements through a wise selection of vegetables. Vegetarians can correctly argue that the vegetable options allow the avoidance of both the cholesterol inherent in all fish, and the possibility of mercury contamination found in many of today's fish. They also rightly point out that given today's and tomorrow's world population it is simply impossible for everyone to be consuming fish twice a week, regardless as to whether it is farm-raised or wild.

Finally, a few words about omaga-3 eggs are in order. Several companies are now marketing eggs that contain omega-3 fatty acid. They achieve this by feeding their hens a diet of canola oil and other types of non-animal fats. Hens raised on these diets indeed produce eggs with lower saturated fat and higher levels of omega-3 fatty acid (three to six times that of normal eggs). This undeniably is a good thing and on the face of it makes for a wise selection. However, these eggs often can cost twice as much as "regular" eggs and the amount of omega-3 fatty acid they yield is very modest. Each egg contains 100 to 200 mg of omega-3s. That quality of omega-3 fat is found in just one-and-a-half teaspoons of salmon (a 3-ounce serving of salmon yields more than 1000 mg.). Clearly the advertised benefits of these eggs are being deceptively exaggerated.

CALORIC BALANCE

In closing this chapter on nutrition it is appropriate to emphasize the necessity of balancing the intake and expenditure of calories. Let us first address the imbalance of taking in more calories than what are burned up through basal metabolism and physical activity. In America, it is by far the more widespread of the two. When it occurs over a period of time excessive body fat and its concomitant health problems are the consequence. Something in the range of a third of children and two thirds of adults are now classified as overweight or obese. Those figures are two to three times as high as what they were 20 years ago. Ten percent of the population has developed type II diabetes and unless better caloric stability can be established the projections are for that number to rapidly increase to one third.

Reducing the disparity of intake to expenditure can of course be accomplished by burning more calories via more physical activity, reducing the calories consumed, or a combination of the two. The previous chapter clarified how physical activity and lean muscle mass contribute to the consumption of calories and weight loss. The take-away theme was that upgrading exercise would not quickly lower the amount of body fat, but that a persistently active lifestyle would in the long-term yield tangible dividends. Also, adhering to an active lifestyle was thought to be eminently feasible in that everyone should be able to find physical activities that they found enjoyable and which enriched their lives.

On the calorie intake side of the equation, modest restriction of one's normal consumption of food is a sensible, effective strategy. Reducing or eliminating non-essential foods should be the first priority. Even slight changes can produce big changes. If a daily soda (140 kcal) were removed from the diet it would result in a savings of 14 potential pounds of fat by year's end; or lowering one's butter allotment by just one tablespoon (100 kcal) would mean 10 fewer pounds. Significant long-term calorie savings could also be gained by minimizing the quantity of more nutrient rich foods. Economizing on serving sizes and eschewing seconds can be done without compromising nutritional requirements. In fact, animal studies have shown that by reducing caloric intake by as much as 30 percent, while maintaining nutritional balance, results in pronounced health benefits and lengthened life spans. The animals display obviously greater fitness, have lower cancer and cardiovascular problems, and live an amazing 40 percent longer. A small but increasing number of people has enthusiastically taken these findings to heart and have adopted this sort of Spartan lifestyle. Data gathered to this point has found these followers to be experiencing exceptionally good health. More time will need pass before duration of life figures will be available. Of course, making such draconian cuts in diet is something most of us would not eagerly contemplate doing. How many of us would really want to perpetually live in a half hungry state and never have the option of at least occasional indulgences? But surely these findings contain a lesson for everyone. They appropriately remind us that unnecessary consumption of calories is not good for us. Nor is it good for society. Surely we all have a civic responsibility to maintain our fitness to the best of our ability and hence lead as productive lives as possible. Control of health care cost is contingent upon everyone doing so. And there is the issue of resource consumption. Enormous energy and natural resources are expended to raise, process, and package and transport foodstuffs. Certainly it is ethical to exercise temperance and to put no more on our plates than is necessary.

One other effective avenue for decreasing calories is to change the types of foods eaten. Eating more whole grains and fruits and vegetables means large amounts of complex carbohydrates (4 kcal/g), modest amounts of protein (kcal/g), modest amounts of fats (9 kcal/g), and a huge increase in fiber (0 kcal/g). When such a diet is compared to a similar sized Standard American Diet (SAD), with its abundance of fats and simple sugars, a very real caloric difference is evident. The fatty and sugary fares carry a costly calorie hammering with little of the bulk and filling effects inherent in fibrous foods. Meats and dairy products are compactly full of fat calories and offer no fiber. Think of the satiating differential between a potato (130 kcal) and a donut (270 kcal), or an apple (65 kcal) and a "Miniature Snickers" candy bar (95 kcal). Accustoming oneself to lower calorie options of commonly eaten foods can also attain significant savings. Compare whole cows' milk (146 kcal/cup), soy milk (127 kcal/cup) and non-fat cows' milk (87 kcal/cup). If someone where drinking an average of just two cups per day, the move from whole cows' milk to soy milk would be a difference of 4 pounds in a year's time; the move from whole cows' milk to non-fat cows' milk would be a difference of 13 pounds.

The most effective weight loss programs are ones in which individuals lose about one pound per week. Doing so means that a person must to take in approximately five hundred fewer calories than he/she burns each day. Five hundred calories, times 7 days, will equal the 3,500 calories in one pound of fat. Although adjustments of this size are real and require a degree of fortitude, they are generally manageable. When patiently followed the desired weight eventually is lost and a new lifestyle is established.

The most common weight loss error is the adoption of diet plans whose purpose is to drop weight fast. It is normal to be impatient and wish to make rapid progress. People become enthused and begin skipping meals and/or limiting themselves to extremely small portions. This type of behavior will definitely work in the short run. The problem is with the long run. When the semi-starvation phase is over the dieter typically returns to his/her former eating practices that created the problem. They have not inculcated a sustainable routine. Furthermore, there are other reasons for avoiding crash diets. They often do not meet all nutritional needs because of their severely restrictive nature. Mineral and vitamin deficiencies are a real risk, energy levels are naturally low, and often lean muscle mass is cannibalized as well as fat cells. Finally, going through feast and famine cycles, so called yo-yoing, is not good for a variety of metabolic reasons. Copious statistics verify that nearly everyone who engages in rapid weight loss diets will within a year or two have regained more than initially was lost.

Anorexia

Although taking in too many calories and gaining excess body fat is the all too usual American problem, there exist the small but dangerous counter phenomenon that warrants attention. Anorexia is an eating disorder where people develop a fear of being overweight and as a result engage in excessive exercise and/or eat far too little. These starvation practices usually begin in young people around the onset of puberty. It is most common in those who are involved in activities where thinness is especially valued, such as dancing, theater, and distance running. Approximately one percent of teenage girls have been classified with the condition. Although it is less likely for boys to display these behaviors, they do account for 5 to 10 percent of the cases.

Sufferers from anorexia are very skinny but paradoxically are convinced that they are overweight. The medical risks include osteoporosis, irregular heartbeat, fatigue, depression, and skin problems. Anorexia is especially serious because without treatment it generally worsens and can become life threatening. In fact, nearly 10 percent of anorexics die as a result of their obsessive behavior. It is imperative for them to receive medical help. When individuals display these symptoms the recommended procedure is to gently express concern and to help them secure professional help.

CHAPTER COMPREHENSION CHECK

1. What approximate percentage of total calories should come from complex carbohydrates? *55-60*
2. What is the difference between simple and complex carbohydrates? What are good examples of each? *simple-sugar bad   complex-grains*
3. What kinds of nutrients do complex carbohydrates provide? *vitamins, minerals, fiber*
4. What is meant by *hyperglycemic*? What foods could be so classified? *too much sugar*
5. What has the research found regarding "the sugar high?" *its a myth*
6. Fats should consist of approximately what percentage of total calorie intake? *20%*
7. How many calories are delivered by each gram of fat, protein and carbohydrate? *fat-9 protein-4 carbo-4*
8. How much fat is the typical American consuming (percentage-wise)? *35%*
9. What approximate percentage of calories should be coming from unsaturated fats? *20-25%*

10. What nutritional roles do unsaturated fats fulfill? cell construction
11. What foods are rich in unsaturated fats? grains, fruit veggies
12. Which nuts are considered to be healthier than others? cola, coconut, palm
13. What are the vegetable exceptions that are high in saturated fats?
14. What approximate percentage of calorie intake should come from saturated fats? 10
15. Which foods are high in saturated fats? What are the health consequences?
16. What is the meat exception to the high level of saturated fat that animal products normally yield? Fish
17. How much of a reduction in fat occurs in moving from whole milk, to 2 percent, 1 percent, skim and soy/rice milk? page 82
18. What approximate percentage of total calories should come from trans-fats? less than avg
19. What effect do trans-fats have on the body? Where do they primarily come from?
20. What are *partially hydrogenated oils*? another name for trans fats, Animals, raise LDL
21. When is margarine better for you than butter? All the time
22. How much cholesterol intake should we be striving for? Which foods have it and which foods do not? none - animals have
23. What effect does high cholesterol have on our bodies? arteries clog
24. What is the difference between low-density lipoprotein (LDL) and high-density lipoprotein (HDL)?
25. What is considered an acceptable cholesterol level? How often should we have it measured? 140-200, 5 to 10 yrs
26. A deck of playing cards would be equivalent to approximately how many ounces of meat? Eating 8 ounces of lean (skinless) chicken would raise your cholesterol level how much? 3 oz   10 points
27. What is the story regarding eggs and cholesterol? What is the recommended consumption of eggs? yolks hurt it, whites don't
28. What effect do complex carbohydrates have on LDL levels?
29. What effect does exercise have on LDL levels? To what extent?
30. Protein should make-up approximately what percent of total calorie intake? 6-20
31. To what extent are plant-based proteins capable of meeting protein requirements?
32. Do Americans typically get enough protein in their diets? Do they get too much?
33. What is the effect of getting too much protein in our diet?
34. What is the story on high protein diets? Why might they seem effective in the short run and what about the long-term consequences?
35. What is the recommendation for fiber intake and what is the normal intake of Americans?
36. Where does and does not fiber come from? What role does it play?
37. What is the *8X8 Rule*?
38. What *is* hyponatremia? How common is it?
39. What is the story regarding bottled water? What are the arguments against using it?

40 Soda typically contains approximately how much sugar? What is the recommended daily consumption allotment?
41 What is the story on zero calorie soda drinks?
42 What is the story on Juice and fruits drinks? What is the recommended daily consumption allotment?
43 Is coffee and tea good for us?
44 What is the stance of most nutritionist on multivitamins?
45 Where does vitamin B12 come from? Why is it not now considered a barrier to vegetarianism?
46 What is the role of calcium? What foods provide it? Why are plant-based sources of calcium considered preferable to animal-based sources?
47 What is the recommended limit to milk and dairy food servings per day? Why?
48 Where does most of the salt in our diet come from?
49 What role do Omega-3 Fatty Acids play? In which foods are they found?
50 Is purchase of Omega-3 eggs considered a wise economic choice?
51 Effective weight loss programs recommend loosing how many pounds per week? This could be done by lowering our calorie intake by how many calories per day?
52 What is *anorexia*? What are the symptoms and causes?
53 What percent of *anorexics* die as a result of their obsessive behavior?

[CHAPTER 5]

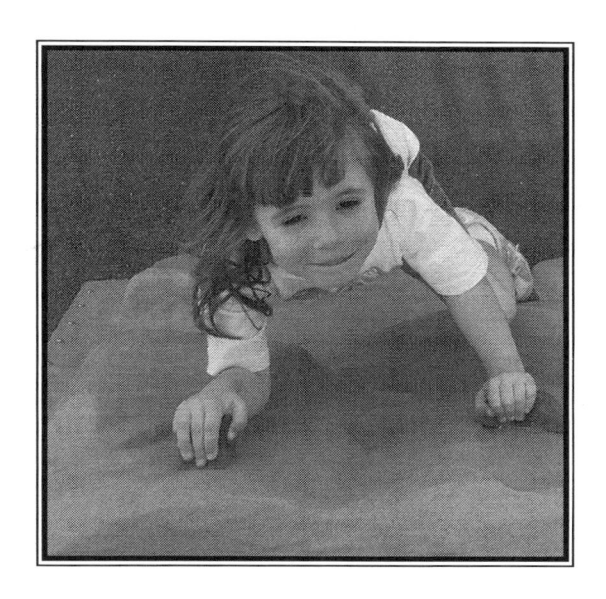

INSTILLING HEALTH AND AFFECTIVE BEHAVIORS

INSTILLING HEALTHY BEHAVIORS

Teaching Self-Responsibility
Selecting the Behavior
Recognizing the Benefits of the Behavior
Doing the Behavior in School
Tracking/Reinforcing Beyond Class Behavior
Going Multi-disciplinary
Changing Nutritional Practices

INSTILLING AFFECTIVE BEHAVIORS
Awareness Talks
Reflection Times

CHAPTER COMPREHENSION CHECK

> *"The great aim of education is not knowledge, but action."*
> ~ George Herbert

> *"Teaching Kids How to Behave is More Important than Any Other Skill."*
> ~ Anonymous

This chapter is broken into two main sections. The first section addresses what teachers can do to develop good health habits in their students. This will be done by explaining four instructional steps involved in teaching self-responsible actions: (1) selecting the behavior, (2) recognizing the benefits of the behavior, (3) doing the behavior in school, and (4) tracking/reinforcing the behavior beyond school. Additionally, the criticalness of working with the entire school in a multidisciplinary manner is introduced, along with some specific ideas for changing nutritional practices.

The second section is devoted to teaching good affective domain habits. The case is made that getting students involved in different types of physical activities and games has great potential for teaching affective behaviors such as perseverance, cooperation, and respect. The techniques of "awareness talks" and "reflection times" are explained.

INSTILLING HEALTHY BEHAVIORS

Teaching Self-Responsibility

Taking children out to exercise and play games is good for their physical fitness and motor skill development. If they enjoy those games, and appreciate their improved fitness and motor skills, we can be sure that they will continue to regularly participate outside of school. Telling your students that they should adopt the lifestyle that incorporates The Healthy Eating/Vegetarian Food Pyramids and The Activity Pyramid will be sufficient for them to do so. OKAY, WE CAN STOP RIGHT THERE AND GET REAL! We know that if we wish to make major habit changes, and that is our ultimate goal, we will need to do much more than expose students to activities and/or tell them what they should do. They will need to be fully convinced of the benefits of the new practices and they will require guidance and sustained encouragement in initiating those changes beyond school. Ultimately they must realize that they alone must be accountable for these exercise/health behaviors and then take that responsibility.

What must be done to establish this self-responsibility in young people so that they will independently adopt and maintain good exercise/health practices? Let us look at four important instructional considerations: (1) selecting the behavior, (2) recognizing the benefits of the behavior, (3) doing the behavior in school, (4) and tracking/reinforcing the behavior beyond school.

Selecting the Behavior

Although you may see many exercise/health behaviors in need of alteration, and for which you would love to affect a change, it will be best if you, at least initially, narrow the field of possibilities to a few and then focus on one at a time. Perhaps with experience you will become more skilled and can accomplish more ambitious goals, but keep in mind the truth that habits are not easy to change, and changing just one habit can demand a lot of time and effort. Mark Twain said, "Habit is habit, and not to be flung out the window by any man, but coaxed downstairs a step at a time." One of the lessons I have learned from many years of teaching is to avoid rapidly covering large amounts of information. I have found it better to reduce the scope to the most important concepts and behaviors and then relentlessly teach them from many different angles.

It also a good idea to begin working on habits that are "relatively" easy to change, that is, ones not necessitating major lifestyle changes. Consider these examples: drinking more water, doing sit-ups, buckling your seat belt, flossing your teeth, drinking less soda, or adding a fruit to each breakfast and lunch. Notice that none of these call for a major time commitment, they are not particularly onerous, if at all. Nor do they require any equipment or items that should not be readily and inexpensively available.

From a list of these simpler kinds of habits, it is suggested that you select those that are particularly relevant to you. They should be ones which you either have already established in your life and benefited from, or ones for which you are determined to begin following along with the children. Be sure you are beyond a mere contemplation stage and are resolved. With this level of commitment, your enthusiasm is bound to show and make you a more convincing teacher to be emulated. I like to remind myself of the quote, "If you don't model what you are teaching, you are teaching something else."

Of course your selection decision should also take into consideration which habits you suspect the children are following and not following. Giving a simple survey of their practices might be usefully enlightening. Figure 5.1 provides a survey that can serve as a starting point from which to prioritize, select, or make additions.

Figure 5.1 Physical Health Practices Survey

Scoring:

    1 = almost never (less than 10% of the time)
    2 = Occasionally (approximately 25% of the time)
    3 = Often (approximately 50% of the time)
    4 = Very often (approximately 75% of the time)
    5 = Almost always (90% or more of the time)

Exercise

_____ 1. I do some kind of movement activity or sport at least 60 minutes every day.
_____ 2. I do some vigorous, sweat-producing exercise at least 3 times per week.
_____ 3. I do some sit-ups at least 2 times per week.
_____ 4. I do some dynamic stretching activities/exercises on a regular basis.
_____ 5. I walk or bicycle as a means of transportation whenever possible.
_____ 6. Unless I have a heavy load, I walk stairs rather than ride the elevator or escalator.

Nutrition

_____ 1. I eat at least three fruits everyday
_____ 2. I eat at least 2 vegetables everyday
_____ 3. I eat whole grain bread instead of non-whole grain
_____ 4. I drink at least 3 glasses of water every day
_____ 5. I drink soymilk or non-fat cows' milk instead of milk containing saturated fat
_____ 6. I drink no more than 12 ounces of soda per day
_____ 7. I eat no more than 8 oz of meat per day (size of a deck of playing cards)
_____ 8. I avoid eating hot dogs/sausages more than once a month

Personal care

_____ 1. I wear my seat belt and/or shoulder harness while traveling.
_____ 2. When I travel on a motorcycle, bicycle, or all-terrain vehicle, I wear a helmet.
_____ 3. I wear a brimmed hat in sunny weather to protect my skin
_____ 4. I apply sun-screen in sunny weather to protect my skin
_____ 5. I wear sunglasses in sunny weather to protect my eyes
_____ 6. I brush my teeth every day for at least 2 minutes.
_____ 7. I floss my teeth everyday.
_____ 8. I get 8-9 hours of sleep every day so that I feel well rested
_____ 9. I wash my hands before leaving the restroom and before eating
_____ 10. I use my elbow to cover my coughs so as to not spread germs

> **STAGES OF CHANGE EXERCISE MODEL**
>
> This model classifies exercise habit formation into five distinct stages. What stage would you assign to yourself? Can you think of friends, family members or acquaintances to place in each stage? I know I am not totally convinced that someone truly has the exercise habit until he/she has continued all the way through the winter months. Then I know they might be more than summer soldiers and sunshine patriots. Data shows about half of those who start an exercise program will drop out within 6 months to a year.
>
> Using this model to understand where a friend or student is can be useful. It could help you better see what might be the best approach to help him/her move toward the next stage. When individuals stall at one of the lower levels, or move backwards, I like to think of it as a relapse rather than a collapse. The same steps are approached again, perhaps with a different strategy.
>
> *Stage 1: Pre-contemplation:* the person is not even thinking of exercising.
> *Stage 2: Contemplation:* the person is thinking of exercising. He/she might say things like he/she should or might begin to exercise sometime.
> *Stage 3: Preparation:* the person is making plans to begin exercising. Maybe some shoes or clothing was bought, a membership bought, or a specific beginning exercise date has been set.
> *Stage 4: Practicing:* the person has been engaged in regular exercise for less than 6 months.
> *Stage 5: Maintaining:* the person has been engaged in regular exercise for more than 6 months.

Recognizing the Benefits of the Behavior

Although usually not sufficient, recognizing the benefits is a *sine qua non* for behavior change. No one is going to be disposed to endure the effort of behavioral change unless he/she is totally convinced of the benefits to be derived. Therefore, it is our duty to make sure the children appreciate what is to be gained. Good exercise and health practices are going to yield their most pronounced pay-off years down the road and particularly late in life. While we should be informing our youngsters of these delayed consequences, and encouraging them to adopt a more long-term perspective toward their wellbeing, we need to be mindful of the limitations of children's life perspectives. They tend to be most influenced by more immediate consequences. As a result, as much as possible we need to be also showing them the short-term payoffs that they might value. Here are a couple of examples.

Suppose you have selected the behavior of "doing abdominal exercises three times a week." You begin by explaining why having strong abdominal muscles are good for them. To make the to-be-derived benefits as applicable to the children's present day interests as possible, you might stress how strong abdominals play an important role in their favorite sport skills and in an attractive postural appearance. You could show them the active and stabilizing function those muscles play in activities such as throwing, serving, and various gymnastic and dance skills. As for posture, you could contrast the attractiveness of a proudly erect posture to that of a slouching, sagging one. In addition to these immediate effects, maintaining abdominal strength will have long-term consequences. Neglect of the stomach muscles might see adults suffering from permanent structural problems and low bad pain. While it might be worth while to inform the children that 50 percent of adults will experience low back pain, you can see that this later-in-life disability may be too remote and a less powerful motivator than images of today's successful sports performances and better personal appearance.

A second exercise/health behavior example is "doing three or four aerobic workouts per week" as prescribed by The Activity Pyramid. In Chapter 1, an impressive list of benefits was shown to be produced by aerobic fitness. Remember the powerful long-term effects on heart attacks, strokes, cancers, diabetes, bone density, compressed morbidity, etc. Our explanations of why we should aerobically exercise should include these reasons. But what are all the various attributes which children might be able to gain now or in the not so misty future? Recall the quality of life factors such as having more endurance for sports, feeling better, sleeping more soundly, having more energy, losing weight, being more alert and thinking better, effectively coping with stress. And what about learning to appreciate the vigorous moving experience for its own sake? We would be wise to comprehensively stress all these salient kinds of things. Who knows what justification might become the motivator for some child?

There is final point that might be worth making regarding the recognition of the benefits of good health/exercises practices. Thus far the discussion has focused on what information the teacher should put together to argue the case. Another approach would be to have the students do their own research. Undoubtedly you will regularly be having your students engaged in reading and writing in content areas. My point is that you not forget the content area of health and fitness. This would be a great way to have children learn more about the benefits of sound health and exercise habits. I am sure their research would find a great amount of information that would be interesting and relevant to them.

Doing the Behavior in School

Some of the behaviors you have earmarked for change can be easily begun in school while others may not. It should be apparent that it is a good idea to begin doing the activity in school if possible. If you can develop the skill through actual doing, and can perhaps even develop it into a routine or habit in school, you will be one step closer to moving it to your final goal of extra-school continuance. For best understanding of the manner in which we might do this, we will continue with our example of, "doing abdominal exercises three times per week."

For this particular habit you need not only know reasons for doing it, but you also need to know a number of things about how to do it (This is true for most behaviors, but not always to as significant a degree; consider the less technical skills of using seat belts, wearing bike helmets, washing hands.). Before having the students begin abdominal exercises, you would begin with a good demonstration. When demonstrating sit-ups you might point out errors such as failing to have your knees bent or coming up too fast in a jerking motion. You might also show them any good alternate ways of exercising the abdominals; putting your feet on a chair or bench and doing crunches would be a possibility. Showing a variety of ways of doing the activity should increase the likelihood they will find the one best suited for them. You might discuss not only the technical quality of the sit-up but also the issue of quantity of exercise. Here you would need to be communicating your exercise physiology knowledge, namely *The F.I.T. Principle* and how it relates to overloading the muscles on a regular basis (to near exhaustion, two or three times per week).

As they begin exercising, you could check for proper technique and give encouragement. If possible, it would not be a bad idea to have them perform on a soft surface to avoid any unneeded discomfort during their beginning exposure. You hope their initial experience will not be "Ouch! That was uncomfortable and painful." Rather, you should be striving for a general class feeling that the activity was not hard, or at a minimum, not too unpleasant. It would be desirable to reach a class consensus that the effort involved was reasonable and well spent?

Having done the activity in class once, twice, or sporadically is good, but continuing to do the activity on a regular basis carries much merit. Actually doing sit-ups and/or crunches three times per week would solidify a routine mentality. It would do two other things as well. It would make clear the seriousness you attached to this activity by giving you repeated opportunities to make your argument. Furthermore, with practice the students' performance might progressively become more comfortable and improved. When they incur some gains they will have a greater vested interest. You could tell them they should be proud of the steady work done and the stomach fitness achieved.

Tracking/Reinforcing the Behavior Beyond School

Great! We now know why and how to do the activity and we have even practiced and improved upon it in school. This is in many instances where instruction ends. The assumption is that now the children will integrate this behavior into their lifestyle and live happily ever after. In fact, we are stopping one difficult and most crucial step short of what is needed. We cannot expect that consistently doing an activity under a teacher's tutelage will invariably translate into the same self-directed behavior in the home and community environment. Far from it, the stage may have been set for the child to begin incorporating abdominal exercises into his/her life, but we are a long way from winning the war of establishing a self-initiated, self-sustained habit. This reminds me of a clever response Winston Churchill made following an early World War II battle victory. He gave this tempering admonition to those who were excitedly optimistic. "Now this is not the end. It is not even the beginning of the end. But it is, perhaps, the end of the beginning."

After we have established an in-class routine for say, sit-ups, it is nearly imperative to incrementally get the children doing it on their own outside of school. I see it as a weaning process moving from teacher-led to self-directed behavior. You must unequivocally convey the message that if they wish to remain fit they will have to begin to take responsibility for it. They must comprehend that you will not always be around to dictate when it is time for them to do sit-ups. Tell them that the only way they will be fit in the long run is if they are self-directed. They must know that over the holidays and during the summer months the *reversibility principle* will operate to nullify any hard won gains; and what do they expect will happen next year and beyond when you will no longer be there is lead them?

A specific *Behavioral Weaning Procedure* regarding sit-ups would be to inform the class that, because of many other things demanding attention, there will only be time enough to do in-school sit-ups once or twice a week instead of thrice-weekly. The ramification is that either they lose the fitness gains made or they agree to start supplementary exercises outside of school. Perhaps you could begin by asking and getting everyone to agree that they will do a set of sit-ups over the weekend. They understand you think this is an important assignment and they know you will not be forgetting to check with a show of hands on Monday to see how many remembered.

When you are counting hands on Monday you might decide to record and post the percentage of students in compliance with the weekend assignment. Next you might decide to set a goal of more of the class achieving it next time. Maybe you could get peer pressure working for you by developing an *esprit de corp* in the class where everyone is reminding and encouraging each other. This would also be a good time to address the barriers, psychological or physical, which may have accounted for some of the non-compliance. For instance, some may have simply forgotten. This being the case, you could lead a discussion about things to help remembrance. One suggestion would be establishing a regular time for the exercise, another would be when you first get up or as soon as you get home from school. This discussion session might also be a good time for you to *Personalize Behavioral Practices*. Do you not think it might be influential if you could say that you successfully remembered to do your sit-ups by always doing them in conjunction with some other established routine, or that you do yours as a cool-down to your regular jog, etc.?

The ideal *Behavioral Weaning Procedure* will progress until the students have eventually assumed complete self-responsibility. This does not mean that your task will ever be completely done (remember how the *Stages of Change Exercise Model* differentiates between practice and maintaining stages). You would be continuing to track

Instilling Health and Affective Behaviors

the students' performances during periodic check-up activities and/or discussions throughout the year. Adherence to behavioral changes are bound to drop-off over time and reminders and encouragement spread out over as long a period of time as possible is helpful. The last day of class would be a good wrap-up time for congratulations and wishing them well with all the exercise/health behaviors initiated during the year. Figure 5.2 provides a sample "Summer Activity Challenge." You will see that in it I have personalized my behavioral intentions and provided different categories of activities that will contribute to my activity. Such a plan could serve as a template for an exercise in which the children write their plans and then discuss them with the class.

Figure 5.2. Summer Activity Challenge

Imagine that it is at the end of the school year. Perhaps you have some reading suggestions and other pursuits you are encouraging the students to continue. Since you have been working with the children's health habits would it not be a good idea to help them plan for the coming vacation time. Research data shows that during the summer months most children watch much more television, get less activity, and gain more body fat. Here is an example of a summertime physical activity challenge you might help them fill out. It lists four categories of activity.

1. Lifestyle activities: *always taking stairs if less than five flights; bike or walk to store whenever possible; walk the dog each day; etc.*

_____
_____
_____

2. Physical work: *help with household chores, neighborhood help, etc.*

_____
_____
_____

3. Sports and active recreational activities: *swimming lessons, sports, hiking, etc.*

_____
_____
_____

4. Exercises: *aerobic exercises, sit-ups, dynamic stretches, etc.*

_____
_____
_____

Health AND *Fitness* An Elementary Teacher's Guide

I recently heard of an even further extension of this concept. A teacher was explaining how she always has had her third graders write essays about their life goals, and then, nine years later, mailed them their papers. Over the years, many of her students have given splendid testimonials of how fun it was to receive those letters. Additionally they were impressed by the teacher's continued concern for their wellbeing. Anyway, I thought her practice was an admirable one and wondered if her procedure could also be employed as a truly long-range check-up. Image the letter including the message, "I sincerely hope you, like I am, are still finding time to do those health habits we worked on."

As indicated before, the sit-up example we have been following is a behavioral change that, while by no means easy, might be easier to make than would be some others. Doing aerobic exercises would require a much greater lifestyle change because it requires more time, it is more physically demanding, and it might require more attention to facilities and equipment. Many dietary behavior changes would pose special problems because certain kinds of foods would need to be procured. If we wished children to eat *5 a Day* (fruits and/or vegetables) or drink non-fat milk, or soymilk, it would be essential to involve parents in the process. The parents must understand why these changes are desirable if they are going to be supportive in purchasing and making the foods available.

In Figure 5.3 you will find two homework assignments that attempt to inform and involve families in behavior change. They also exemplify an incentive system. Taking the extra step of designing an assignment of this kind could be well worth the effort. In the next section of this chapter we will be going into more detail regarding how to involve of parents and others for a variety of purposes.

Figure 5.3. Family Homework Assignments

AEROBIC EXERCISE/ACTIVITY - ACTION PLAN

This week you can earn TWO POINTS in this section by exercising 3 times.
* Choose any exercise or activity that will raise your heart rate, get you breathing deeply and maybe perspiring. Remember the 1-10 *Perceived Exertion Scale?* You should be at least a 5 or higher on it. You need to be at that level for at least 20 minutes. It is okay if you are playing a game or sport with rest breaks or periods of lower intensity activity, but you must accumulate a total of 20 minutes at the higher intensity.
  - You must do this 20 minutes of vigorous exercise/activity at least 3 times during the week. You can choose to do the same activity or try something else. Doing the same exercise/activity has the advantage of allowing you to do what you most enjoy and getting more skillful at it. This is called *specificity of training*. Switching to different exercises/activities is called *cross training*. It has the advantage of adding interest through variety; it also better

Instilling Health and Affective Behaviors

insures that you are exercising a variety of muscles and allows them more time to rest and recover it they are sore and feel overused (remember the *Overuse Principle*).

Write down the days you will exercise and what you will do (running, swimming, biking, basketball, soccer, elliptical trainer, skateboarding, dancing etc.).

Which day_____ What I'll do _____
Which day_____ What I'll do _____
Which day_____ What I'll do _____
Signed: _____ Date: _____

You can earn TWO BONUS POINTS if you get an adult to exercise three times this week too.

* Remind the adult to exercise at about a 5 on the 1-10 exertion scale.
* If the adult is not used to exercise, he/she might not be able to keep up with you. They shouldn't force themselves to go too fast. Tell your adult that it's best to start slowly and build up speed gradually.

Name of adult_____

YOUR SCORE

Now add up your "Exercise" score, and ask a parent to sign this sheet for you.

I certify that _____ has earned _____ points in the "Race to Health."
Signed: _____

LOWERING SATURATED FAT IN-TAKE - ACTION PLAN

You can earn FOUR POINTS in this section. You get two points if you make a change for a week. And you earn two bonus points if you can get an adult in the family to make a change too.

Your plan will be to drink soymilk or a non-fat version of cows' milk:

--------------------GOOD NEWS---------------------

If you already drink soymilk or nonfat cows' milk you have just earned two points without even trying.
WRITE A BIG "2" HERE for your fast and easy points.

Everyone else should get their points the old-fashioned way, and earn them:

FOR TWO POINTS you will drink soymilk or non-fat cows' milk for one week. The idea is give it an honest try and see if you might accustom yourself to liking it. You may find you want to change forever.

Health AND *Fitness* An Elementary Teacher's Guide

> Moving away from whole or 1% and 2% versions of cows' milk means that you will be getting a lot less calories and saturated fats in your diet. Both non-fat milk and soymilk provide the calcium and other vitamins that our bodies need. The couple of advantages in moving to soymilk is that it contains fiber that the cows' milk doesn't have, and it also has the environmental and ethical advantages of a vegan diet.
>
> Sign up: I promise to drink _____ milk for one week.
> Signed:_____ Date:_____
>
> Now, for your TWO BONUS POINTS in the "Race for Health", get an adult in the family to promise to drink milk with less fat in it for a week.
> Name of adult:_____
>
> *If everyone in the family already drinks soymilk or nonfat milk cows' milk, you get your two bonus points anyway.*
>
> YOUR SCORE
>
> Now add up your FAT score in the "Race to Health", and ask a parent to sign this sheet for you.
> I certify that _____ has earned _____ points in the "Race to Health".
> Signed:_____

Before leaving this topic of developing self-responsibility, one more suggestion is in order. I explained in this chapter how the teacher might record and track student behaviors. Would it not be a worthwhile idea to teach children to document their own exercise/health accomplishments? The concept of journal keeping and portfolios is probably not a new one to you; you know that they can serve many valuable educational purposes and you may already have many ideas about how you intend to use them. What I am proposing is the idea that you could have your fourth, fifth, and sixth graders assume responsibility for managing their own personal fitness education portfolios. These initially would not have to be elaborate compilations but they could grow and include such things as weekly logs, individually designed exercise and health practices programs, family homework assignments like those discussed above, contracts (see Figure 5.4), graphs, and personal fitness scores.

Figure 5.4. Fitness Contracts

STUDENT FITNESS CONTRACT

We, the _____ family, promise that we will adopt an active lifestyle for the coming month of _____. We acknowledge that general physical activity is very important to the health of all family members. We promise to participate in some kind of physical activity 6 or 7 days per week throughout the month. The daily activities will normally be at least an hour in length. They can be done in a continuous block or divided.

Achievement of this contract will be recognized by the physical education department and published to the school and community.

Family members: _____

This promise was witnessed by _____

OPEN-ENDED STUDENT FITNESS CONTRACT

For the coming term I will select a component of physical fitness on which to work (body composition, aerobic fitness, anaerobic fitness, muscular strength/endurance or dynamic flexibility). At term's end I will write a 1000 or more word report that will contain: (1) Why is this chosen component is important to you and people in general, (2) What are *The F.I.T. Guidelines* as they relate to developing this component of fitness, (3) What was the activity plan you followed (fully explained activities and times), and (4) What was your reaction to the experience (difficulties, lessons, plans for the future).

Sign _____
                Student

Sign _____
                teacher

Sign _____
              parent or guardian

Going Multi-disciplinary

We have already dwelt on how difficult it is to change habits; not only must the students be convinced tangible benefits will follow, they are likely to encounter many barriers to establishing and maintaining a self-directed routine. This can really seem like a daunting task when you realize that you are just one force out of the many influential forces shaping the children's lives; and often those others can be giving very powerful counter messages. Many children may be coming from homes in which the parent(s) does not value, model, or encourage commendable exercise/health practices. The students' close peers, with whom they so passionately wish to fit in, may be living inactive lifestyles supported by a diet mainly of "big gulps" and French fries. They may even be getting mixed messages from school personnel and policies. You have been laboring to have them eat according to the food pyramid while other teachers are constantly providing them with snacks and treats that are loaded with empty calories. They are being recruited for school fund-raising campaigns to sell candy and cookies for band trips or sports equipment. Machines are glowing in the hallways displaying enticing candy and soft drinks. Students are regularly being served school lunches that contain high amounts of sodium, saturated fat, and sugar. Almost three-fourths of school lunch items exceed the U.S. dietary guidelines for fat; ninety percent of the surplus foods bought by the government for school lunches are butter, cheese, whole milk, beef, pork, and eggs.

The school may also be providing a number of subtle messages that physical education is not really something to be taken seriously and to be done everyday: it is treated as a frill being scheduled only once or twice a week, it is taken away for misbehavior or failure to complete other academic assignments, it is commonly the preempted activity of choice when special events are planned. Would these things be done if in our heart of hearts we believed exercise/health was an integral element of the educated person?

So what do we conclude? Do we despair of swimming against a sea of opposition? Do we continue climbing the climbing wave alone? No. If we honestly want to make a difference in the health of our children we cannot give up, and fighting the fight alone might be noble but is not apt to be fully effective. There is truth in the African proverb, "It takes a village to raise a child." To be effective we need help, and be assured that help can be found if we seek it. You are not the only person in your school and community who is worried about children's health. There are citizens, parents, fellow classroom teachers, physical education specialists, administrators, health care workers, school lunch personnel, university faculty, and others who are already convinced of how critical an issue this is, and if asked, would be eager to work with you for this cause. Beyond them, there are many more who would be readily receptive to this viewpoint if provided some information and leadership. After all, everyone wants to do what is best for children.

The question is how do we recruit all this aid that will permit us to employ a ==Multidisciplinary Team Approach== to behavioral change? As you may recall from the Preface, the federal government has already mandated that schools do precisely this. ==The Child Nutrition and Reauthorization Act== (Public Law 108-265: Section 204) requires every school district that participates in the federal school meal programs to establish a wellness policy. It states that a committee must be organized and consists of such people as classroom teachers, physical education specialists, administrators, school lunch personnel, parents and community members. They are required to meet regularly and set yearly wellness goals and assessment procedures.

If you truly want to instill good health habits in children you will want to make this desire known when you interview for your first teaching job, and once on board you will seek to serve on the school's wellness committee. Some schools might have a vibrantly functioning group. If so, it will be a joy to fall in and coordinate your efforts. Others schools could very well be lax in implementing the law. A committee may never have been formed or attempts to maintain one have languished. What might you do if this is the situation you encounter? Once you have gained the imprimatur of the administration you could gather a group of interested individuals. They should be a diverse group as prescribed by PL 108-265 but the size would not need to be large. Three or four representatives might be most manageable and enough to get few ideas or initiatives going.

At the initial meeting you probably would have to do little more than explain some of your concerns and then ask for comments and ideas. It is hard to forecast what directions ensuing discussions may take, and what suggested courses of action planned. The possibilities are endless. For example, the school lunch director may think of an idea for coordinating some lunch offerings with an instructional topic you are planning; the physical education specialist might see how he/she could include a lesson or two reinforcing a certain topic the group feels to be important. Maybe the group could plan a special event like a health fair; the administrator would agree to organize some short, school-wide exercise breaks at certain times during the day. The group might come up with some acceptable alternate treats which the other teachers could agree to (frozen yogurt certificates, jello-fruits, juices, low-fat cookies, etc.). A parent or community member might know and contact some guest speakers for your class or the school. These speakers might represent both genders and a variety of ethnic groups; they could be fitness instructors, marathon runners, triathletes, bicycle club representatives, hiking club representatives, health care professionals, physical education professors. Sometimes it can be useful to have fitness conscious middle school or high school students/athletes visit you class; the testimonials of these near peers can have an influential modeling effect.

Another potentially useful avenue for some members of the committee is to research and contact national organizations that are interested in promoting health. Here are two organizations with programs designed to help elementary schools:

U.S. Department of Health and Human Service: Their Centers for Disease Control and Prevention (CDC) has great materials for how to start and run a "Kids Walk-to-School Program."
(www.cdc.gov/nccdphp/dnpa/kidswalk.htm).

* *The American Alliance of Health, Physical Education, Recreation and Dance* (AAHPERD). (www.aahperd.org). This is a big organization with an extensive web site. Here you will have a wealth of information in such areas as coaching, recreation, health, physical education, and adaptive physical education. This is where you will find all the particulars of the *Fitnessgram and Activitygram.* From AAHPERD you will find linkage to the state organizations who might be able to have people come to your schools. They could help with events such as "Jump Rope for Heart" and "Hoops for Heart."

The *Multidisciplinary Team Approach* could also be instrumental in establishing lines of communication between you and the parents. Parents are a critical link and some partnership must be formed to join home and school. If you adopt some of the homework and portfolio ideas presented earlier, you will be starting in this direction. However, more can be done. Parent/ teacher conferences and PTA presentations are of course one approach to pursue and they should be taken advantage of. Another approach is a newsletter. Although writing a newsletter requires significant time and effort, the returns can be significant. It would be great if they could be published as much as three or four times a year, that at least could be a goal. Remember, you do not have to do it all yourself, you have a team and hopefully that team can be delegating responsibilities to others. The newsletter, just like your committee projects, could take many forms. It certainly could explain some of the concepts you and the school are attempting to teach the children. It might contain listings of student accomplishments. Fitness facts could be a regular section: articles in magazines and newspapers might be good material sources for this. Furthermore, the newsletter might be a means of getting information from home; it could be surveying the parents regarding their health practices and it could be a venue for soliciting their ideas and volunteered assistance. In a recent Louis Harris survey 6 in 10 parents said that they would be willing to volunteer to supervise school and after school activity programs for children. Finally about the newsletter, I would not think of it solely as a communication to the parents, I would hope it was suitable for the children to read, and you would be sending it to faculty, staff, administrators and other professionals.

The above discussion has taken the perspective that you, with the aid of a wellness committee, might write a separate newsletter devoted entirely to exercise/health issues. The possibly exists that you already have been planning to communicate with parents via a regular comprehensive report on all your academic goals and projects.

If that is the case, your exercise/health newsletter could be conveniently attached and integrated with the overall report.

Changing Nutritional Practices

In previous chapters we have learned three things about nutrition. (1) We learned what constitutes good nutrition, (2) that nutrition is absolutely essential to good health, and (3) that the *Standard American Diet (SAD)* is almost diametrically opposite to what should be eaten. The task facing us is a daunting one. If good health is going to be achieved it means that society must make the transition to an eating style that is far outside the cultural norm. This sub-section is devoted to providing a few specific ideas for changing eating habits. How can we get people to prefer healthy foods over the unhealthy ones to which they are habituated? No life-long change will result until that is achieved. Before considering what we need to be specifically doing for elementary school children, let us set the stage by looking at food preferences in infants and toddlers and how they can be shaped.

Although infants and toddlers have a naturally higher preference than adults for sweet and salty taste, food preferences are almost entirely a function of acculturation. This is clearly evinced when we consider the hugely different preferences between cultures that have individually developed in different environments. Think of the gooey squiggly things some Eastern societies find delectable but which we find revolting. And conversely, they and other cultures can be repulsed by the likes of our roast beef and potatoes. The fruits, vegetables, gains, and meats that an environment affords are what people eat, and what people eat is what they come to like. These preferences begin even before birth. Flavorful compounds from a mother's diet cross the placenta into the amniotic fluid, which babies in the third trimester swallow at the rate of a quart a day. Babies develop preferences for these foods long before they actually eat them. Similarly, during lactation, flavors pass from the mother's bloodstream into breast milk. For example, babies whose moms drink carrot juice or eat fruits while breast-feeding have been found to like carrot and peach baby foods better than formula-fed infants.

Most young children are naturally picky eaters. They are biologically programmed to be wary of new foods until they know they are safe to eat. This *food neophobia* peaks between 2 and 5 years of age, when a newly mobile child would otherwise be at greatest risk of ingesting, say, colorful but toxic berries. The degree of caution varies greatly among children and it applies mainly to bitter foods (think vegetables), since bitterness often indicates poison. So what must moms and those caring for toddlers do to overcome this pickiness and thus inculcate a preference for the richly varied diet that will be needed? The answer, we should not be surprised, is to persist in providing this healthy, richly varied diet. That is not normally being done for most young children. Currently, on any given day, 25-30 percent of infants and toddlers ages 9-24 months do not eat any fruit and 20-25 percent do not eat vegetables. This is patently wrong. Fruits, vegetables, whole grains and legumes should constitute the baulk, if not the entirety, of every meal. Nutrition counselors advocate regularly offering a wide variety of small helpings. The toddlers should not be forced in eat it; they should be permitted to spit it out if they want. But persistence is key. Young children often need to try a new food 10 or 15 times before they will accept it. Most moms give up after three to five times.

It is also recommended that the children should ever be bribed to eat something. Promising ice cream as a reward for eating broccoli only fuels the suspicion that there is something wrong with the broccoli. The adults should be eating a nutritious meal and a separate meal should not be fixed for the child, it only reinforces their biases. If the child has a friend who is a good eater, he/she should be invited to dinner. Peer influence is profoundly powerful.

Finally, if the meals we feed toddlers consist of healthy fare it obviously means that we are not providing them that which is unhealthy. But this point is so important that it must be said for emphasis sake. We must stop providing formative minds and bodies with hotdogs, sodas, chips, cookies and other such brethren! The majority of loving adults are unthinkingly guilty of this behavior. Today, French fries are the most commonly consumed vegetable for infants and toddlers 15 to 24 months. This is flat-out wrong and even a form of abuse. Putting these foods in the hands of the very young is not only bad dietary practice in the immediate sense, doing so is establishing preferences that they will need to battle in elementary school and throughout their lives.

The specific suggestions for instilling good eating habits in elementary school children are fundamentally the same as those advanced for the infants and pre-schoolers. Like the young ones, elementary aged children must be persistently exposed to healthy foods and not be surrounded by unhealthy choices. But now, achieving such a situation is more difficult. We don't have nearly the total control that the early care providers had. School children live in a *toxic eating environment* flooded with enticingly sweet, salty and fatty foods. These products are relatively inexpensive, exceedingly convenient, and marketed craftfully by the enveloping medias. Furthermore, most of the children's early eating history has largely solidified a preference, and the conformist societal pressure to eat as do their peers and models is overwhelming.

What are we and the schools to do when so many overwhelming forces are aligned against us? Despair and acceptance is not the answer. The health of our children is at stake. Rather, we must resolve ourselves to determined effort. And although the task of changing the children's eating habits will not be easy, we need recognize that elementary teachers are in a frightfully powerful position. At this stage the children are still far more receptive to new ideas and ways than what they will be later in their lives. Try presenting a new idea, nutritional or otherwise, to your children, your peers, your parents and your grand parents; the odds are that you will encounter increasingly greater resistance the older the people are.

Although we cannot control the children's entire nutritional environment we can at least make the schools' a healthy one. This means gradually changing the school meal offerings that are characteristically too high in saturated fats and proteins, and too low in complex carbohydrates. They must eventually become replete with fruits, vegetables, grains, legumes, seeds, and nuts; and they must seriously reduce the meat, dairy, salt and simple sugars. It also means eliminating these offerings from food dispensers, school parties, special events, and fund raising enterprises. There is a counter school-of-thought that opposes the idea of creating a uniformly healthy milieu. Subscribers to this view hold that at least some unhealthy options should remain available as the nutritious fare is increased. The theory of this approach is that since we ultimately want children to become self-responsible decision-makers they must be given opportunities to make choices. However, while wise selecting is undeniably a final necessary step before anyone achieves a completely self-actualized lifestyle, most nutritionists would strongly argue against expecting children to make correct choices when they are confronted with highly seductive food to which they are already accustomed. Even adults, who appreciate the value of healthy foods, are likely to succumb under such tempting temptations. In other school disciplines we have had no difficulty in the rejecting the legitimacy of serving up the bad with the good. School libraries do not carry comic books and vacuous novels along side quality literature; likewise, the better course seems to be to remove the nutritionally vacuous junk food and systematically immerse the school in that which is healthy.

> "I can resist anything except temptation." – Oscar Wilde

The presence of a sound eating environment must also be accompanied by nutrition instruction. The steps of the *behavioral weaning procedure* introduced earlier in the chapter are an effective guide: selecting a few simple behaviors, showing the immediate benefits, doing the behavior in school, tracking it beyond. Examples of simple behaviors that could be initially targeted might be adding a fruit, vegetable or non-dairy milk to the daily diet. Following presentations and discussions of the benefits of eating this particular food or food type the school would be sure to have it regularly available in the lunch menu and/or as a snack item. And of course, some formal or informal means of outside of school continuance would be tracked and discussed.

Finally, two basic instructional/philosophical points are critical if nutritional habits are going to be revamped. First, we must not push. When we preach and push children, or anyone, to do something that they are not ready to do, we will probably get the opposite of the result that is wanted. It is better to non-aggressively present the advantages of a practice, be open and encouraging to discussion and research of it, and then quietly go about modeling it. Secondly, we must be sure that the message is not one of going on a self-sacrificing "diet" but instead it is of gradually and genuinely changing preferences from unhealthy foods to healthy ones. Many people cannot presently conceive of a richly varied, enjoyable diet that contains either no or limited amounts of meat, dairy products, fried foods and sugary/salty foods. We need to teach that living on a plant-based diet actually affords the greatest variety of colorful, flavorful foods with more options available today than ever before.

CHANGING HABITS IN THE AFFECTIVE DOMAIN

Being concerned about the social and emotional behaviors of children is not new. Consider this statement, "Children today are tyrants. They contradict their parents, gobble their food and tyrannize their teachers." That statement may sound like a contemporary lament, but Socrates made it over 2000 years ago. Nevertheless, many educators and people in society strongly feel that teaching appropriate affective domain behaviors is needed today, more than ever. Many think we are seeing a surge of social pathology as a result of our fast-paced, mechanized times and an increase in dysfunctional families. Don Hellison is a well-respected physical education teacher who has had extensive experience in teaching social and emotional values to children with behavioral problems. Figure 5.5 shows the *Personal/Social Responsibility Model* he developed over many years of hands-on experience. Like me, many teachers have used and found the model to be effective in codifying social and emotional goals. As can be seen, it advances a system for defining specific levels of children's social and emotional functioning. It provides an ultimate goal of helping children become caring people and it spells out what that entails. Also, understandable interim steps to reach that goal are outlined.

Figure 5.5. Personal/Social Responsibility Model (Six Levels of Affective Development)

Level 0: Irresponsibility - students who are unmotivated and undisciplined. Their behavior includes discrediting or making fun of other students' involvement as well as interrupting, intimidating, manipulating, and verbally or physically abusing other students and perhaps the teacher. They make excuses and blame others for their behavior and deny personal responsibility for what they do or fail to do.
Level 1: Self-Control - students who may not participate in the day's activity or show much mastery or improvement, but are able to control their behavior enough so that they do not interfere with other students' right to learn and the teacher's right to teach. They do this without much prompting by the teacher and without constant supervision.

> *Level II: Involvement* - students who not only show self-control and respect for others, but are involved in the subject matter.
> *Level III: Self-Responsibility* - students who learn to take more responsibility for their choices and for linking these choices to their own identities. They are able to work without direct supervision, eventually taking responsibility for their intentions and actions.
> *Level IV: Caring* - students who are motivated to extend their sense of responsibility by cooperating, giving support, showing concern, and helping.
> *Level V: Outside-of-Class Caring* - students who apply the upper levels outside the program - on the playground, at school, at home, on the street.

In this section we will look at some ideas on how to use Hellison's model to habituate desirable personal and social behaviors in our children. But before we consider two specific instructional practices, awareness talks and reflection time, it is worth reminding the reader that the physical activity setting is uniquely suited for teaching affective skills.

We can divide physical activities into *three instructional approaches (individual, cooperative, and competitive)* and identify the separate contributions each can make to the affective domain. The *individual approach* is where everyone works independently and non-competitively on his/her own. Maybe everyone is given a ball and practices dribbling skills; everyone has a hula-hoop and practices different spins; or everyone independently works on some self-determined physical fitness skills. This type of environment is effective for learning motor skills. Everyone can practice at the same time and learn at his/her own rate. Also, performing in this manner is relatively stress free since classmates are busy with their own tasks and hence are not scrutinizing and making judgments of others. As for affective domain development, independently working on motor skills and physical fitness can teach valuable lessons about perseverance and self-responsibility. And if tangible progress can be made in skill development, as it more quickly can be made in many physical skills compared to reading and writing and other academic achievements, we should be able to anticipate improvements in self-esteem. I have long questioned the efficacy of the common practice of unconditionally telling children to think better of themselves. I have never noticed doing so to help elevate a child's or adult's confidence and self-esteem. However, over the years I have unmistakably seen many instances of children deservedly thinking of themselves far more positively after working and mastering a motor skill or improving their fitness; simply learning to juggle some balls or doing an extra push-up was sufficient.

The *cooperative approach* is where partners, small groups, or the entire class attempt to work together to accomplish a physical goal. These kinds of activities are also good for learning physical skills and hence self-concepts. This is because their partners are encouraging and often helping support their performance. Of course, encouragement and teamwork are just the kind of higher-level affective interactions we want. I have seen it to be so strong and spontaneous in physical settings. While you may or may not be able to get the children to praise each other's art work or science project, I bet I have witnessed more vociferous, genuine congratulations and high-fiving when a group of children has succeeded in carrying a giant earth ball from one end of the gym to the other, or when a group completed a physically challenging team-building task in a few seconds less time.

The *competitive approach* encountered in games and sports is eminently attractive and exciting to most children. These experiences result in emotionally charged and highly interactive situations which are filled with opportunities for teaching social responsibilities such as leadership, teamwork, fair play, emotional control and physical and verbal conflict resolution. Think how much cooperation can be learned in volleyball where the bump, set, hit sequence is so integral to the sport. Think of sports that are sometimes associated with violence, where trash talking and in your face attitudes have become common (i.e. basketball, hockey); would not experiences in these kinds of sports provide opportunities to confront and discuss these values? Think of two students playing a racquet sport in which they are responsible for making the line calls and other infractions on their side of the court. If an opponent made what was thought to be a bad call, what should be done? Complain? Retaliate? Abide by the call and never show any resentment? While this sort of ethical dilemma could be posed in the classroom for discussion, think how much more real and testing the actual game behavior would be. To make appropriate affective decisions in win-loose situations of perceived importance is not easy, and is a true test of ethical fiber.

Each of the *three instructional approaches* can be an invaluable teaching tool for affective growth. However, we cannot expect that mere participation in them will automatically produce the desired behaviors. We have already made the point that, even after long periods of participation, children still might not have learned the affective skill of self-responsibility. All that has happened is that they have become accustomed to the instructor making all the decisions regarding when and how to perform or exercise. I have known extremely fit young and old students and athletes who ceased training when their instructor or coach was no longer attentively standing over them. Those individuals had not internalized the self-actualizing discipline to continue on their own. Nor can we expect games and sports experiences to automatically yield better social-emotional behaviors. In fact, there exist troubling sport psychology research data which shows that in certain youth sports programs, namely boys' football, hockey and wrestling, the children became more egocentric and developed a greater acceptance of rule violating behavior and violence. Furthermore, their more egocentric viewpoints were shown to generalize beyond sport specific situations to everyday decision-making. Surely we all are aware of instances of poor ethical displays in competitive games and sports. Because of the glamorization and ever-presence of professional sports, it sometimes seems that winning at all cost has become the prevailing ethos and that emotional control and playing by the rules is not the norm (see Figure 5.6 for consideration of *Five Philosophy Levels of Competitive Sports*).

Figure 5.6. Five Philosophy Levels of Competitive Sports

very altruistic perspective	*Philosophy 1: concern for the success of opponent* *implications*: might entail intentionally loosing in some situations *Philosophy 2: sport as a physical challenge* (purpose is to see who is physically best) *implications*: playing one's best to win, but playing by the rules, calling own infractions, and even helping competitors with advise and encouragement *Philosophy 3: sport as a physical & mental challenge* (purpose is to see who is physically and mentally toughest) *implications*: playing one's best to win, playing by the rules, calling own infractions, but not helping competitors with advice and encouragement, psyching out strategies are acceptable *Philosophy 4: winning is paramount* *implications*: bending rules and doing most anything to win is acceptable, but you do not intentionally cause physical harm
very egocentric perspective	*Philosophy 5: winning & aggression paramount* *implications*: it is a all-out battle, survival of the fittest

People hold different views of the purpose of sports. The philosophy that a person subscribes to dictates whether or not he/she will find certain practices acceptable and good. When people have different philosophies they naturally will disagree on which specific behaviors should be taught or condoned. The spectrum of philosophies presented above can be thought of representing a continuum moving from an extreme altruism (looking out for others) to extreme egocentrism (looking out for yourself).

One of the first tasks of teachers and coaches should be to determine which of the five they accept, making sure they have sound justification for their selection being in the best interest of the children. Once you know which philosophy you believe in, it will make it much easier to be consistent in your feedback and to know how to respond to the many dilemmas that will arise.

Whether or not children learn better or poorer affective behaviors is going to be mainly determined by the instruction they receive in conjunction with their physical participation. If we wish these physical activities to be the positive affective lessons that they can be, we need to talk to the children beforehand to make them aware of what constitutes good and poor behavior. And then, during and following activity we must help them reflect on what happened. Let us look at these two fundamental techniques for moving the children up the personal-social responsibility levels.

Awareness Talks

Awareness talks occur before physical activities are begun. It is where you explain your affective behavior expectations. It could be as simple as setting forth a succinct philosophical message. An example might be, "Always do your best and be respectful!" Once the students concur with such an adage it can be used throughout the year to deal with any behavior, good or bad. Whenever students are hustling and staying on task they will be reinforced for doing their best. Whenever they are unkind to others or are careless with the equipment they will be reminded of being respectful.

The process of using *awareness talks* to move children along the levels of the *Personal/Social Responsibility Model* is slightly more complex but could be worth the effort. For the students to comprehend and visualize the model, it would be good to have a posted chart to which you could refer. The chart should be kept simple, but you might wish it to contain examples (see Figure 5.7 as one possibility). Make sure you go over a couple of examples that will be applicable to the present situation and the immediately ensuing activities or game. For instance, you might start by a congratulation of everyone for being good quiet listeners as you have been explaining the levels; can they see that they are all exhibiting a level one behavior? Or you might say that the game to be played today will require the finding of new partners in a rapid fashion; what level would you be exhibiting if you avoided someone and were unwilling to work with anyone in class? You could ask them if they see why that is a level four behavior?

Figure 5.7. Affective Levels Self-Evaluation Form

LEVEL	DESCRIPTION
Zero:	I did not respect the rights and feelings of others
I:	I did not participate in all the activities today (but I did respect everyone's rights)
II:	I participated in all the activities today (and respected everyone's rights)
III:	I participated in everything and worked on my own (and respected everyone's rights)
IV:	Besides doing all the other Levels, I helped someone (or more than one person)
V:	I did Level IV, and I intend to try some things from the Levels outside of class

Instilling Health and Affective Behaviors

Certainly all levels do not need to be introduced at once. For first and second graders it may be appropriate to focus on only the first two levels. With more mature students you could begin to focus more on levels three and four. My feeling is that it is never too early to start with *awareness talks* as long as they are brief and in language children can understand. Also, be careful about thinking the children are not yet mature enough to deal with the higher levels and are not ready to take much decision-making responsibility. It may be true that they are not, but on the other hand, they never will get to higher levels until we give them some of those opportunities and communicate those expectations to them.

Reflection Times

Reflection times are when you get the children to think about the affective behaviors displayed in class. Sometimes it is a *teachable moment* worth stopping everyone in the course of activity to focus on some affective behavior, good or bad, which has just occurred. Although you are creating a small disruption in the physical activity, an opportunity may offer too much relevancy to pass up. Imagine this happening in your class. A child attempts to do a cartwheel and crashes awkwardly. A couple of students laugh at him/her, but another goes over and offers to get behind and spot the next attempt. You might say right then, what behavior did the spotting child display? What about the laughing students?

I knew a teacher who felt it was well worth the time to occasionally stop everyone so as to point out some affective behavior. Just as we sometimes might *spotlight* some students to demonstrate good motor skill performance, he would halt all activity to briefly recognize some person(s) who was modeling a commendable socially responsible behavior. He also had instituted a time-out hand-signal which, if anyone was especially troubled by someone's behavior, he/she could use it to stop the action. Obviously the students needed to realize making these time-outs must be used judiciously so that activity would not be constantly interrupted. He believed that the students learned to use this responsibility appropriately and that it did get the class to analyze their behavior as soon as a problem was developing.

During the cool-down period at the end of class is probably the best opportunity to regularly reflect on and reinforce what has taken place. Having the students sitting in a circle is conducive for such a discussion. This provides an opportunity to make some brief comments and to ask questions. You might have the students say the number that best represents their level that day. Or you could have them hold up fingers to show their level. I heard it reported of one teacher that she had a very simple system for using the levels concept. She had her levels chart located right at the entrance to the gym. When the children came in they tapped the level at which they intended to function that day. Then, they tapped it again on their exit. She reported that normally the system ran by itself and simply served as a means of the children being reminded and then self-monitoring themselves. But the teacher did say that she would often notice how they were scoring themselves. If she saw any zeros or ones on the way in, it might warn of somebody having a bad today and to watch out for him/her. Also, if discrepancies existed between the student's exiting self-score and what the teacher thought the score should have been, she would call these students aside for a brief discussion.

One more note. Refection time does not have to be entirely limited to the class. If you have been making use of logs and journals to record amounts and feeling about physical activity, perhaps journal assignments could also be made relative to affective experiences. Figure 5.7 is a form that could be used in the journal for self-evaluation purposes.

CHAPTER COMPREHENSION CHECK

1. What are the 4 instructional steps involved in instilling self-responsible actions? *pg 108*
2. What are two or three things good to keep in mind when selecting a behavior to work on?
3. What are the five stages (and their characteristics) of *The Stages of Change Exercise Model*? *pg 112*
4. Which more effectively influence children, explanations of the long-term benefits or explanations of the more immediate quality of life factors?
5. What is the *Behavioral Weaning Procedure*?
6. What is the *Personalize Behavioral Practices* concept?
7. What is meant by employing an "Active Summer Challenge?"
8. What does going *Multi-disciplinary* mean?
9. How soon do food preferences occur?
10. What are some innate food preferences of babies and young children? *sweet salty*
11. At what age, and why, are children characteristically picky eaters? How best is this pickiness countered?
12. Young children might need approximately how many offerings before they accept a new food? *10-15*
13. Is forcing or bribing a child to eat something ever considered an effective habit forming practice? *no*
14. What is meant by a *toxic eating environment*?
15. Which theory does the author support: (1) providing a school environment in which both healthy and unhealthy foods are available, so that children learn to make self-responsible choices? (2) providing a uniformly healthy food environment? What reasons were advanced?
16. What are the stages and characteristics of the *Personal/Social Responsibility Model*? *127-128*

17. Why is the physical education setting an ideal environment for teaching affective domain skills?
18. What is considered an effective way to improve a student's self-concept?
19. What are the 3 basic instructional approaches to teaching physical skills and what affective domain skills are each best suited to teach?

   Individual
   cooperative
   competitive

20. What are the *Five Philosophy Levels of Competitive Sports*? What are the implications of each? Pg 130
21. What are *Awareness Talks*? When are they used and for what purpose?
22. What are *Reflection Times*? When are they used and for what purpose?

[CHAPTER 6]

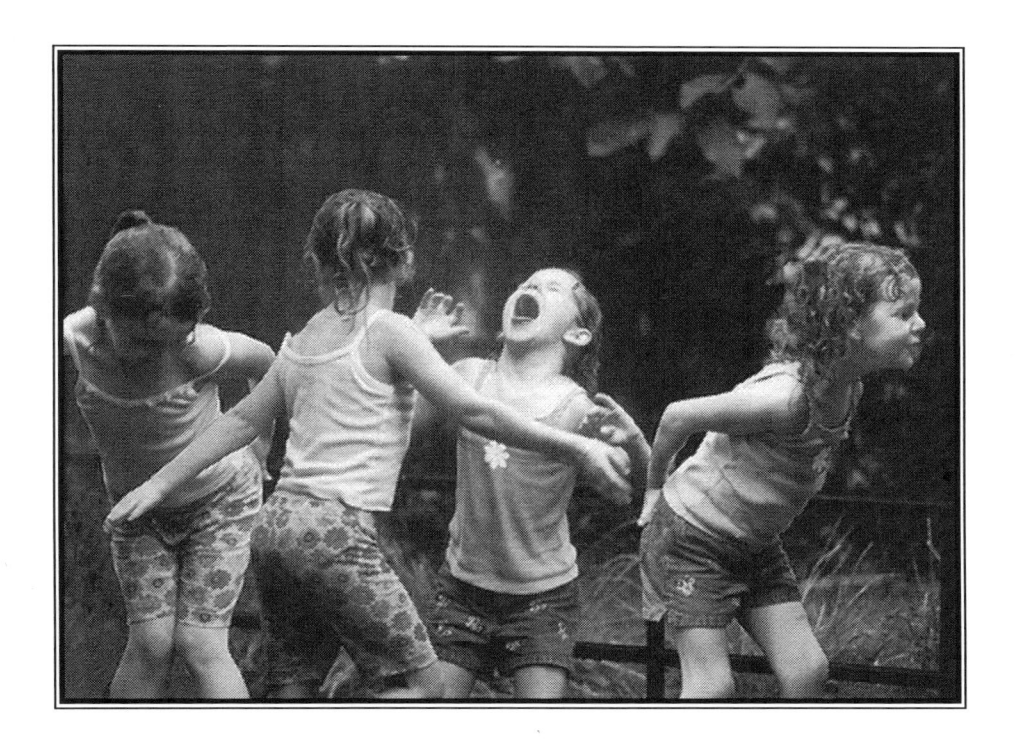

GETTING CHILDREN TO ENJOY PHYSICAL ACTIVITIES & CONDITIONING EXERCISES

ENJOYMENT OF PHYSICAL ACTIVITIES

Exposure to a Wide Variety of Activities
Facilitating Successful Perceptions
Teaching Perseverance

ENJOYMENT OF CONDITIONING EXERCISES

Sanctioning All Intensity Levels
Setting Self-Performance & Process Goals

CHAPTER COMPREHENSION CHECK

"*Stop thinking of exercise as more of that self-improvement stuff and start thinking of it as rescue: private time, a tranquilizer (and energizer), an antidote for the poisons of modern life... Exercise: how badly that term fails to capture the excitement and reward that hard use of the human body can bring.*"
~ John Jerome

"*Such is the constitution of man, that labor may be styled its own reward. - Nor will any external incitements be requisite if it be considered how much happiness is gained, and how much misery escaped, by frequent and violent agitation of the body.*"
~ Samuel Johnson

When I speak of *physical activities* I am referring to a continuum of movement experiences; highly organized competitive sports would be at one end, informal endeavors such as leisurely walking or gardening would be at the other. Normally we participate in these because we enjoy something about the activity itself. Any physiological conditioning benefits we might incur from these activities may be important to us, but are generally secondary to our intrinsic interest in the activity. On the other hand, I am defining *conditioning exercises* as movement endeavors that are done not primarily for the fun of the activity itself, but for the physiological benefits that will be derived. We might do conditioning exercises so as to facilitate the ability to play sports better and lessen chances of injury. Or we might do them simply to improve or attempt to maintain general physical capabilities for everyday healthful living and appearance. Calisthenics would normally fall into this category as would weight training and stretching exercises. Clearly, in using these definitions, there is no fixed demarcation between *physical activities* and *conditioning exercises*. Many people might jog and participate in aerobic dance classes solely for physical benefits and would quit if they thought their fitness would not suffer too much. But there are others who might come to enjoy doing these same activities for the rhythmic feelings, the sheer joy of moving, the psychological rewards, and for social reasons.

If we expect people to lead active lifestyles that will promote their health, it is essential for them to have at least one, but better yet, a range of physical activities they enjoy. Surely finding and integrating physical activities into one's life is best achieved at young ages. Children will normally choose to be active given the opportunities and encouragement. But if movement skills and habits are not learned and enjoyed during the childhood years the likelihood increases that such a lifestyle will become foreign to them and adoption will be more unlikely.

In addition to participating in *physical activities*, people eventually need to realize that incorporating *conditioning exercises* into their lives may be necessary if they wish to maintain well-rounded, balanced health. Most activities will not develop or maintain all of the important components of health. Also, as we age, exercise becomes more essential for safe and successful continuance of the activities we enjoy. Did you ever hear the adage, "I do not play sports to condition myself, rather I condition myself so I can play sports." This may be slightly over stating the role of conditioning, but it does have some validity. Finally, we should be aware that adults typically will find it difficult to devote as much time to physical activities as they were able to when younger. The mature demands of work and family will typically abbreviate the perhaps long hours of youth spent at the gym or playing fields. Encountering these time constraints will necessitate a greater reliance upon time efficient conditioning exercises. In my younger years it was not uncommon for me to play sports for two or more hours most very day. Now I must assiduously schedule my time in order that I can meet my goal of about an hour a day; and because of that reduced time, I feel it has become more necessary to concentrate that activity and devote much of it to balanced conditioning rather than more leisurely physical activity.

It is probably unnecessary to put much stress on *conditioning exercises* when working with primary level children. At this stage we hope that the children will be becoming accustomed to being active, enjoying moving and performing movement skills, being creative and explorative, and playing simple non-competitive games. It is probably too early for them to be much concerned about doing specific activities for fitness reasons or attempting to do exercises in a prescribed manner. Telling children to exercise for the sake of "staying healthy" simply isn't very effective. Long-term health is about #63 on a child's priority list. Fun is #1. However, during the intermediate grades, while major emphasis should still be directed at exploring enjoyable *physical activities*, some introduction to *conditioning exercises* would seem appropriate. Children at this age are beginning to play sports more vigorously and thus it is important for them to begin to understand the need for achieving minimal levels of fitness to do those sports successfully and safely. While I do not favor children being heavily involved in weight training and long demanding steady-state aerobic workouts to achieve high levels of performance in a specific sport, the learning and practicing of some level of conditioning exercises makes sense. They should be starting to appreciate activities for the indispensable contributions they make toward cardiovascular, musculoskeletal, and body composition fitness. It is not too soon for them to learn that they need to begin taking care of their bodies. I would like to think that when they wake-up in the morning they are beginning to plan when during the day they will be getting some physical activity and/or doing some conditioning exercises.

ENJOYMENT OF PHYSICAL ACTIVITIES

There are three things teachers can do which will contribute to children enjoying regular physical activity. (1) They need to encourage and expose children to a wide variety of activities. By so doing it is hoped the children will encounter those activities which are well suited to their unique physical abilities and temperament. (2) When students are experiencing a new activity the teacher must attempt to ensure that they will be reasonably successful or, more importantly, perceive that they are successful. This is because the students normally will want to continue participating in activities in which they feel competent and often will not remain with those where they see themselves incompetent. (3) The children may also need to be taught a certain degree of perseverance. Many physical activities require serious practice before the skills can be effectively performed. Individuals who have not learned to persevere may give up during the early difficult goings.

Below we will separately discuss ideas for how you might accomplish these three things.

Exposure to a Wide Variety of Physical Activities

If children are not exposed to a wide variety of activities many of them may not discover those they would find most rewarding. The breadth of activities encountered in and out of school is in some cases quite narrow. Not uncommonly curriculums may only emphasize a few different team sports. While these sports will be attractive to many students they are not necessarily the best solution for decreasing the hypoactivity of American children. When you think of all the diverse kinds of movement activities everyone should be able to find one, if not many activities, he/she would enjoy doing on a regular basis. In support of this view, we should realize that most people probably have some movement abilities that would allow them to be fairly successful at certain types of activities. Research tells us that there are many kinds of relatively specific motor abilities and that it is wrong to think of people as being either athletic or not. This is known as the *Specificity of Motor Abilities Hypothesis*. The implication of this concept is that different types of activities and sports draw on different abilities. For example, children who do not have the abilities and/or temperament to excel at basketball or soccer could do very well and enjoy rollerblading, dance or swimming. Cross-country jogging or yoga may fit the hidden talents of others. Even people with severe physical disabilities might still have other abilities that allow them to skillfully participate in certain movement skills; sight impaired individuals have been Olympic track performers and wrestlers; people who have lost significant use of their legs have won national championships in archery, gymnastics, and many others sports.

Although most sports require some degree of ability to perform well, it is important to make the point that it is not necessary for people to be athletically gifted in order to live an active life. I think this is a lesson of which all young people need to be made aware. I have a number of friends who would not be considered athletic at all, and yet they regularly enjoy moving and are healthy as a consequence. They do things like walking, cycling, inline skating, backpacking, and lifting weights. Walking probably has the greatest carryover potential of any activity for keeping many Americans active. We must dispense with the idea that "walking is wimpy." It probably is the most transferable of all long-term activities and to my mind we should be regularly walking kindergarteners, twelfth graders, and everyone in between. What if you established the routine of taking your class on a daily walk? You might not have the skills or abilities to run and jump rope but you can successfully walk and, barring a serious disability, so will all your students. You would be role modeling an active lifestyle right alongside your kids. Any academic subject you might be teaching in the classroom could be reinforced on the walks. Many of the children may have never experienced 10 or 20 continuous minutes of exercise before reaching the sixth grade. A healthy practice, like a fun walk, could become etched in a kindergartner's mind for life. Figure 6.1 charts some reasonable walking distance guidelines for the younger children. Also, refer to Chapter 12 for a number of "Walk/Run Activities." Be sure to look them over. They can be so fun and easy to do by all, and yet so beneficial. I like to spread the Latin proverb, "Before super walk a little, after super do the same."

Figure 6.1. Walking Distance Guidelines

	To start with (miles)	Later in the year (miles)
Kindergarten	1/2-3/4	1-1 1/2
First Grade	3/4-1	1 1/2-2
Second Grade	1-1 1/2	2-3
Third Grade	1 1/2-2	3-4

Undoubtedly there are things that will limit your ability to introduce many other activities to your classes: your knowledge and skills, your facilities and equipment, your preparation time. However, it might make a big difference to some, if each year you could have your class participate in at least one or two new things beyond what they normally encounter in their traditional curriculum. If actual participation is unmanageable, it may be worthwhile discussing and listing various activity possibilities. An enthusiastic talk from you might be enough to get some of the children to give it a try outside of school. You could personalize and explain the different activities you and your friends like to do. Also, ask the students what kinds of activities they do to be regularly active and praise them for it. I have known many children and adults who as a result of unsuccessful attempts at a limited range of activities have concluded that they were "not athletic" and did not enjoy sports. A little timely encouragement from you could make the difference. Inviting guest speakers from the community and various clubs might be effective. Many local individuals and groups (bicycle clubs, karate clubs, volts-marchers, etc.) are ready and eager to introduce their favorite activity. Also, many sports and recreational organizations have programs and representatives available for school presentations.

Facilitating Successful Perceptions

Encouraging and providing children the opportunity to participate in a wide variety of activities, that range from light-paced experiences to vigorous will result in most of them finding some movement experiences enjoyable. But another reason some will not find activities enjoyable, even when an activity is potentially suited to their likes and abilities, is how well they can initially do the skill or how well they feel they are doing (of course this is more of a risk in the games and sports requiring more skill and fitness). In Chapter 8 you will be given many ideas about how to design the learning environment to make skill performance easier and more successful. For now, let us address the basis upon which children form perceptions about their successfulness. This is important because even though they may be reasonably accomplishing a task, they still could be dissatisfied with their performance and hence discontinue its pursuit. Being overly self-critical of one's performance, along with being too tenderly sensitive to what others may think, is arguably the greatest cause of failing to pursue a new activity.

Normally children in the primary grades judge the goodness of their performance on the feedback they receive from significant adults, most commonly their parents and teachers. They want the adults' attention and if they are given praise for their performance they will accept it and conclude they are doing good. Since most parents and teachers are supportive and encouraging, young children typically have high self-concepts of their abilities. It is not uncommon to hear remarks such as, "I am the strongest boy in the world, feel my muscle!" "I can run fast!" "Watch me!" Children enjoy most activities at this stage because they are told, and faithfully believe, that their performance is good. The obvious recommendation for teachers hoping to further these attitudes is to be liberal in their praise of the children's attempts. We should be encouraged by the extraordinary influence we have at this stage in the child's development, but it is also a weighty responsibility. Sadly, the powerful influence of adult feedback can be all too well documented in those children who have had abusive and unsupportive parents or teachers. Young people in such environments often have extremely low perceptions of self-worth and capabilities. Of course, it is doubly important for us to give encouragement to individuals who have had this kind of debilitating background.

> ## A WORD OF CAUTION ABOUT CONDITIONAL PRAISE
>
> I stand by my recommendation to praise children for their early performance efforts as a means of facilitating their successful perceptions. However, we must always be watchful that in employing operant conditioning techniques that we do not unintentionally undermine the inherent motivation to enjoy an activity. Consider this story of an old man whose sleep was disturbed each Saturday morning by the regular early morning pick-up baseball games of the neighborhood kids. One Saturday he goes to the sandlot and tells the kids how much it warms his heart to hear them playing their game. In fact, he likes it so much he gives them a twenty-dollar bill and asks them to be sure to come back next Saturday and hoop it up. Of course, the next Saturday the games are started early with everyone in full throat and vigor. As the games are finishing the old man comes out and again praises all of them. But this time he says he is a little short of cash and gives them a ten-dollar bill. The players are still pleased and promise to return in seven days. Events are much the same during the third week but the old man now can only afford to part with five dollars. The enthusiasm of the children in not nearly as great but they take it and plan on meeting again. Finally week four arrives as do the kids and play occurs. The old man appears and maybe you guessed it, while he enjoys the games he announces that he is out of money and cannot longer pay them. When he asks if he can plan of their return the following week one of the children pipes up, "No way, I am not coming to play for nothing!" And other voices of rebellion agree.
>
> Our highest objective is for the children to be *intrinsically motivated* I think it is fun to walk, or run, or play sports and that is the long-term attitude I want the children to develop. When we continually make our praise and rewards contingent on performance some children might become controlled by it, as were the children in the story of the old man. They see that they are doing the activity for those things, not for the activity itself. They are *extrinsically motivated* and when the rewards are gone, they see no further reason to do the activity for its own sake. Perhaps the best approach to avoid this undermining of intrinsic motivation is to always begin and continue to stress the inherent worth of the activity. Remember to convey the expectation that the activity is interesting and fun to do; that you or others like it and look forward to doing it. As for praising and rewarding performance, try to do so only when you think some individuals are encountering difficulties and are not yet seeing the enjoyment of it. Hopefully, as they continue you may be able to fade the use of rewards and praise. The lesson is that if the students are having a good time just doing it, let it sell itself. That is where we want to end up.

As children move into the intermediate grades their basis of reference begins to change. They typically are no longer wholly accepting of elders. Now you might hear, "Come on Dad try, you are letting me win!" Teachers are less likely to hear, "Watch me!" Increasingly the children become more aware of the performance of their peers and begin to value their acceptance above all else. They become more realistic, discovering themselves to perhaps not be the strongest or fastest. The feedback peers give each other is sometimes not as kind and diplomatic as it should be. This social comparison process results in an inevitable lowering of self-concepts for some. This is a major factor in why children are no longer quite so unanimously pleased with new activity endeavors and why large numbers begin to be less enthused with sports programs and may completely drop out. Everyone cannot be a first-place winner, and if enjoyment is viewed as being contingent upon performing as well or better than others, one's activity options are unnecessarily limited.

The appropriate role for the teacher at this stage in the children's development, as well as later, would seem to be to attenuate or soften this social comparison process. Some believe that many overzealous parents, teachers and coaches do just the opposite. They create *hyper-competition* by always keeping scores, recording ranking and giving special recognition to top performers. Charts are posted depicting which skills have and have not been accomplished by whom. The intent of these efforts is to provide extra incentives to make the children strive harder and be happier with awarded successes. The danger is that many are taught to think even more along social comparison lines. Also, we would argue that the students who will receive the most positive recognition are going to be the top performers who are oftentimes least in need of it. They are more likely already sold on the activity. On the other hand, the message provided to a large number of other students, whose liking for the activity could go either way, is a discouraging one. These tender growing shoots see that social comparison is to be valued and that, in this instance, they are only average or sub par. Euphemistic scales ranging from good to above average to great should not be expected to disguise this reality from them.

The implication to be drawn is not that we should never put children in competitive sports and other social comparison situations. These activities can be excitingly fun and they have the potential of teaching many lessons. However, there also are good reasons for having the children participate in physical activities and exercises where the focus is on self, rather than inter-student comparisons. Learning to direct attention to one's own physical performance is a more necessary lesson than always worrying about beating or being beaten by some else. A quote made by the well-published physician and running enthusiast George Sheehan aptly captures this spirit. He said, "I run against the absolute best I can do. The other runners hold no terrors for me. I am not diminished by those ahead of me nor am I enhanced by those behind. I have moved from an antagonistic relationship with other runners to an agonistic relationship with self."

Regardless of how socially competitive the learning environment is, the feedback you habitually provide is also a factor in whether or not social comparisons will be promoted or reduced. Its intent should be to direct the students' attention toward their own performance and its progress. You want the students to realize that enjoyment is found in doing and self-improvement and is independent of others. This means that as children are sampling new activities and accessing their performance, you should try to avoid saying things like, "How many reached 20?" "Did you win?" "Who could do it?" Rather, say, "If you gave it your best, you should be proud of your effort and progress." "Lets see if everyone can do more than last time." "Don't worry about what others are doing, be your best." "Sure it is difficult, that is part of the challenge and fun." "Did you have fun?" "Did you learn?" If through persistent feedback we could sway them to adopt some self-performance goals rather than thinking only of social comparison goals where they are concerned about who is better than whom, enjoyment of activities should be open to many more people. I have known numerous people to truly enjoy participating in sports even though their level of play was much below average. It did not much matter to them, and indeed why should it. Pleasure was in the doing and the benefits were just as rich.

Also, because the feedback the child gets from the other children is coming to have such great valence, we need to emphasize their social responsibility of helping and caring for each other. Ralph Waldo Emerson said, "I pay the schoolmaster, but 'tis the schoolboys that educate my son." Being laughed at or criticized by peers can be devastating to one's feelings about their skills or appearance. We simply cannot permit such to occur. We need to be constantly rewarding good interactions and informing them of why unkind behaviors are hurtful.

Teaching Perseverance

Perseverance is one of the important moral lessons that participation in physical activities is well suited to teach. Many physical skills cannot be accomplished immediately, but if continued effort is put forth, rewarding, tangible results will soon occur. What can we do to help children persist long enough at an activity, to get through the rough going, and experience the joy of achievement? This is an important question because persistence is characteristically low in many children. They simply have not learned the necessity of working and delaying need gratification. I have had many children make a few attempts at a task and then say quite resignedly, "I don't like this." "I can't do it, I tried but I can't do it."

There are a number of things we can do to facilitate persistence. To begin with, when introducing a skill make clear to the students that it may well require lengthy practice before they will be completely successful. Tell them it will take some people longer than others. When a skill is being demonstrated either by you or another skilled model, be sure to explain how much practice was required to reach this level of proficiency. Whenever I give a competent demonstration of a gymnastic stunt, a throw, a jump-rope skill, I make it a point to explain that thousands of trials and often years of practice have gone into its mastery. If possible I also give a brief account of the initial difficulties and frustration. In fields of endeavor as diverse as chess, sports, and music, there exist what is known as The Ten -Year Rule. A substantial body of evidence suggests that elite performers require about 10 to 12 years of regular quality practice to acquire the necessary skills and experience to perform at an international level. The very best violinists have spent over 10,000 hour in "deliberate practice" (deliberate practice is defined as an effortful activity motivated by the goal of improving performance). The average intermediate level violinists have spent "only" 8,000 hours. Estimates are that basketball players have performed over one million shots before they get to the professional level. The lesson is clear, if your kids want to be like Mike, they have to "Practice, practice, practice." "But, hey! what could be more fun?"

PERSONAL PERSEVERANCE STORY

This discussion of perseverance brings to mind a personal experience. A number of years ago I decided to take a watercolor class through the city's recreation department. I had little knowledge of my abilities in this area but I figured it might be fun to try something new. The first night the instructor gave a slide presentation of his painting career. We all knew that he was an excellent professional painter and the slides of his later works confirmed that in all our eyes. He also showed examples of some of the paintings when he was beginning art school over twenty years ago. These early works were not at all impressive and he good-naturedly admitted that to be the case.

I struggled throughout the eight weeks of class. My paint ran where I did not want them, my colors were muddy, and my shapes were unerringly distorted. Many times I thought about quitting and I noticed that about two thirds of the class members had done so by the last night. That last night of class, the painting I was doing turned out a good bit better than my previous ones. I was cautiously proud of it and my instructor and remaining small band of classmates were kindly congratulatory. That little success and timely encouragement was enough to keep me painting following the cessation of the class. I have continued to pursue this hobby over the years and have derived much reward from it.

Although the instructor and student praise was important, I believe that the early slide show was an indispensable key to my continuing to paint throughout the class and beyond. I wanted to skillfully paint like he did, but my performances were so inferior to his demonstrations. What has kept me going to this day was recalling the weakness of his beginning efforts. I convinced myself that maybe my attempts were not all that discouragingly bad; my messes were about as good as his, and it took him twenty years to get where he was today.

Today, when I am teaching physical skills, especially to children, I attempt to apply this valued lesson learned from my art instructor. I don't rely upon praise alone, I make it a habit it let beginners know how much time has gone into the skills I or others are demonstrating. And if I cannot give them visible evidence of how much weaker initial attempts were, I can at least attempt to describe some of those difficulties.

As the children are engaged in the activity you need to keep reinforcing the persistence theme. Rather than directing verbal reinforcement toward best performances, habitually look for effort and publicly recognize it. Those who truly tried hard are deserving of all your kudos, regardless of their level of performance or even if they did not improve. Those who easily succeed do not need much praise and are not necessarily deserving of it. When you see effort flagging tell them you have confidence that they eventually can get there. When you hear the dispirited, "I can't", and you regularly will, apply *The Yet Principle*. You cannot do it 'yet' but you will if you keep trying. William James said "Effort is the measure of a man." We must teach children this precept.

Finally, we can foster stick-to-it-ness by helping the children detect any performance improvements that may be occurring. Sometimes the students will not know that their technique is becoming more fluid and efficient, or they may not remember that their performance outcomes were worse than what they have now become. For some skills, assessment and/or charting might lend credence to our encouragement or make you aware of advances being made that you had not detected. Plotting out the number of times targets have been hit over a week, two weeks, or over a much longer time frame could make for a good exercise. This could be done for individuals or groups. Repeated recording of times needed to get through an obstacle course or the number of minutes and seconds of successful rope jumping would be other examples. In a later chapter the idea of having students keep portfolios will be introduced. These graphs of performance over a period of time would make a nice project.

ENJOYMENT OF CONDITIONING EXERCISES

Is it possible to get children to actually enjoy *conditioning exercises*? If we adhere to the definition presented at the beginning of this chapter, physical conditioning exercises cannot really be enjoyable, if they become enjoyable they are no longer conditioning exercises but pass into the realm of *physical activities*. This sort of desirable transition is sometimes feasible. I know people, myself included, who over a period of time doing exercises such as swimming, jogging, and stretching have actually reached a point of truly enjoying those activities. So much so that they would do those activities even if no physical health benefits were concomitant. Hopefully a high degree of liking would develop for some of your students. More probably for most students it is unrealistic to expect that physical *conditioning exercises* will be actually relished. They will remain *conditioning exercises* and may not become especially enjoyable *physical activities*. But recognizing this reality does not mean that most people need to view exercising with loathing or even dislike. I know many people who have learned to accept exercises as a not unpleasant aspect of their normal routine. Indeed, virtually all those people who have developed the habit of exercising over an extended time period seem to have achieved this status. If exercise is truly onerous to somebody, it is the exceptional person who would long persevere at it. Let us look at two things we can do which may help to make exercise enjoyable, or nearly so.

Sanctioning All Intensity Levels

One factor strongly related to the enjoyment of exercise is how strenuous it is. Generally, although the relationship does not apply to everyone, the more strenuous the exercise the less pleasurable it is perceived to be. There is a wealth of evidence showing lower intensity exercise programs such as walking and hiking are rated as being more enjoyable than jogging, aerobic dance, step aerobics, and aerobic swimming activities. As a consequence, the more vigorous exercises are not maintained nearly as well. Less than a quarter of the population are successful in long-term adherence to these more heart thumping pursuits. This evidence should teach us that if we place all, or even most of our instructional emphasis upon high intensity exercise, we are doomed to be unsuccessful with many children. Most people simply will not subscribe in the long run to a strict "no pain, no gain" philosophy.

My recommendation is that we sanction all intensity levels of exercise: vigorous, moderate, and light. All are good for you and you need to find those with which you can be comfortable. We should not give up on promoting maximally strenuous efforts and we should attempt to explain both the special physical and psychological health benefits they confer. Many children are very energetic and can become quite enthused about exercise given the encouragement and right environment. Likely you will have students who are eager and receptive to moving at high levels. A goal for these children is to keep them interested and to accustom them to regular practices. Brutus Hamilton, a former track coach at the University of California had this to say about the joy to be discovered in pushing the body to its limit. "It is one of the strange ironies of this strange life that those who work the hardest, who subject themselves to the strictest discipline, who give up certain pleasurable things in order to achieve a goal, are the happiest men and women. When you see 20 or 30 runners line up for a distance race in some meet, don't pity them, don't feel sorry for them. Better envy them instead."

THE PAINFUL JOY IN VIGOROUS EXERCISE

According to Shakespeare, "There be some sports are painful." Scott Martin, a competitive bicyclist, poetically explains it this way. "To be a cyclist is to be a student of pain. Sure the sport is fun with its seamless pace-lines and secret single-track, its post-ride pig-outs and soft muscles grown wonderfully hard. But at cycling's core lies pain, hard and bitter as the pit inside a juicy peach. It doesn't matter if you're sprinting for an Olympic gold medal, a town sign, a trailhead, or the rest stop with the homemade brownies. If you never confront pain, you're missing the essence of the sport. Pain is a big fat creature riding on your back. The faster you pedal, the heavier he feels. The harder you push, the tighter he squeezes your chest. The steeper the climb, the deeper he digs his jagged, sharp claws into your muscles. Without pain, there's no adversity. Without adversity, no challenge. Without challenge, no improvement. No improvement, no sense of accomplishment and no deep-down joy."

Some of your students will find it more difficult to savor vigorous conditioning. These children need to be of special interest to us because it is they that are often at greatest risk of becoming sedentary. In their case I do not feel that unremitting admonishments to push harder and pick-up the pace is the best route to follow. Research has found that being forced to exercise during childhood may have potentially negative consequences for later activity. Our message might rather be that it is okay to do less vigorous exercises. It should be one of finding what is comfortable for you so that you can make it a regular part of your lifestyle

I heard someone once go so far as to say "exercise is that gentle pastime in which we coax subtle changes from our bodies." This mild philosophy may not produce great athletes but of course that is not our purpose. It could greatly profit many of the more sedentary people. They need to develop the attitude that exercise is not something to dread doing. It is something we do for ourselves, not to ourselves. Faster, longer, higher might be a good creed for Olympic athletic achievements but can be burdensome to some.

Setting Self-Performance & Process Goals

I pointed out earlier that *physical activities* might be enjoyable to more people if social comparison worries were minimized. I believe the same applies to physical conditioning. The actions of many teachers would suggest they believe just the opposite. They employ many practices that socially compare the fitness performance of students and then provide rewards to the better performers. For example, they will ask which students were able to do 30 or 35 sit-ups, they may provide normative data on a running test, they may display charts and graphs depicting individual performances, and extra praise, rewards, or even better grades are given to the higher performances. They justify these practices on the grounds that they will provide extra fun and motivation for the students to improve their fitness. The students meeting those standards will be receiving extra positive vibes, the students not achieving them will be motivated to strive harder to reach those levels and achieve awards in the future.

My view is that the incentives based on comparisons of social outcomes do not always work in this manner. There is no question that rewards to those students achieving standards will act as an extra incentive. However, a couple of questions need to be asked. Firstly, are extra incentives all that important to those already performing at the upper end of the class? Most of these people are frequently already sold on fitness. Secondly, more often than not, good outcome fitness goals are not as much the result of effort and practice as they are of natural ability and early maturation (this issue will be discussed more fully in Chapter 10). If this is the case, we may be rewarding some who are not deserving because they are not necessarily developing the lifestyle practices for which we are striving. They are getting the message that, "Hey, I am fit, therefore I must be doing all that I need to."

As for the other students whose outcomes are below par, it is very questionable that they, in response to this information, will work harder, catch-up, and receive positive recognition for doing so. Undoubtedly this happy scenario could be true for some, however, there will be many more others that will receive the poor information and simply be discouraged by it. They will feel bad and wish only to avoid all thoughts of conditioning exercises in the future. They will feel it is impossible for them to reach the standards of others. And what of the students who are motivated to labor diligently so as to catch-up? Because of the overriding significance of developmental rates and genetic differences, physical fitness outcomes in children are in only very small part due to effort and lifestyle. Consequently, many, no matter how conscientious their effort, simply will not perceptibly close the performance gap with their peers. This means that we may be setting impossibly difficult goals for them. If this is the case, we are guilty of one of the great sins of teaching. We in essence are setting the children up for failure, and failure isn't fun. In some individuals it does not take too many such experiences before they acquire the attitude of *learned helplessness* towards not only about exercise but perhaps other aspects of their schooling and life as well.

The alternative to encouraging *social comparison goals* is to get people to direct their focus primarily upon maintaining or improving their own performance. Here we are again advocating *self-performance goals* as opposed to *social-comparison goals*. *Self-performance goals* tend to be more realistic for all the children. The top students should have challenging goals as well as the lowest. Such goals are more under their control and thus less stressful and threatening to many. The criterion now being taught is based upon their own relative performance. The teacher makes it a habit to say things like "Who was able to do as many or more than last time?" "You all know how long it took you to complete the circuit yesterday. Set what you think would be a good time for you today." Striving for your "personal best" or "maintaining your fitness zone" would be typical directives.

When students set goals of doing 25 sit-ups, touching their toes, or jumping rope for three minutes, they are striving for a certain standard of performance. Although these personal-referenced *self-performance goals* may be reasonable ones for their individual abilities, even here there is still some inherent stress. Some people may find always having to work towards criteria is onerous and adds an unpleasant aspect to exercise. When someone exercises, is it always necessary to be counting and timing oneself and worrying about those scores? "Feeling the need to always do better." The answer is no. What about simply having *process goals* that simply specify doing a certain amount of exercise without concern for meeting any criterion? I, and many of my friends who maintain satisfaction with chronic exercise, generally operate this way. Our goal is to do certain amounts of exercise: getting a minimum of five aerobic workouts in this week, dynamically stretching each day this week, weight training two or three times. Notice that when thinking this way people do not need to be monitoring and being concerned about how fast they are running or how far they are stretching.

They can cut a workout a little short on some days they do not feel their best; at least they are disciplining their lives and consistently exercising. Why worry and bother. Are they not after all doing what is reasonably necessary? Will fitness therefore not take care of itself? Will conditioning not be more enjoyable?

CHAPTER COMPREHENSION CHECK

1. What is the difference between *physical activities* and *conditioning exercises*? How much emphasis should be placed on these across the elementary school years?
2. What are 3 things teachers should do to help *children enjoy physical activity*?
3. What is the *Specificity of Motor Ability Hypothesis* and what are the implications it has for the eacher?
4. What are the following: Conversational Jogging, Time Estimation Run, Card Run, The Straw Walk?
5. What was the moral of the Conditional Praise story in which the old man pays the children to play?
6. Normally primary level children judge the quality of their performance on feedback from whom? What about intermediate level children?
7. What is the concept of *hypercompetition* and how might teachers contribute to it?
8. What is the difference between *self-performance goals* and *social-comparison* goals?
9. What is the *Ten-Year Rule*?
10. What is the *Yet Principle*?
11. Why should we be promoting all levels of exercise (light, moderate, and vigorous)?
12. What is the motivational consequence of rewarding students on the basis of social-comparison performances?
13. What is the concept of *Learned Helplessness*?
14. Which goals are more under the students' control, *social-comparison*, *self-performance*, or *process goals*?

[CHAPTER 7]

MANAGEMENT TECHNIQUES

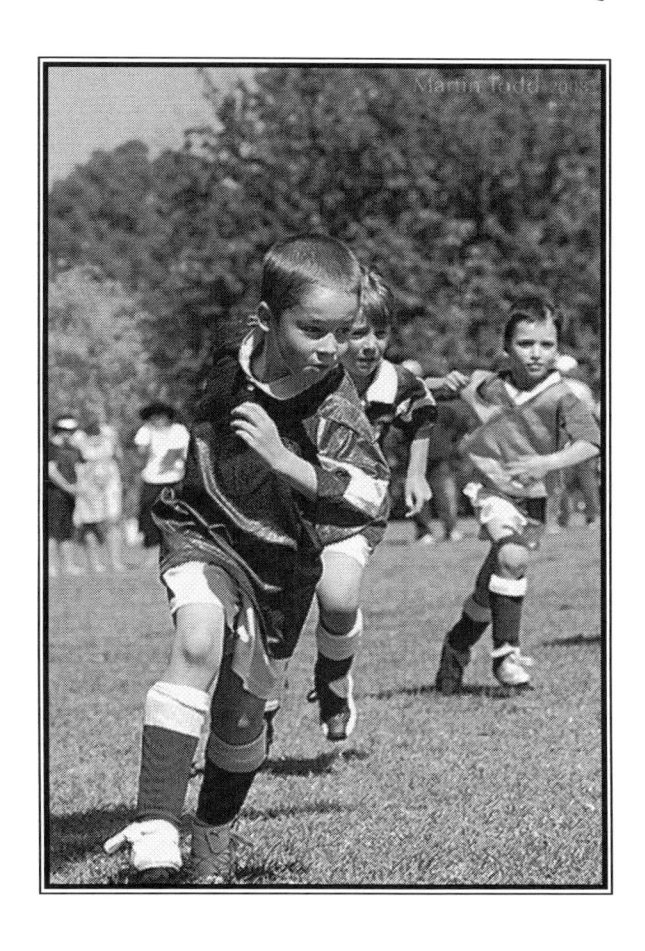

EASTABLISHING CLASS RULES

STARTING CLASS

OTHER MANAGEMENT TECHNIQUES

Communication Styles
Passive Communication
Aggressive Communication
Assertive Communication

MANAGEMENT GAMES

CORRECTING MISBEHAVIOR
Removal of Positive Consequences
Six-Step Discipline Plan
Exercise as Punishment
Group Punishment

CHAPTER COMPREHENSION CHECK

> *"Education is a painful, continual and difficult work to be done by kindness, by watching, by warning, by precept, and by praise, but above all – by example."*
> ~ John Ruskin

> *"I love kids, but love well behaved kids better."*
> ~ Anonymous

"If I can't manage I can't teach." Teacher candidates put a huge effort and resources into obtaining their degrees and gaining employment. Yet approximately one half of them will quit school teaching within two to three years. The major reason for this high attrition is an inability to establish a manageable teaching environment. Every teacher encounters difficulties in doing so. Some struggle and eventually develop the needed management techniques, others are unsuccessful and teaching becomes frustratingly impossible. Those who become successful class managers have not all found the same invariable magic formula. Their techniques range widely with their personalities and school circumstances. What works for one might be unsuitable for another. However, that does not mean that there are not specific pedagogical techniques and procedures that they have learned and which have contributed to their success. It is my belief that anyone can become a good teacher if he/she really, I mean really, wants to. It will require much effort for some, and yet more effort for others, to know these techniques and learn to incorporate them into their unique styles.

This chapter will introduce many of these techniques known to be associated with effective management. Most can be applied in both the classroom and the playing-fields, some will be specific to the activity areas. When you have children participating in movement activities, management procedures become particularly important for a number of reasons. Those environs often have many distractions to which children are especially susceptible. You will have more difficulty making yourself heard because of generally poor acoustics, the greater dispersion of the students, the high noise levels of the activities, and the great excitement and laughter of the students. The children face greater inherent physical risk during movement activities and thus you must be able to quickly start and stop the action. Finally, because the children often experience high levels of physical and psychological arousal as they participate in games, undesirable behaviors will inevitably result unless good control structures are in place to prevent or quickly correct them.

> **THE TEACHER'S POWER AND CLASS CLIMATE**
>
> Haim G. Ginott (1922–1973) was a teacher, child psychologist and psychotherapist, who worked with children and parents. He pioneered techniques for conversing with children that are still taught today. This quote is taken from his book *Teacher and Child*.
>
> I have come to the frightening conclusion.
>   I am the decisive element in the classroom.
>   It is my personal approach that creates the climate.
>   It is my daily mood that makes the weather.
>   As a teacher, I possess a tremendous power to make a child's life miserable or joyous.
>   I can be a tool of torture or an instrument of aspiration.
>   I can humiliate or humor, hurt or heal.
>   In all situations, it is my response that decides whether a crisis will be escalated or de-escalated and a child humanized or dehumanized.

ESTABLISHING CLASS RULES

Most educational authorities recommend that class rules be a short list of simply worded positive statements. They should be carefully established at the very beginning of the school year. The teacher might choose to have a prepared listing that is introduced and discussed with the students. Or the teacher may engage them in the process of democratically formulating the rules. This latter procedure has the potential advantage of creating a high level of student ownership and hence more willing compliance. Regardless of which approach is taken it is important that everyone understands the rules and ascents to the necessity for them. Once the rules have been written they should be posted where they will be frequently seen. Try not to exceed three to five rules; more than this makes it difficult for students to remember all the details and makes you appear overly strict. In addition, too many rules make students engage in rule-specific thinking. A youngster may believe it is acceptable to chew gum in the multipurpose room because the rule says, "No gum-chewing in the halls." When students think in a rule-specific fashion, they do not learn to think about right and wrong and the spirit of the rule; rather, they often look for exceptions to the rule.

   The following are examples of appropriate general rules that cover a wide range of behavior:

   Stop, look, and listen. This implies freezing on signal, looking at the instructor, and listening for instructions.

Take care of equipment. This includes caring for equipment and distributing, gathering, and using it properly.

Respect the rights of others. This includes behavior such as not pushing others, leaving others' equipment alone, not fighting or arguing, and not physically or emotionally hurting others.

The following list of rules is useful with young children in an activity setting:

Be a mover.

Be kind.

Be safe.

Although you have introduced the rules, discussed the need for them, and even gained good student concurrence, you should not expect that everything will run smoothly ever after. The behaviors that the rules are specifying are skills that must be practiced and learned. As immediately as possible after the children are exposed to the rules it would be good to begin this practice. Let us say that you have three class rules: (1) good listeners, (2) fast reactors, and (3) friendly people. You explain a simple tag game of some sort. Before starting the game you insert the comment about how you are pleased that everyone was good listeners and how that is allowing us to get started playing this fun game. After the game has been in progress for a short period you give a clear stop command. As everyone comes to an immediate halt you enthusiastically congratulate them on their fast reaction skills and applying the class rules. You might also remind them of how important that is for safety. After they again have played a brief while you stop them and comment proudly on their running and dodging. Everyone stayed under control and did not crash into anyone else. You tell them that that is part of being "friendly people." You also mention that behaviors such as rescuing people who have been tagged are instances of "friendly people" and this makes the game enjoyable for everyone. The point being made here is that you are concentrating on teaching and reinforcing the application of the class rules. I believe that this should be the primary purpose of the teacher during the first week or two of physical activities sessions. The other fitness and motor skill goals might be considered of secondary importance at this stage. If the children first learn the class rules you will be able to accomplish all other content goals much better over the year. Also, it will make life infinitely easier on you and the students.

The task of working on the class rules does not end after the first week or two. Even if you get your class off to an excellent start, the phenomena of *slippage* will occur. This is where the students will drift or slip away from adherence to the class rules unless they are periodically reviewed and reinforced. For instance, part of being fast reactors was the expectation that the students would stop immediately on your command. During the first weeks the students were faithfully stopping within 3 to 5 second but later on you noticed that you and the class had to wait significantly longer for some to settle down. This is *slippage* and the best course for you to take is not to allow it to continue and invariably grow worst. If you do not deal with it now, you will have to deal with an entrenched and larger problem later. The recommended course to take is to avoid becoming angry with the group or any individual. Rather patiently await the full attention of the class and say something like, "We seem to be starting to forget one of the rules. We are not being fast reactors and stopping quickly. Remember how we agreed that we needed to do so for safety reasons and because it would permit us to have more time for fun activities. Let us start this activity again and when I give the command we will impress ourselves with an instantaneous stop."

It is not enough to share your rules with students. If it is true that "it takes a village to raise a child," it makes sense to ensure that all parties know and understand your rules. A newsletter to parents at the start of the school year explaining your approach to class management and listing your rules and consequences will set the appropriate tone immediately. Parents rarely complain about their child being disciplined if the routines, rules, and consequences are clearly identified in advance.

You should also share your rules with other teachers who work with your class, such as the music teacher, librarian, etc. This ensures a consistent approach to rules and consequences throughout the children's school day. Sharing your rules with administrators is also helpful. When you and your principal have the same understanding of rules and consequences, it is easier to work together to achieve common goals.

STARTING CLASS

When children are taken into a gym or other play space they naturally are excited by the environment and the prospect of physical activity. If little teacher control is present, they in all probability will begin racing about and screaming and shouting. Experienced teachers have found two basic procedures effective for avoiding this problem. One is to simply have a clearly established policy of the children moving to a set area and sitting down to await instruction. The other method is that of *instant activity*. The concept of *instant activity* is where the children know they are to engage in activity as soon as they enter the area. The activity could be in the form of a routine such as jogging a few laps and/or completing certain exercises or activities. As soon as those activities have been finished they know to move to a prescribed area and sit for the lesson's instructions. Another instant activity regimen is where the students know that when entering the area they will encounter written directions. These directions might be posted near the gym entrance, or in the case of classroom teachers, given to the students prior to leaving the classroom. The prescribed activities might be conditioning in nature or they may be skills that are related to the previous or ensuing lesson. Figure 7.1 offers a couple of examples of instant activity assignments. Notice how the directions can be written so that all the students will not be assigned the same task. This procedure might be desirable because it makes better use of equipment and space. Also, it instills the habit of all the students reading the instructions for themselves rather than just following the lead of what the others are doing.

I particularly like the idea of *instant activity* instructions for three reasons. Firstly, the students are learning to read directions and become self-learners. Secondly, it directs them immediately into purposeful activity. And thirdly, it serves the management goal of releasing some of their pent-up energy and thus makes them better listeners for the beginning of class.

Figure 7.1. Instant Activity Directions

1. Everyone find a personal space and practice a set of sit-ups and 3 different dynamic stretches we have learned.
2. If your last name begins with A-L get a ball, find a personal space and practice your stationary dribbling skills.
If your last name begins with M-Z get a partner and one ball, find a space and practice your passing skills.
When the music stops, put the balls away and sit your squads
3. Draw a playing card from the stack, look at it, and put it back.
   Hearts and Diamonds: get a hula-hoop and see how well you can spin it around your, waist, wrist, and neck.
   Clubs and Spades: get a rope and see how well you can jump with a forwards and backwards spin; and on one foot.

Another small but possibly useful point to consider is the arrangement of the children when beginning the lesson. Simply having everyone sitting in a group is probably the most used formation. Being close together makes it easier to hear and sitting reduces shuffling and bumping. However, having the students assigned to *squads* has some advantages. With the students sitting in straight lines of about six per squad you can often utilize those divisions to quickly form teams or make station assignments (having an even number of students per squad is a good rule). Also, with squads you can have student leaders. Squad leaders can be given duties to help you in many ways. I believe in child labor. They can help with the distribution and collection of equipment, assignments, and exams. They might be given the charge of monitoring and recording their group's effort. Whatever the role you might see them fulfilling, it is probably a good idea to have a system where most everyone has the opportunity to qualify for this coveted leadership role.

OTHER MANAGEMENT TECHNIQUES

There is a variety of other management techniques which experienced instructors have found particularly useful in the physical education setting. The first technique is simply that of *teacher movement*. You may have been already taught the educational benefits of moving beyond the front of the classroom and circulating between the desks. Moving about the play area while games and practices are in progress will make a big difference in keeping all the children on task. Not only will it enable you to provide more direct verbal reinforcement but also it puts you in a position to provide personalized demonstrations and feedback. Timely physical guidance help can also be offered in the form of helping someone through the correct throwing action, spotting a gymnastic landing, or repositioning hands on an racket or club.

When you are engaged in teacher movement and drifting about the area, it is good to be near the perimeter most of the time. This better permits you to have general supervision of all the action. It also lends itself to your employing the *back-to-the-wall principle*. This principle states that when you wish to address the class you should position yourself at the perimeter of the group. Your back should not be to any of the students because they will not be able to hear you as well and they more likely may be off-task while out of your sight. This must sound like such an obvious technique but I find beginning teachers often do not think to do it and encounter poorer student responses as a consequence.

Another management technique is what I have coined the *When I say... Principle*. The idea here is to preface your instructions with "When I say go," "When I say begin," "When I say walk," etc. This procedure avoids the inevitable rushing of some children to begin an activity before you have finished your explanation. For example, suppose you wished the children to get a piece of equipment from a supply box and then, without swinging the implements, spread out in a personal space. If you began these directives by saying "Get a piece of equipment and then..." That likely is as far as you would get before at least some of the students would be drifting or hurrying to the supply box. With the ensuing movement and noise it would not be unusual for the remainder of your message to go largely unheard. This confusion and unwanted behavior could have been avoided if your instruction had begun with "When I say walk, we will get the equipment from the box and then..." The forethought of attaching this one small but significant preface might save you one small but significant headache.

Yet another technique for heading off potential or incipient management difficulties is the use of *proximity control*. As an example, you are beginning to instruct the class and you suspect that a given individual may not be the best of quiet listeners, or perhaps he/she is already talking out of turn. You exercise *proximity control* by happening to move in the direction of that student or danger zone. The intent of your getting closer to the student is to correct behavior without disrupting your instruction or having to say anything negative. Just by being closer to the student will hopefully be enough. My experiences have been that if the students are used to you floating about during the lesson it will not be apparent to them that you are engaged in exerting attention to a particular misbehavior. Of course, we are not saying that your looming presence alone will nullify every problem, but if you'll abide the pun, it is a good first preventive step in the right direction.

Music can also be used as a management tool. It can energize activities and make movement more fun. Simply having a collection of upbeat music ready for use can create a major difference. Many of the best physical education instructors I know use music as a matter of course, some even when outside. Often they have established it as a management cue; the children know that they are to be engaged in activity when the music is playing and to stop and listen when the music stops. If you do find yourself using music extensively, acquiring a remote control on-off devise might be worth the investment. Some good physical education specialists have even discovered the significant benefit of regularly using a microphone system. Not only does this make their instructions vastly more dominant and effective, it also saves on the stress of having to project in a loud voice.

Communication Styles

Finally, one other major point needs to be made regarding the establishment of a well-managed class. All of the above techniques will help you build a positive class environment, but the manner in which you regularly communicate with students is over-ridingly critical. If you do not establish yourself as a caring person, yet one who is unmistakably in charge, difficulties are likely. In the following subsections I have outlined three communication styles. The first two are all too common and lead to trouble. The third is that which we need to develop.

Passive Communication

A passive teacher hopes to make all children happy in order to avoid all conflict. Directly or indirectly, the passive teacher is constantly saying, "Like me. Appreciate what I do for you." Many passive teachers strive to behave perfectly themselves and in turn hope that their students will behave perfectly. When children behave like children and go off task, these teachers often let the behavior slide. This gives children permission to continue to misbehave, and they typically do so until the passive teacher "can't take it anymore." The teacher then loses his or her composure and lashes out at the class in anger. When the anger subsides, the passive teacher tries to make up for the outburst and again starts the cycle of letting things go and trying to be liked. This cycle is repeated throughout the school year.

Passive teachers typically exhibit other characteristic and unproductive behaviors.

* They often turn over power to students, particularly the least-cooperative students. For example, passive teachers might say, "We are not going to start the lesson until everyone is listening!" Students may hear, "We don't have to start the lesson until we finish our conversation."

*They ignore unacceptable behavior and hope it will disappear. Ignoring seldom causes behavior to disappear; rather, it becomes worse over time.

* They often say threatening things but fail to follow-through, saying, for example, "If you do that one more time, I am going to call your parents." When there is not follow-through or it is impossible to follow-through, the words are empty and meaningless and students soon learn disrespect for the teacher.

* They ask questions that elicit meaningless information, for example, "What did you do that for?" Or "Why are you doing this?" Or "Don't you know better than that?" None of these questions elicit useful information, and the teacher soon becomes frustrated and angry with all of the "I don't know" responses.

Aggressive Communication

Aggressive teachers come on strong in a desire to overpower students. To them, communication is a competition they must win at all costs. A common trait with aggressive communicators is their frequent use of the word *you* in statements, which keeps students feeling defensive and attacked. Examples are "you never listen to me," "you are always the one in trouble," "you are the problem here."

Aggressive communicators tend to view students' behavior as a personal attack. As a result, they may label the person rather than deal with the behavior. That's why aggressive communicators commonly use the words *always and never*. These are labeling words. They make students feel as if they are intrinsically bad people who cannot change their continually unacceptable behavior. This often causes students to become alienated from the teachers, from learning, and even from themselves.

Many aggressive teachers speak as if they are omniscient. For example, they may say to a student, "You think that because you got away with that last year, you can do it in my class." Obviously, no one knows what another person is thinking and to imply that one does undermines mutual respect and trust. On the other hand, aggressive communicators typically don't reveal how they feel about things, and they are unwilling to express their own thoughts and feelings. If students never know how a teacher feels, it is unlikely they will develop much empathy for their instructor. A guideline to keep in mind is this: Any statement about the student's feelings or thoughts, rather than your own, will give your communication an attacking and aggressive quality.

Assertive Communication

An assertive teacher does not beg, plead, or threaten. Rather, he or she expresses feelings and expectations in a straightforward manner. Assertive people are not afraid to say what they want and do not worry about what others will think of them. Teachers who want to be liked are quite concerned about what their students think. An assertive teacher wants what is best for students and doesn't worry about what they think. Assertiveness comes across to students as a "no-nonsense" approach that is clear, direct, and very specific (requiring little interpretation to be carried out). For example, an assertive teacher might say to a student who has been talking out of turn, "It upsets me when you talk while I am talking." This teacher is expressing feelings and identifying the unacceptable behavior. The teacher would then continue with an assertive statement that expresses the acceptable behavior, for example, "That is your second warning; please go to time-out."

An excellent way to make messages more assertive is to use the word *I* instead of *you*. Talking about your own feelings and emotions will make the messages sound much more reasonable and firm. For example, say, "When you are playing with your equipment while I am talking, it bothers me and makes me forget what I planned on saying. Please put your equipment down while I talk." Assertive messages identify the behavior that is disruptive or annoying, state how you feel, and direct the student to behave in a proper manner.

MANAGEMENT GAMES

Management games can be used in many ways to facilitate adherence to class rules. Among other things, these games can make it fun for the students to quickly follow your commands to begin an activity, stop an activity, find a partner, and form a circle or other formation. They can help you rapidly pick teams or gain the students' undivided attention when they are off-task. Below I have listed some such games that have been effectively used by other teachers and myself.

Back to Back: The teacher has the children locomotoring around an area and when the "back to back" command is given, everyone finds someone with which to get back to back. Everyone should pair with the nearest free person (it is not being a "friendly" person if you avoid anyone). Those who cannot find someone are told to go to the center where the "lost and found" area is located. To solve the problem of someone being left out, I sometimes join in the action when there are an odd number of students. This game can be varied in many ways. Different body parts can be called out: toe-to-toe, biceps to biceps, elbow to back, knee to knee to knee (three people).

Numbers can be shouted out with the understanding that groups of that size are to be formed. How about integrating math problems: 5 minus 3 or 12 divided by 4.

Silent Shapes: The teacher calls different shapes and groups of students attempt to position themselves in that formation as quickly as possible: the number 7, the letter S, a square, a circle, a trapezoid. The task is easier for smaller numbers of students but eventually it is hoped that the entire class could be able to correctly arrange themselves. You can see how their being able to do this would be a usable management tool for you. You want to play a circle game and they can quickly form it. You call out the number 11 and they are there ready for a two-sided game. The game is called Silent Shapes because they are not allowed to say anything as they make the shapes. For fun and increased activity, I usually have them perform the version called *Moving Silent Shapes;* this is where I specify that a movement such as jogging or skipping must be maintained throughout.

Shipwreck: The teacher is the captain of the ship and the children are the sailors. The sailors must ensure a taut ship by carrying out all commands with alacrity. Orders of "bow," "aft," "port," and "starboard" sends the sailors scurrying to those sides of the ship. "Sharks" has them rush to the center to cover their heads. "Leaky ship" has everyone madly pumping out the water with push-ups. A partner activity is called to "abandon ship"; here two people sit facing each other, with their feet touching, do a rowing exercise. All right, you can take it from here. The idea is to instill the habit of responding to the teacher and making it fun. I have heard of this same game played with a variety of interesting themes and activities: Christmas, Halloween, Star Wars, Cowboy & Cowgirls, Travel time.

Popcorn: The teacher calls popcorn and everyone must start jumping up and around as if they were popcorn being popped. On the "sticky popcorn" command each is to pop over to somebody, stick shoulder to shoulder and keep popping. This is of course a quick way to form partners for a subsequent partner activity. If you wished groups of 4 or 8, "stickier popcorn" and "super sticky popcorn" should produce the popcorn ball sizes you desire. Sometimes it is fun to have them all stuck together and then have everyone melt into a gooey mess.

Code Words: All that is involved here is having designated code words for various desired formations. For instance, I have used the code word theme of "Fruits and Vegetables." Whenever I said "bananas" the students were to go bananas and spread out so each had some personal activity space. When I said "potatoes" they knew to sit down. "Celery" meant stand-up. "Kumquats" meant pairs and "grapes" directed everyone to come and sit in a clump in front of me. You might find that a list has a tendency to grow. I once began to make a remark about a "potato" which was lying down as I was talking. His clever riposte was that he was a "mashed potato." Immediately a popular new word was added to our class lexicon.

Attention Getters: The above games were primarily designed to produce fast responding to the teacher's commands. Occasions sometimes arise then the students' attention is elsewhere and they may not be mentally set or focused on you. It is at these times that a clearly recognizable attention getter is an asset. Of course, a shouted "Stop!" or whistle blast may serve this purpose but there are other more effective fun ideas. A good procedure is to give some well-known distinctive signal to which the students have a set response. I knew one teacher who would forcefully say, "Are you ready!" and this cued the students to give an arm pump and shout "You bet!" Even if a given student did not catch the teacher's signal the shouted response of the other students would be distinctly heard and understood as a cue to pay attention. Another teacher used a unique hand clapping pattern (slow, slow, quick, quick, quick) which the students could not help but notice and to which they would have to respond which a practiced unison clap. How about this one for generating a fun student response? Whenever the teacher said, "Where am I?" the students rapidly recited the following poem while simultaneously touching the corresponding body parts, "Here I am! Head, shoulders, knees and toes, ankles, thighs, heart and nose!" Can you not see how this practice would have the effect of drawing everyone into the chant and away from what they were doing? At its completion all eyes and minds will be on you.

 101 Ways to Pick Teams: A common physical education situation is the lining-up of the children and the picking teams. I am sure we all remember that. Quite likely you may have counted off by 2s or 4s. Or maybe captains were designated and they in turn selected who would play for them. Both these time worn methods have shortcomings. Neither is very rapid. Counting off is oftentimes confusing to the younger students and sometimes there is even some shuffling of positions in the hopes of being counted on the same team as a best friend. As for selection by captains, I call this the slave market approach. I have heard many adults say that the thing they recalled and hated most about physical education was the sinking feeling of being picked last. Even Ann Landers has received many testimonials of this kind.

 Here are some concepts that should provide you with 101 or more ways of almost instantaneously breaking your group into the number of teams you want. (1) Simple body gestures or positions could be used; "Clasp your hands together. Okay, everyone who has his/her right thumb on top step forward." Or "Cross your legs. Okay, those with their left leg in front take three giant steps forwards." Or "Inspect your finger nails. Those whose palms are turned upward move over here." (2) Specifying different actions or shapes will work; "Swimmers think about doing either the back crawl or front crawl. When I say swim, do four strokes. Okay, ready swim." Or "Think of making either an X shape with your body, like this, or an O shape like this. When I say shapes, go. Ready, shapes." (3) Favorite things can work. "Think which you like best, crunchy or smooth peanut butter. Okay, smoothies over here." Which movies, books, sports, colors, etc. (4) The names of the students can be used. "Anyone whose first name begins with A through L..." "All whose first name has four letters or less..." (5) Birthdays are known by even the youngest. Winter people with birthdays in December, January, and February, form a snow drift on this line..."

By now you must have the idea how you can get to 101 or beyond. When your initial division tactic does not yield equal divisions don't panic, it's easy to move a few students from one team to another. A quick survey of clothing is one sure way to do it. Those in this group wearing shorts, hats, red, belts, rings...

CORRECTING MISBEHAVIOR

By far it is best to head off behavioral problems before they happen. Successfully doing so is the lion's share of the battle. Throughout this chapter, and scattered elsewhere throughout this book, I have offered ideas that should serve this purpose. Nevertheless you know that problems will arise. Handling these problems is the number one concern of beginning teachers. I do not have all the answers for what you may face but can describe a few procedures that have been useful to other teachers and myself.

In your education courses you undoubtedly have or will be introduced to a number of the most current recommended approaches. Whichever procedure you adopt for classroom management should be carried over into the gymnasium and playing-field setting; consistency has the advantage of producing clearer expectations for both teachers and students. To my mind, it is ideal if the entire school has a coordinated assertive discipline plan. If your school has such a plan, I suggest you give your full effort to supporting and working with others to make it the best it can be.

When misbehavior first occurs I would prefer to deal with it positively, without any element of punishment. One such procedure is the *reprimand*. If done in a caring and constructive manner, reprimands serve as effective reminders to behave acceptably.

* Identify the unacceptable behavior, state briefly why it is unacceptable, and then explain what would be desired or acceptable behavior. For example, say, "You were talking while I was speaking, which bothers other students and me. That is unacceptable behavior. I expect you to be respectful and listen quietly when someone else is speaking."
* Avoid labeling. Ask the person to stop the misbehavior and do not comment on the person. For example, avoid telling a student "You are always causing problems in this class."
* Don't reprimand in front of other students. Not only does it embarrass students, it also can diminish their self-esteem. When students feel belittled, they may lash out in a manner more severe than the original misbehavior.
* Reprimand softly. Studies show that soft reprimands are more effective than loud ones.
* After reprimanding and asking for acceptable behavior, reinforce it when it occurs. Be vigilant in looking for the acceptable behavior because reinforcing such behavior will cause it to occur more often in the future.

Another positive discipline approach is *Positive Overcorrection*. If a reprimand has been delivered and a mis-behavior reoccurs, the student is asked to *do-over* the incorrect behavior in the appropriate manner. For example, if a student ran into the gym and slid across the floor, he or she would be required to go back to the gym entrance, walk into the gym, and take his or her assigned place quietly, and maybe have to do it more than once if you thought further reinforcement and practice might be needed. The same could be done for the entire class if they entered in an unruly manner.

Beyond the use of *Positive Overcorrection* is what is known a *Restitutional Overcorrection*. In *Restitutional Overcorrection*, students are required to restore the environment that they have disrupted with their unacceptable behavior. For example, if any students left their recess equipment strewn in a disorderly mess about the playground, they would be required not only to pick up the equipment that they were using, but also to clean the rest of the playground and/or equipment area. Or if a student defaced a wall in the gym with magic markers, he or she would be required to clean that wall as well as all the other walls in the gym. The idea behind this procedure is that the student will learn not to engage in inappropriate behavior by experiencing the inconvenience of restoring the environment.

What if *overcorrection* does not work and some type of further discipline or punishment procedure is required? Two approaches are worth consideration. One is that of *Removal of Positive Consequences* and the other is a *Six-Step Discipline Plan* that incorporates the *Time-Out Concept*. Elementary children usually are eager to participate in movement activities and a warning or short denial will serve as a strong incentive. Even if removal from certain physical activities might not be adverse to a particular child, very likely there are other greatly valued activities that will be. In such a case, the disruptive child needs to know that some of the time-out can be carried over into a more attractive, future activity.

Removal of Positive Consequences

Removing positive consequences is an approach commonly used by parents, so many students are familiar with it. The approach is to remove something positive from the student when misbehavior occurs. For example, students give up some of their free time, lose points toward a desired goal, or are not allowed to participate in an activity that is exiting to them. For removal of positive consequences to be effective, students must value the removal activity. A few key principles should be followed when using this technique.

* Be sure that the magnitude of the removal fits the crime. In other words, children who commit minor infractions shouldn't have to miss recess for a week.

* Be consistent in removal, treating all students and occurrences the same. Teachers are behaving unfairly if they are more severe with one student than another for the same misbehavior. In addition, a student penalized for a specific misbehavior should receive the same penalty for a later repetition.

* Make sure students understand the consequences of misbehavior *before* the penalties are implemented. If students know what the consequences will be, they are making the choice to accept the consequences when they choose to misbehave.

* It is helpful to chart a student's misbehavior to see if the frequency is decreasing. Regardless of the method used, if the behavior is not decreasing or is increasing, change methods until a decrease in frequency occurs.

Six-Step Discipline Plan

Of all times when clear communication is required, during discipline is the most critical. In clear and certain terms, the student must understand what they did wrong, what the consequences are, and that repeating the behavior is not acceptable. The intent of this discipline plan is to be firm but humane. Discipline should be delivered in an unemotional, but caring manner. Having a well thought out and rehearsed discipline plan will aid teachers in avoiding making rash judgments. A sound discipline plan provides calm and maintains the dignity of the teacher and the student alike in a difficult situation.

Step 1. Introduction of Class Rules & Consequences: The students first are introduced, both verbally and visually, to the class rules/expectations, consequences, and time-out procedures. Student understanding and acceptance is important.

Step 2. Proximity Control: As we learned earlier, students rarely act up when the teacher is near. Wise teachers use their presence to prevent or put an end to misbehavior by moving close to the problem. Never yell across a room at a kid. If a behavior persists even after step one, move toward the problem while continuing to give instructions. Remember that since you always move in a random pattern and teach from all locations, this will not seem a big deal. Most kids will not even know that you are moving for any other reason. Often the student who is the object of this movement does not even realize it until you are standing right next to him or her. Of course, as you get close, the student usually stops the misbehavior in the hope that you will not notice it. Finish your instructions and start the class on the next activity.

Step 3. Quiet Verbal Warning: If the behavior does not stop, despite you standing next to the student, a quiet verbal warning is warranted. Get the rest of the students engaged in the next activity. Since you are already standing next to the offending student, you simply issue the warning, "Sally, you were talking while I was talking. Your voice needs to be off. This is your warning; next time I will ask you to go to time-out." Do not debate. Identify the inappropriate behavior, state your expectation, remind the student of the consequences to follow, and *walk away*.

Step 4. First Time-Out: After giving a warning, sending a student to time-out or dealing with a negative situation, find other students whose behaviors are exemplary and give them some positive reinforcement. This helps dispel the cloud of negativity from having to deal with the misbehaving student.

If you need to send someone to time-out, here is how to do it. Recall that the student has already received a warning. Change your proximity to be near the student. Engage the rest of the class in activity. State your case and inform the student that the consequence is to go to time-out. For example: "Sally, this is the second time I have had to talk to you today. Please go to time-out." Do not debate. Then, and we cannot stress this enough, walk away. At this point many teachers want to stare them down, take them to the time-out area, or in some other way force them to comply. This is a mistake. A wise teacher will walk away. Reengage the class and give some positive reinforcement to other students, but remain subtly aware of the misbehaving student. The student has a decision to make. Most often, the student makes the right one and goes to time-out. The first time-out offers a chance to self-evaluate, correct the behavior, and return to participation when the student is ready to behave appropriately.

A common practice is to place time-out stations in each of the four corners of the instructional area. Time-out means time out from reinforcement; that is, it does not serve as a deterrent if the youngster is reinforced when placed in time-out. The physical location for time-out should provide *as little* reinforcement as possible. For example, imagine that a student who is not participating properly is told to sit in the hallway for time-out. Friends pass by, and they converse. Now the student not only gets to avoid participation, but gets to visit with friends. Note that being a spectator at an athletic event is an enjoyable experience for which many people pay money. Sitting on the side of the teaching area and looking on as a spectator may be more reinforcing for a student than participating in class activities. Therefore, if you put someone in time-out, make sure he or she is not facing the class and interacting with peers. Instead, position him or her facing away from the class, perhaps in front of a list of levels of responsibility or rules and consequence.

Step 5. Second Time-Out: Please keep in mind that if your class is managed well and you have consistently followed the discipline plan, the need for steps five and six will be minimal. Use the same procedure to send them to time-out a second time by saying, "Sally, this is the third time I have had to talk to you today, please go to time-out for the remainder of class or until I invite you to return. Come see me after class." The difference now is that the chance for self-management has passed and the student must remain there until invited to return. The next element is critical: the student must return and talk with you before reentering the activity or leaving the class. Do not debate. Validate the child. Let the child know that, even though he or she has not behaved well today, you know that tomorrow is another day and you are sure that better behavior will follow. Tell them you respect them, love having them in class, and enjoy getting to know them. At this point, the consequence is brought to a conclusion, and nothing is left hanging over the student's head. The child can take away no ill feeling because of what you have just said.

A suggested length of time for the time-out is about 5 minutes, although the average length used by educators has been tracked to be 12 minutes. Some pedagogues recommend that the periods should be shorter for the younger students and longer for the older.

Step 6. Student-Teacher Conference: If step five is rare, step six almost never occurs. After repeated attempts have been made to improve behavior through use of the plan, a teacher may hold a student-teacher conference. In this conference the teacher may opt to do any of the following: (1) call a parent for a parent-teacher conference, (2) inform the principal, (3) send the student to in-school suspension or have the student removed entirely from the class.

Exercise as Punishment

For as long as I can remember, physical education authorities have been admonishing against using exercise as punishment. The reasoning is an easily understandable one that goes like this, "If we want children to learn to value and enjoy exercise we cannot associate it with something that is disliked and to be avoided." I know many people who have said that they want no more of running, push-ups, or doing other similar exercises because they remember being punished with them years ago in school or the military. But in spite of the logic of not using exercise to punish, and in spite of educators delivering this message over the years, many teachers and coaches still rely on it to one degree or another. They probably do so because it has become a tradition modeled by many in the field, because it is easy to use, because it will generally produce some quick-term results in curbing undesirable actions, and because the instructor has not developed a clear set of time-out or other alternative procedures. I can only add my voice to the chorus of authorities who advocate other punishment avenues. If we keep our ultimate goal of developing enjoyment of activities and exercise in mind, we simple must find other ways. I knew a coach once who had his players so convinced of the importance of hard work and training that he was able to effectively punish individuals by not permitting them to participate in some of the conditioning drills. They had to sit and watch and miss out as the rest of the team improved themselves by determinedly running stairs and the like. While achievement of such an ethos may not be realistic in your teaching environment, it does epitomize the kind of attitude for which each of us should be striving.

It is also worth noting that those who employ exercise as a punishment tool are putting themselves, their school, and the district at legal risk. Doing so is a violation of corporal punishment laws. And if a child should happen suffer an injury, physical or psychological, that teacher will be defenseless against any charges that might be filed. Also remember that it is a well-established fact that children who are physically punished by parents or teachers are more likely to act abusively toward others.

Group Punishment

Much that has been said about exercise as punishment can also be said about whole class punishment practices; both have long been discouraged by those in higher education but they continue to be frequently used by practitioners. Those using group punishment feel that is a potent tool because it results in classmates putting pressure on the truant children to conform to class rules. Counter-argument would be that although it can sometimes be effective, at other times the offending student or students will rebel and lash out at their not always so diplomatic, criticizing peers. My feeling is that creating such a situation is hardly conducive to the establishment of a friendly class milieu where we wish children to learn to help and positively encourage one another. Here again, use of it is probably indicative of a failure to develop and apply a sounder technique along the line of the fore-mentioned time-out procedures.

CHAPTER COMPREHENSION CHECK

Why are good management techniques especially important when teaching activities?
What should be the primary goal for the first-day class lessons?
Approximately how many class rules are suggested and should they be extremely specific or more conceptual in nature?
Should class rules be shared with others besides the students? Why?
What is *slippage* and what is the best way to deal with it?
What is the concept of *instant activity* and why might it be useful?
What are a couple uses *squads* could fulfill? What would make for a good size?
What is the concept of *teacher movement* and why might it be effective?
What is the *back-to-the-wall principle*? Why is it useful?
How is the *When I say... Principle* used and why?
What is the concept *of proximity control* and how might it be effective?
Why might the investment in a good sound system serve a helpful management role?
How is the *Back-to-Back* game played?
How the concept of using *Code Words* operate and why might it be useful?
How do *Attention Getters* operate?
What did the author have to say about the practice of having captains pick-up teams or having the student count-off by 2s, 3s, or 4s? Why?
What are the three *communication styles*? What are the characteristics or implications of each?
What is a *reprimand* and how can it most effectively be delivered?

How does *Positive Overcorrection* work? *Restitutional Overcorrection?*
What is meant by *removal of positive consequences* and how might it be implemented?
What are the six steps of the *Six-Step Discipline Plan?* What are the particulars of each step?
When requiring a child to *time-out,* what is a recommended length of time?
Where might *time-out* locations be placed and how might reinforcement be controlled for?
What are the author's and the legal profession's views on using exercise as a punishment?
What are the author's views on the effectiveness of punishing the entire class when one or a few of the students misbehave?

[CHAPTER 8]

TECHNIQUES FOR TEACHING MOVEMENT SKILLS

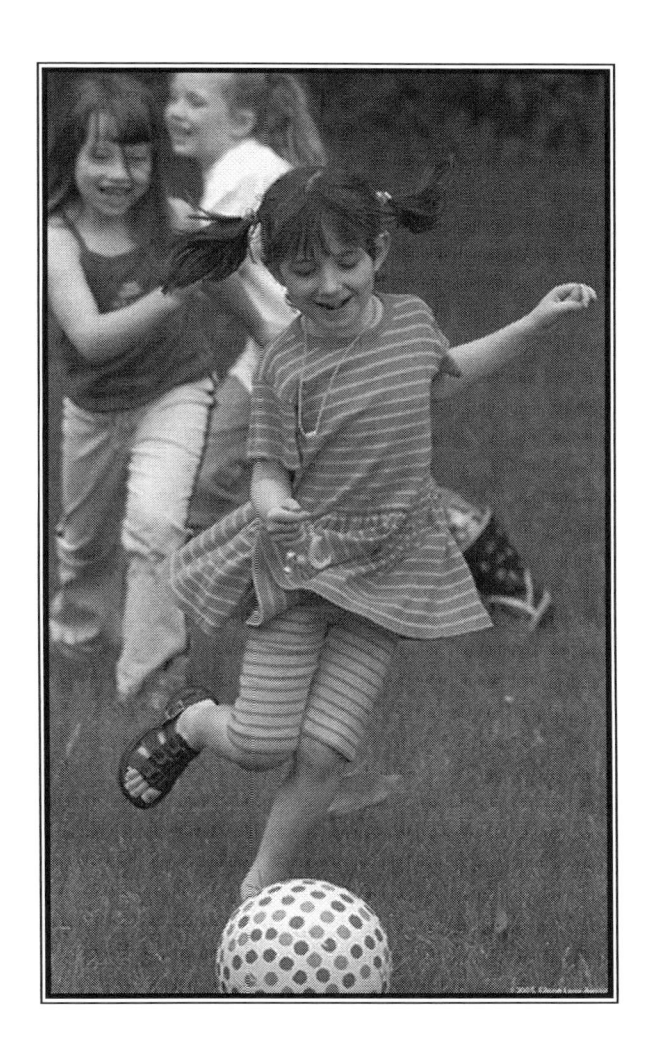

INTRODUCTORY INSTRUCTIONS & DEMONSTRATIONS

PRACTICE

FEEDBACK

REVIEW

CHAPTER COMPREHENSION CHECK

> *Improvement depends far less upon length of tasks and hours of application than is supposed. Children can take in but a little each day; they are like vases with a narrow neck; you may pour little or pour much, but much will not enter at a time.*
> ~ Jules Michelet

> *If, in instructing a child, you are vexed with it for want of adroitness, try, if you have never tried before, to write with you left hand and then remember that a child is all left hand.*
> ~ J.F. Boyse

I strongly believe that education is a most worthy profession and, as I have stated before, I believe most anyone can become a good teacher if he/she really, really works at it. Regardless of your personality and background, if you have the desire, and persevere at developing effective teaching procedures, you will be able to make it happen. In this Chapter you will be introduced to some teaching skills that master teachers regularly demonstrate. If you practice these techniques you will see things falling into place, violate them and potential problems will be likely. The procedures offered specifically pertain to teaching movement skills but you will see that many of the concepts are generic to teaching regardless of subject.

A theme stressed throughout this book is that we need get children regularly moving and ensure that it is an enjoyable experience. Having the attitude that a person likes to be active is even more important than how athletically skilled he or she is. I have a number of adult friends who are not particularly skillful and yet they still regularly enjoy physical activities and exercise. Conversely, I know former athletes who now are quite sedentary. Nevertheless, data shows that people who acquired good movement skills when young tend to remain more active than do those of low abilities. The purpose of this chapter will be to introduce you to some teaching techniques that will help children learn movement skills safely and successfully.

ARE GREAT TEACHERS BORN OR MADE?

Are great teachers born or made? It may seem strange to still be wrestling with this question after centuries of debate. As teacher education research continues to increase our understanding of the teaching process, it seems more and more clear that good teaching (including those vaunted intangibles) can be broken down to a discreet set of skills and abilities that are quantifiable ,(b) transferable, and (c) masterable.

To think differently calls into question the existence of teacher education programs. If teachers are simply born to teach, why then do we have teacher education programs? Would we not be as well served to line up 1,000 hopeful teachers and watch them teach? Those who were able to demonstrate that they were indeed born with the gift would be given jobs, and the rest would be encouraged to look elsewhere. Instead, new teachers can learn by watching, practicing, and eventually mastering the skills, styles, personality traits, and other factors that constitute a great teaching persona. To make this happen, we must examine excellence in teaching and find out what the best teachers are doing and why it works. Then the teachers should be taught to incorporate the knowledge, skills, and dispositions into their own teaching personas.

This position validates the notion that most people who strive to be better teachers can succeed if they put forth the effort. This means practicing, much as you would practice a sport skill. If you are not the most positive person, watch those who are, then practice. If you do not smile much, practice. If you are not good at telling stories, practice. If you are not good at disciplining kids in a way that shapes desirable behaviors in a kind but firm way, practice. If you are wasting time with sloppy transitions, practice. If you are not good at modeling, practice. If you are not good at giving clear and concise instructions, practice. It will take years to become a master teacher. But we are, after all, in the learning business.

INTRODUCTORY INSTRUCTIONS & DEMONSTRATIONS

To better insure that students will be attentive to your instruction and demonstration you should consider the following preliminaries. Firstly, if at all possible, have the students seated. They are often naturally fidgety and it will be unlikely that unseated children will refrain from shuffling feet and bumping others. Secondly, if they have been given any implements such as balls, bats, paddles, rackets, hoops, or jump ropes, get those things out of their hands. A good procedure is to always establish a *Home Position* at the very beginning. For instance, the children know that on the "stop" or "home position" command, they are to place the ball at their feet, stand inside the hoop, stand on the jump rope, etc. Without *Home Positions* there will be some inevitable juggling and swinging of things. It is so much better to have a positive environment and thank everyone for remembering the correct *Home Position* rather than having to nag them about being still. Thirdly, attempt to have the students facing away from the sun and distracters. Of course, looking into the sun will make it harder to see your demonstration. Distractions are common in the gym and on the playground and children are particularly susceptible to them. Finally, before beginning to give instruction regarding the skill, it is often good to remind yourself of establishing an *Anticipatory Set*. This means setting the stage for the skill you will be teaching. Make the skill sound interesting by being enthusiastic. Explain why this skill will be fun to learn and the possibilities to which it may lead. If it is a sports skill, present a reason why possession of this skill is prerequisite to successful enjoyment of the game.

Most knowledge could be taught in an environment that is much more conducive to learning than a gymnasium or playing field. Classrooms are more suitable for engaging in cognitive learning. They are more comfortable, provide fewer distractions, have more instructional aids, and expectations for student knowledge gains are already present. Any instruction done in the gym and playing field is advisedly kept short. I have what I call The Two-Minute Warning. If my talk is much longer than two-minutes I am likely covering more than what will be retained in long-term memory. A useful procedure is to stress one Learnable Piece. This means that with each instructional bout you are focusing on one observable objective that everyone should be able to accomplish or review. For example, suppose you wished to help the children with their overhand throwing. Decide what might be one important aspect of the throw you would like all to have. Maybe "stepping forwards with the opposite foot to your throwing hand" or "following through across your body" would be the Learnable Piece. These would be good because they are do-able and worthy of practice by all, and they are specific things both the students and you should be able to monitor. The point is that you should not attempt to accomplish indeterminable, grandiose things in one day; "Today we are going to learn to become good volleyball players" or "We will get good at jumping rope." These things will not be accomplished in many periods let alone one period, and you and the students may not be clear on what denotes good serves and rope jumping, and what specific actions are required. A better developmental, less frustrating, approach is to learn one thing at a time and then to build off of that in future lessons. This gradual adding to a previous day's learning is called Scaffolding. One day we have an objective of leading with the opposite foot and the next day, if they seem to have mastered that aspect, we add the next objective/learnable piece of the cross-the-body follow-through.

    Demonstrations are the best way to convey movement skills. They, like pictures, are indeed worth a thousand words. The most essential thing about a demonstration is that it shows the skill correctly performed. If you can do the skill reasonably well that is great. You should not feel that it must be done with great power and precision, as long as it is done with fundamentally correct form. If you cannot do the skill correctly there likely will be a student in class who can. If none of your students can, it may be worth the effort to see if you can recruit the services of someone from outside of the class. Even if you can do the skill it is not a bad idea to supplement your demonstrations with student demonstrations. When the students see others of their age and gender successfully performing, it can effectively convince them that they too might be capable. Remember that good demonstrations do more than provide information of how the skill is executed, they serve to convince that mastery may be within their means. This believing that you are capable of accomplishing a specific task is called self-efficacy and having it is an extremely important determinant in attempting, persevering, and mastering skills. I would like to make one more point about your modeling of motor skill; don't feel inadequate if you cannot demonstrate some skills. Admit to the students that you have not yet learned to perform a skill and make it an opportunity to convey the message that physical skills require lengthy practice and no one can be expected to master them all. Remember the point we made in Chapter 6 regarding *The Ten-Year Rule* and the huge amount of practice that sometimes is required.

Even the best of demonstrations may not result in a full conveyance of desired information. There is much going on during a demonstration so it is not to be unexpected that important aspects of the movement might go undetected. The student may have been watching the feet, the arms, the face, the implement, or simply might not have been vigilant and paying attention at all. There are a number of procedures that could help. Firstly, make sure you have cued the key elements; "Watch the feet, notice how I step with the foot opposite the throwing arm." Concepts need to be given labels if they are to be stored in memory. Experienced teachers have learned this and often use catchy, vivid cues to abet the retention process (see Figure 8.1 for some examples). Secondly, demonstrations should be performed a number of times at both full and slow speed. Doing the skill at full-speed should serve to represent the actual patterning and timing. Surprisingly it is common for instructors to not repeat or even give a full-speed execution. Adding a slower-motion performance is obviously good in that it sometimes can make it easier to see. Thirdly, changing your position, or that of the onlookers, so that the skill will be viewed from more than one perspective, might yield a clearer image. Finally, if the skill has a rather dramatic outcome like achieving a target or distance goal, be aware that the children will be easily distracted and may attend to the goodness of the outcome instead of focusing upon relevant parts of the technique. When this is the case, a good policy might be to first perform the skill and allow the students to initially view the outcome of the movement. It can be motivating to see how far the ball can be kicked or how accurately it can be shot. But then, to better insure attention on the movement objective, remove the target by shooting or kicking against a wall or without a target; or even doing the skill without the implement such as pretending you are kicking a footbag or serving a ball.

One last point should be made regarding demonstrations. The influences that our in-class demonstrations have are all pretty minor in comparison to what we demonstrate at other times throughout the school day and beyond. When the children see us shooting hoops in our free time it conveys a doubly effectual message. We are showing that this activity is something we truly value and voluntarily choose to do. Is it not surprising that this might spur greater approach behavior in the students? And on the other hand, if we never participate in some of the other activities, even though we promote them in our lesson plans, is it not conceivable that this lack of modeling might reduce or undermine our message. Children learn a lot more from us than what we introduce in plan lessons. This is known as *Incidental Learning* and it is well that we keep it in mind. If we wish children to try different activities beyond class, we are wise to demonstrate beyond class.

Figure 8.1. Vivid Cues for Learnable Pieces

Learnable Pieces	Vivid Cues
When running, have the elbows bent and the arms swinging forwards and backwards in opposition to the legs.	"pumping steam engines"
When dribbling a basketball, let your fingers give with the ball, don't slap it.	"pet the kitty"
When catching a ball, eyes on the ball, arms extended in preparation, and elbows bending to absorb force.	"look, reach, give"
When fielding a ground ball, get in front of the ball and use both hands.	"make a tunnel"
During aerobic exercise, keep the feet constantly moving.	"happy feet" "ten toes clubs"
When swinging, follow-through high.	"air the armpit"
When doing a backward roll, stay tightly Tucked.	"knees near nose"

PRACTICE

It is best for skill practice to begin as soon after the explanation-demonstration as possible. You want the explanation, image and verbal cueing fresh in their minds. As soon as practice commences you should always alert yourself with the *SOS question*. This means that you judge the appropriateness of the practice by asking three things in this order: Is everyone Safe? Is everyone On-task and active? Is everyone being Successfully challenged?

Of course, safety needs to be the first concern of any movement experience. Look to see if the children are adequately spaced from each other and from dangerous obstacles such as poles and walls. Make sure they are not performing on a hard abrasive surface if they are at high risk of falling down. Are they adequately under control and watching out for others? If you can foresee a real potential for accidents it is your duty to immediately stop the action or make alterations. Just use your good judgment. The law expects you to be *reasonably prudent*.

Is everyone On-task and active? For practice to be effective it is imperative that all the children get to execute the skill many times. Of all the variables that effect the

Techniques for Teaching Movement Skills

learning of motor skills, by far the most powerful determinate is simply how many times the skill has been attempted. Minimal skill development will result if only a few children are performing and the rest are standing in lines waiting turns. In the past, when the students of physical education teachers have been observed it has not been unusual to find that they are only active 10 to 30 percent of the time or even less. We should be able to do much better than this. A good rule of thumb is to strive to have children actively engaged in movement for at least a *Fifty-Percent Minimum Activity Standard*. Meeting or exceeding this standard is easier when teaching some activities as opposed to others. It should not be difficult to keep everyone performing at near 100 percent when teaching aerobic activities and circuit training. Instruction in gymnastics and softball skills present more of a challenge, but still can be done with good planning.

Having enough equipment for everyone, or at least for every two or three students, is critical for high participation rates in many activities. What would you do in your classroom if you had only a few textbooks, computers, microscopes, paint brushes, etc.? Would you form lines and expect students to fold their arms and serenely wait their turn to read the book or use the equipment? Obviously that would not be educationally sound. You would either go to lengths to get more equipment or you would design your instructional approach so that students would have other stations at which to work until the needed equipment was not in use by classmates. Having and acquiring balls, racquets, jump ropes, hula-hoops, beanbags, beach balls, balloons, for all or half of the students may prove to be a difficult task. Sixty-one percent of physical education teachers report having an annual budget of under $1,000, and of course, classroom teachers will probably not be given movies for this kind of purchasing. However, where there is a will there are indeed ways. An *equipment rule-of-thumb* set by some advocates is to strive for having at least one piece of equipment for every three students. Most schools have sports teams whose equipment could be made available; many children might be able to bring their own items from home; the physical education specialist might have available equipment or avenues of procuring some; many outside organizations would be glad to make a small contribution to this sort of worthy cause. I have known classroom teachers who, through various means, were even able to gather a significant number of more expensive items such as roller-blades, unicycles, bicycles, and tumbling mats. Another point relative to equipment is that it does not always have to be officially correct to be a serviceable learning aid. Different kinds of playground balls might do as substitutes for soccer or basketballs. I have had students make their own beanbags and jump ropes. I once used crunched-up milk cartons for a soccer dribbling lesson and it turned-out great; they were easier to dribble around cones and pass short distances.

If you cannot procure sufficient equipment or space to permit a high rate of practice of the skill, plan other activity stations to reduce downtime. Many teachers have learned that *Circuit Training* is a time efficient teaching method; while some students are learning the new skill others are simultaneously reviewing and practicing other skills at one or numerous locations around the gym or play space. The workstations can be spread out to reduce congested safety concerns and yet you can still have general supervision of everyone. Posting instructions and teaching the students to independently read and carryout the activities can be a good educational process. Figure 8.2 offers an example of instructions for an individual and partner circuit. Notice how different levels can be listed to accommodate differences in ability. Music can be effectively used both as a pacing and motivational tool. When the music begins the students know that they are to be active. When the music stops it is a cue to stop and to move to the next station. The use of music tends to energize and make the activities more fun. I have many CD with breaks placed in the music at 30 second, 45 second, 1 minute, and 2-minute intervals. This saves me from having to watch clocks and blow whistles. I know other physical education specialists with remote control devices for turning the music on and off.

Figure 8.2 Circuit Training & the Long-Slanty Rope

Individual Soccer Circuit	*Partner Circuit*
Sole Trap	Throw-in & Trap
level A. toss ball off wall, allow 2 bounces then trap	level A. short distance line
level B. toss ball off wall, allow 2 bounce then trap	level B. middle distance line
level C. toss ball off wall, trap before it bounces	level C. long distance line
Head	Passing
level A. toss ball above head, and head it	level A. 10 passes
level B. toss ball above head, and head it twice in a row	level B. 15 passes
level C. toss ball above head, and head it repeatedly	level C. 20 passes
Shoot at goal	Dribbling through cones
level A. score goals as you can from the short line	level A. 5 circuits
level B. score goals as you can from the middle line	level B. 10 circuits
level C. score goals as you can from the long line	level C. 15 circuits

Dribble around cones	Corner kicks & goalie catches
level A. strive for 10	level A. 10 ft. line
level B. strive for 15	level B. 20 ft. line
level C. strive for 20	level C. 30 ft. line

The third letter of the *SOS* mnemonic stood for Successful. Is everyone being Successfully challenged? It is not good to have a situation in which the children are experiencing repeated failure. Nor is it good if the skills are too easy and therefore fail to challenge. As a general rule it is best to have a *Learnable Piece* at which everyone initially has something in the realm of a *80% Success Rate*. Because your students will have different experiences, abilities, disabilities and maturational levels, some individualization of instruction will be necessary to achieve this level of success for everyone. To achieve individualization of practice, remember the principle of the *Long Slanty-Rope*. Here is what it is. Imagine you had one end of a long rope held on the ground and the other end pulled taut and raised to a height of three feet. The children's task is to practice their leaping skills. As they are practicing they can choose to jump over the rope at the section suited to their abilities and confidence. Because the rope is an extra long one, all the students can practice at the same time with little interference to each other. Of course, the idea of the *Long Slanty-Rope Principle* is to see if you can organize all your practices, regardless of the type of skill, along the same conceptual lines. There are a couple of avenues for doing so. One way is to modify the equipment for the students. If in a batting practice drill, the students are not successfully hitting pitched balls, a switch to t-ball might be appropriate. If some were still experiencing difficulty, the conceptual rope could be slanted by assigning or allowing the students to select from jumbo or fat bats and larger balls. If the children are having difficulty with badminton striking activities, short-handled, large-faced racket variations might serve. If their volleyball skills are not ready for official volleyballs, what about balloons, beach balls, and lightweight vinyl balls.

Another means of individualization is to set different task criteria. There are many ways of doing this. Setting different target criteria: shooting at different size targets from different distances. Different time criteria can be set: when a teacher tells the students to attempt as many push-ups or skier-jumps as possible in a minute, he/she is using time in a slanted rope manner because the students are being encouraged to set the task difficulty suitable to their abilities. Different technique criteria can also be presented: doing the dribble with the opposite hand, doing the skill switching from forehand to backhand, doing the skill with the eyes up and with toes pointed, doing push-ups either from the knees or toes. Notice that the Figure 8.2 *Circuit Training* example employed a number of the above means of creating different challenges.

Before leaving the issue of having the children practice skills I would like to make the point about the kind of movement skills best practiced during school and outside of school. I have said over and over that most movement skills require a large amount of practice to be mastered. No matter how high of an On-task activity standard you are able to have in your class, the children's skill levels are likely going to be low unless they also practice beyond the lessons you have for them. And due to the great individual differences in learning rates, some of the slower learners can only be expected to make minimal progress in class. Because of this, it so important that we always remember to remind and encourage further practice outside of class or to make either formal or informal homework assignments. Monitoring of typical physical education classes have found that only around four percent of lessons include this kind of prompting and advocacy. Individual movement skills are especially conducive to this. Most of the students can get good exercise outside of class as they practice individual skills you might have introduced to them: shooting baskets, dribbling a soccer ball, practicing jump rope or gymnastic stunts, etc. Skills that require partners and more teammates become more difficult for them to do at home because getting together with friends might not always be possible. If you can get the children to achieve some level of individual skill mastery as a result of outside of class practice, you will be able to focus on more cooperative skill learning. I know of some good youth sport coaches who follow this concept of promoting individual skills beyond practice so that the actual time, when the team members are together, can be spent on developmental games using those skills. Encouraging the students to practice together during recess periods is another out-of-class opportunity. I think recess should be re-named activity-breaks. Non-directed recess results in 65 percent of the children being inactive. Studies show that the children become more active when activity zones are designated and when facilitators are there to encourage practice. Too often, when teachers or aides are supposed to be supervising the playground, they actually spend the time chatting with each other or standing in one place without becoming actively involved. Playground supervisors should be active, energetic, and enjoy encouraging students to participate in various activity zones. Most schools use a "news network," that is, a public address system through which they make school-related announcements. This network would be an idea medium for promoting the activity program and for announcing new activities offered in the playground zones. Announcement could be upbeat and fun to get children excited about practicing skills and learning new ones.

PHYSICAL EDUCATION AND EXEMPTIONS

Physical education classes are unique in introducing students to the learning and practicing of a wide variety of motor skills. *The National Association of Sport and Physical Education (NASPE, 2004) Position Paper* states the following:

"K-12 students should take all required physical education courses and that no substitutions, waivers, or exemptions should be permitted. The unique goals of physical education are the development of physical competence, health-related fitness, cognitive understanding, and a positive attitude toward physical activity so that individuals can adopt and maintain physically active and healthy lifestyles.

Classes and activities that provide physical activity (e.g., marching band, ROTC, cheerleading, school and community sports) have important but distinctly different goals than physical education. Any opportunity for students to participate in sustained periods of meaningful physical activity can be valuable for their health and fitness, but these activities do not provide the content of a comprehensive, standards-based physical education program and thus should not be allowed to fulfill a physical education requirement."

FEEDBACK

As children are practicing skills you can play a helping role in the learning process by providing feedback. Feedback can be divided into two basic kinds: *General Feedback* and *Specific Feedback*. *General feedback* is when the instructor projects encouragement or disapproval about the overall performance of the students. It can be verbal: "Great going today." "Nice job Mary." "Good swing, Jason." "I am disappointed with our behavior today." It can be non-verbal: smiling, head nods or shakes, yawns, folded arms, inattention, high-fives. The function of this sort of feedback is to improve motivation either by rewarding good or punishing undesirable performance. Both verbal and non-verbal feedback are important but some believe that non-verbal messages carry the most weight because they often are perceived to be more accurate indicators of the teacher's true feelings. The teacher may say, "great going" or "you did wonderful" and not really mean it. It is less likely that the teacher's actions and gestures are disingenuous.

It is desirable to establish a warm learning environment in which the positive reinforcers outweigh the negative ones by a high ratio. Hopefully enthusiastic instructions/demonstrations and well-established class rules/procedures will minimize generally poor conduct and efforts. This should free the teacher to be supportive and praising.

It is also believed that for the *General Feedback* to be most effective it should be varied. The *Global Good* is a term used to represent an instructor's repeating of the same general feedback over and over, in this case, good. It is good this and good that, good job, good going, good try. Have you heard something like this before? The repeated mantra may have been a different word or phrase than good but the repetition was unmistakable in its global presence. Overuse of the same words and actions lessens their motivational impact. It is an easy, almost normal trap into which teachers may fall. It is probably wise for every teacher to have a lesson or two videotaped and then to look and listen for excessively common language and movement habits. Awareness is the first step. If you catch yourself guilty of some mannerisms don't despair. As already mentioned, it is expected and normal and it is easily corrected. Simply give thought to some ways that you might begin to increase your repertoire of reinforcers, both verbally and gesture-wise. Figure 8.3 offers a small list of suggestions. Perhaps you can think of some others you could progressively begin to add which might be more in vogue and hip with the culture of your students and which are best suited to your personality. I sometimes have had my pre-service teachers teach a lesson in which they were going to be assessed entirely upon the variety of their feedback, you could think of it as their instructional Learnable Piece. It is impressive how quickly they acquire the skill, especially if they have given a priori thought to the movement and verbal possibilities. It is also striking how improvements in this one aspect of instruction invariably creates a noticeably more enthusiastic learning environment.

Figure 8.3. Varied General Positive Feedback

Verbal	Gestures
super	smiles
terrific	thumbs up
awesome	high fives or tens
stupendous	hand shakes (of all kinds)
great	head nods
wonderful	raised arms

Specific Feedback is feedback that does more than identify if performance was good or bad. It qualifies or quantifies. It identifies what was good or bad. "You didn't follow-through." "Your knees weren't bent." "You watched the ball well." This kind of feedback will be critically important for some to learn skills correctly. Not only can it be motivational like General Feedback, it may convey the information needed to learn the skill and avoid the formation of bad habits. Research indicates that the best teachers give much more Specific Feedback than less skilled teachers. In fact, it is not uncommon for many teachers to give virtually no Specific Feedback at all. Either they are not taking the effort or they do not know enough to provide it.

When the students are practicing it is good procedure for the teacher to move about the area and at some point get close to every student. This better facilitates the ability to give personalized Specific Feedback to everyone. The Specific Feedback given should be kept simple, it is easy to try to correct and help too much. This excess of feedback often ends up confusing the student and results in the phenomenon of Analysis Paralysis. This means that the student is overloaded with so many suggestions he/she cannot incorporate any change. One way to keep your feedback simple is to remember the Learnable Piece and so focus your feedback. When our feedback is related to the Learnable Piece we are employing Congruent Feedback. Here is an example. The class is working on soccer dribbling skills and I have explained and demonstrated the Learnable Piece of "Happy-feet." Happy-feet is a label for remembering to keep your feet moving with quick, short steps. As I move about the practice area I am looking and commenting primarily on this aspect. "Mary, what are we working on?" "Amazingly happy footwork Jim." " Jan, you are moving those feet nicely!"

When giving Specific Feedback recent research studies have confirmed that both children and adults learn and perform motor skills significantly better when they direct their attention towards the movement effect they wish to produce rather than thinking about their own movements. Researchers label this as having an external focus as opposed to an internal focus. It seems that thinking about the muscles and movements only interferes with automatic processing and reflexes that should control skilled movement. The implication for teachers is that we should phase our feedback to direct the learners' attention toward the desired effect and not the body movements that produce it. If the skill involves an implement the focus had best be on it: "Think of the ball arching up towards the basket with backspin." "Think of the racket coming up and over the ball." "Think of the skateboard tilting and swerving to the left and then the right." If the skill does not involve an implement the focus is on something else external: "Think of the water flowing past." Or think in terms of external analogies: "Think of spinning like a top." "Think of the compressing and expanding like a coiled spring."

As stated before with regards to General Feedback, learning best occurs in a mostly positive environment. You might question how you can keep your Specific Feedback positive for students who are not performing the skill correctly. A helpful technique for these situations is the Sandwich Principle. This principle is where you surround your corrective feedback with positive comments about other aspects of performance. In a situation in which a child is not adhering to the Learnable Piece of swinging the bat level this feedback could be offered; "I like your ready position, remember you need to swing level rather than upwards, keep up the good effort." You can notice how these kinds of messages are more sensitive to potential discouragement than correction-only comments might be.

Thus far I have been exemplifying only verbal Specific Feedback. You will find that that will not always suffice. Telling the child he/she is not swinging level will not always remedy the situation. A useful feedback progression is first to tell, then show, and then provide physical guidance. If the swing is not leveled when you verbally commented on the noncompliance it is useful to take the bat and demonstrate the swing again. If they still have not gotten the idea, the final physical guidance step may be required. At this stage you attempt to give them the kinesthetic feel by guiding their bat and or limbs through the proper path. I have found that this final hands-on stage makes the critical difference for some learners and shows that you are truly interested and involved in the process. A cautionary note is worth mentioning here pertaining to physical touching students. We need to remind ourselves that everyone, regardless of age, has a right to their personal space and should not have others touching them if it makes them uncomfortable. Because of this right, we need to be absolutely sure that we do not touch students if it would be unwelcome, no matter how good and innocent our intentions. If you have the slightest doubt about their feelings, be sure to ask their permission before jumping in to help. A simple "Can I help you through a level swing?" would be wise. The issue of appropriate and inappropriate touching and other sexual harassment guidelines will be further covered in Chapter 11.

REVIEW

When we think of review we normally think of the lesson's closure and summary statements by the teacher. Here we are taking a somewhat broader view of the review process. Review is not something that only occurs at the completion of practice, it must also be taking place throughout the introductory explanation-demonstration and during practice.

When a skill is being explained and demonstrated to students, they must not only pay attention to the salient points, they must also review or rehearse those concepts in their minds. If they do not repeat what they have seen or heard, that information will quickly fade from short-term memory and never enter long-term memory. It will go into one ear and come out the other. If this happens they likely will not have purposeful practice even it that practice occurs a fairly short time following the explanation/demonstration. Many teachers of the young have experienced this phenomenon. Research indicates that school children have just as good short-term memory mechanisms as adults and if they rehearse what has been presented to them, are as capable of moving information into long-term storage. However, children sometimes do not acquire concepts as readily because they use rehearsal strategies less effectively than mature learners do.

The instructor can do a couple of things to insure that presented information gets into useful long-term memory. We have already stressed the importance of keeping your message simple and directed at one *Learnable Piece*. The more different things you attempt to explain the less likely any one of those aspects is going to be thought over and repeatedly imaged. The second thing is to develop the habit of ending your presentation with a question such as, "What are we going to think about?" You need to know if what you introduced registered with them and this quizzing may force them to immediately rehearse. Also, the manner in which we ask questions has much to do with whether or not reviewing will be stimulated. The *Effective Questioning Strategy* is a good technique for promoting rehearsal of all the students. It consist of posing the question, waiting at least five seconds or more so everyone has time to mentally consider, and then randomly picking on a student to respond. If the students get used to you always asking questions in this manner they may learn that they must be thinking about what you say because they may be called upon to respond in front of the class. When you throw open questions to the class the same quicker, hand waving children will tend to dominate and the others may feel no pressure to mentally prepare. They may zone out on you.

During practice, the reviewing process continues if you are giving feedback. Instead of always immediately providing *Specific Feedback* you might ask the student to review for his/herself what it is that is to be remembered. Also, you might wish to provide another demonstration for that student, or to stop the whole class and give a repeat demonstration. Just because an excellent demonstration was provided at the beginning does not mean that it was totally grasped or retained. A good means of providing this review during practice is to employ the technique of *Spotlighting*. This is were you stop the class and have them watch a couple of students who are performing well. This provides the review you want for the class and may bolster their *self-efficacy*. It additionally gives those demonstrators a chance to show-off a little and receive some kudos. Having two or three simultaneous demonstrators works well because it allows you to have more children receive recognition and it takes some of the pressure off them as everyone watches.

At the end of the period the traditional summing up review is considered a sound teaching procedure. Final questioning will result in a terminal review and hopefully this will solidify the concept to be transferred into beyond class use. But even yet the review process should not be considered to be over. Reminding yourself to ask review questions at the beginning of next period and periodically throughout the remainder of the year might make a telling difference. If something was worth a lesson's instruction it is worth the students' recalling.

CHAPTER COMPREHENSION CHECK

What is the technique of *home position*?
What is *Anticipatory Set*?
What is *The Two-Minute Warning*? Why does the author think it to be a good guide?
How is a *Learnable Piece* different from some other objectives?
Scaffolding is what?
What is the special advantage in having one of the students' peers demonstrate a skill?
Why might it generally be a good idea to have more than one student demonstrate a skill?

How *is self-efficacy* different from *self-concept*? Why is it so important for the learning of skills?
What is the most effective manner to demonstrate a skill?
What is *Incidental Learning*?
What is the *SOS Principle*?
What is the *Fifty-Percent Minimum Activity Standard*? How well have most teachers been achieving it?
What is the *equipment rule of thumb*?
What is the idea of the *80% Success Rate*? For whom is it recommended?
What is the purpose of the *Long-Slanty-Rope*?
What approximate percentage of physical education classes include specific encouragement to practice of skills beyond class?
Without special encouragement, approximately what percentage of children are physically active during recess?
What would be a good name change for recess? Why?
What is the stance and justification of *The National Association of Sport and Physical Education* regarding permitting exemptions from physical education?
Why is non-verbal feedback commonly considered more powerful than verbal feedback?
What is the concept of the *Global Good*?
What is the difference between *general* and *specific feedback*?
What is the concept of *Analysis Paralysis*?
What specifically is *congruent feedback*?
What is the difference between having an *external focus* as you perform a motor skill, compared to having an *internal focus*? Which is considered more effective and why?
What would be examples of teacher feedback directing focus internally and externally?
What is the *Sandwich Principle*?
Is the use of *physical guidance* recommended in the teaching of motor skills? If so, when?
Children have just as good short-term memory as adults but do not normally take in information as effectively. Why?
What are the steps of the *Effective Questioning Strategy*?
What is *Spotlighting*?

[CHAPTER 9]

MAKING GAMES & SPORTS FUN & EDUCATIONAL

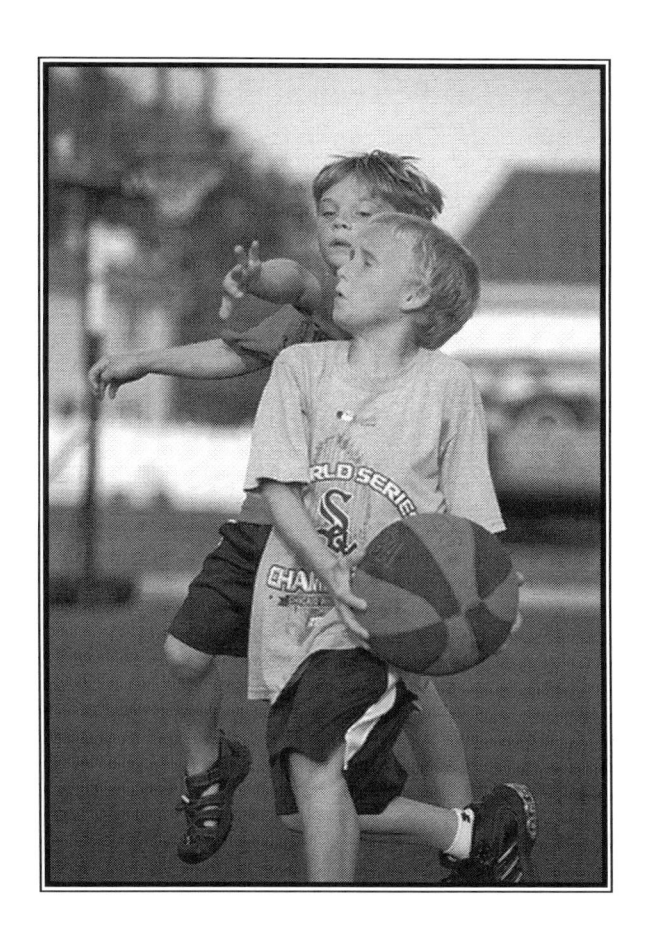

MAKING GAMES FUN AND EDUCATIONAL

Introducing Games
SOS Principle Revisited
Safety
On-Task Activity
Successful

MAKING SPORTS FUN AND EDUCATIONAL

Changing the Rules
Matching Competitors
Changing Equipment and Facilities
Adjusting the Contextual Aspects of Sports
Traditional vs. Games Approach to Teaching Sport Skills
Beyond Traditional Sports

CHAPTER COMPREHENSION CHECK

> "*It should be noted that children's games are not merely games; one should regard them as their most serious activities.*"
> ~ Michel de Montaigne

> "*Happy hearts, and happy faces / Happy play in grassy places.*"
> ~ Anonymous

Most of the children in your classes will be incessantly clambering "Lets play a game!" "Let's play softball!" "Let's play basketball!" Games and sports can be gleeful fun for children and they can be a great avenue for developing motor skills, affective skills, and physical fitness. However, you may have some students who are not always keen to participate; some games and sports may not provide everyone with much activity for motor and fitness development; and sometimes the students can learn poor, rather than good, social-emotional behaviors.

In this chapter you will learn how to introduce, select, modify, design, and organize games and sports so that they can be fun and educational for all.

MAKING GAMES FUN & EDUCATIONAL

Introducing Games

In Chapter 8, we discussed how motor skills might be effectively introduced to learners by means of the concept of Anticipatory set. We said you might improve the students' interest in learning a skill by presenting some reasons how the skill would help them in the sports contest. This understanding should increase their motivation to learn. When you are introducing a game to the students it is also a good practice to create an Anticipatory set or desire to participate. Your manner of introduction can make a big difference. Imagine the dissimilar reactions you might get from second graders in these two scenarios. In scenario one you tell the children they will be playing a tag game. If you are tagged you will run over to a hula-hoop and jump in and out of it three times. This completed, you can re-enter the ongoing tag. In scenario two the teacher is wearing a false face and robe and is wielding something that is supposed to resemble a sword. In a stentorian voice she proclaims herself to be a samurai warrior of the highest order. Stirring music is playing. In "Samurai Warrior Tag" the tagged students run to her and she slams the sword on the ground and yells, "Samurai warrior will save you!" Then she swings the sword along the ground at the students feet and then over their heads, carefully of course. They jump and duck the sword three times and then can join the tag.

The above point being made is that names, themes, music and a little hamming by the instructor can have a major impact on how well games will be received. As another example, a mundane set of "grass drills" might become more exciting when it assumes the challenging name, "THE ONE MINUTE TORTURE TEST!" With a little thought and creativity, a simple tag game can easily become Pac Man Tag, Star Wars Tag, Ninja Turtle Tag, Jurassic Park Tag, Power Ranger Tag, Pokemon Tag, or Good Wizard-Bad Wizard Tag. Notice these names illustrate how quickly some themes become hot or not so hot. If Napoleon was right when he said, "men are ruled by names," how much more true can that not be said for excitable elementary children.

Another useful concept to remember when introducing games is *The Three-Rule Rule.* This means that you can explain your game in three rules or less. If there are only three rules you will be able to explain the game quickly and move right into action. More rules necessitates that your explanation must be lengthier, and as a consequence, the children may become fidgety and in all probability not remember all those rules anyway. Once the game is in progress, you not uncommonly will have to stop the confusion and try to re-start the game. Here is an example of *The Three-Rule Rule.* You have the children positioned in a double circle. Each child is facing a partner so that outer circle child is looking towards the center and the other child outwards. You introduce the "Horse and Jockey" relay like this: the people facing outwards are the horses that will start racing by crawling between the spread legs of their partners (this is rule 1). The horses then make a left-hand turn to race a lap around the outside of the circle (rule 2). When they arrive home they straddle their partner who has assumed a hands and knees position (rule 3). Now maybe, just maybe, if all the children were attentive, and you demonstrated all the actions as you clearly explained them, the game will be understood and properly performed. Of course you may have spiced up your introduction with some *anticipatory set* things like bugle calls, summons for horse to be at the gates, and race music and commentary. But can you not see that even three rules are pushing the information processing and retention capacities of at least some of the students?

The Three-Rule Rule does not mean that you cannot ever play more complex games. It just means that you probably will not be successful if you begin with more than three. Lets stay a bit longer with our example of the horse and jockey game. The next time the horses complete their laps they must give their partners high-tens before assuming the ending straddle position. The time after that they give the high-tens and then do five sit-ups. And so it goes with more and more rules and activities being added on. What we are doing here is employing *The Expansion Principle*. This means that once the game has been played a couple of times in a simple form, and those rules have been internalized, it now becomes feasible to add others. Once the fundamentals of a skill or game is learned you can then elaborate to a more advanced level.

Permit me to reiterate that if all the children are to understand a game you had better demonstrate it, not just explain it. Seeing someone actually going through the legs, seeing the direction of the laps, and seeing the finishing horse position are necessary. Taking the time to show them will save you time. If you believe anything I say, believe this.

SOS Principle Revisited

You remember what *The SOS principle* is, right? In Chapter 8 we said that as children begin to practice a skill you step back and ask yourself three questions in this order: are the children Safe? are they actively On-task? are they being Successful in their performance? In this section we are advocating that you ask those same questions of games. Games will not be fun or educationally sound if they are unsafe, if there is not abundant activity, or if successful performances are not the norm.

Safety

Every game should be initially assessed as to both its physiological and psychological safety. As for physical safety, there is always an inherent risk in any movement game. Even if the game is basically safe, the environmental conditions are safe, and it is being played in an orderly fashion, there is no end to the minor, and even major, catastrophes that are possible. People can fall, collide with others, get hit by implements or balls. These events can result in contusions, sprains, dislocations, cardio-respiratory problems, dismemberment's... Okay! Okay! Now I am exaggerating, but you get the point. Even though inherent risks are a reality they do not prevent us from living active lives. Staying in bed is not the answer. But the games we offer our children must be reasonably safe and the hazards minimized to the lowest possible levels. If we, as *reasonably prudent people* (the legal standard we are held to), can foresee the likelihood of a game causing injuries we must not allow it to continue. It is not worth the risk. Furthermore, once we select a game as having an acceptably low level of risk, we must do whatever we feasibly can to make sure it is carried out in a safe manner.

There is no steadfast, always easily discernible dividing line between games that are safe enough and those that are not. Here are some red-flag activities that might serve as touchstones of sensitivity. What about a "Dodgeball" type game where children are throwing playground or volleyballs at each other. We should be able to anticipate the real eventuality of someone getting hit in the head or some other sensitive place. This would be true even if the instruction were to throw to hit below the waist because errant throws will happen. Teachers who have their classes play these kinds of games feel that they are not overly hazardous and say that only some stings and bruises might result. But detached retinas and damaged eardrums have also sometimes occurred and the courts have not ruled in favor of the teachers.

> **POSITION STATEMENT ON DODGEBALL IN PHYSICAL EDUCATION**
> By the National Association for Sport and Physical Education
>
> NASPE believes that dodgeball is NOT an appropriate activity for K-12 school physical education programs. In a quality physical education class teachers involve ALL children in activities that allow them to participate actively, both physically and mentally. Activities such as relay races, dodgeball, and elimination tag provide limited opportunities for everyone in the class, especially the slower, less agile students who need the activity the most. The students who are eliminated first in dodgeball are typically the ones who most need to be active and practice their skills. May times these students are also the ones with the least amount of confidence in their physical abilities. Being targeted because they are the "weaker" players, and being hit by a hard-thrown ball, does not help kids to develop confidence.
>
> The arguments most often heard in favor of dodgeball are that it allows for the practice of important physical skills – and kids like it. Dodgeball does provide a means of practicing some important physical skills – running, dodging, throwing, and catching. However, there are many activities that allow practice of these skills without using human targets or eliminating students from play. Some kids may like it – the most skilled, the most confident. But many do not! Certainly not the student who gets hit hard in the stomach, head, or groin. And it is not appropriate to teach our children that you win by hurting others.

"Wheelbarrow walks" and "piggy-back carries" might be safe enough activities, but if they are used in a relay race they become much more dangerous. The courts and we can visualize the "wheelbarrow" being pushed onto his/her face by an overeager pusher, or the runner with someone on his/her back losing balance and awkwardly falling. What about having all your students racing up and down a narrow all-purpose area at full speed? If some children have a full head of steam are running towards others moving at full speed in the other direction, there is a real potential for a miscalculated dodge and a literal head-on collision. What about the game of "Red Rover" in which children attempt to run across an area while others attempt to catch and restrain them? This seems like it may be producing some pretty significant body contact for young people who do not have the benefit of training and protective equipment.

As mentioned earlier, once you have deemed the nature of a game to be reasonably safe, it must also be implemented in a safe manner. Safe games can become dangerous if the playing surface is slippery due to gravel, water, or littered with clothing, notebooks and papers. Protruding obstacles such as poles, bleachers, and waste cans need consideration. I am always surprised that some teachers will organize tag and relay type games in which boundary lines are placed within a couple of feet of walls. Have they not thought that some racing child will ineluctably not be able to stop quickly enough? In addition to the physical environment, the manner in which the children participate in the activity can negatively impact its safety. Unruly players can make tidly-winks dangerous. What if the children are not under control as they run and dodge? if they carelessly wield implements? If they are not abiding by the class and game rules? The key to remedying these conduct problems is twofold. Firstly, when the game is introduced it should always be understood that a major purpose of playing the game is to see if everyone can play by the rules and be respectful of other peoples' safety. This means that the teacher might often have to remind the students of this at the inception. Secondly, the feedback the teacher provides at the completion of the game should be congruent to this behavior. The primary purpose of these games is not to see who was the fastest or who won. Winning can be recognized and congratulated but it should not take precedence over enthusiastic praise of fair play and rule following. And of course, if the game is not being played in a safe fashion you need to exert your supervisory role and immediately stop it.

Thus far our discussion has been focused on physical safety, but we should be adhering to the stricter standard of psychological safety. Not only should the children be safe, they should not feel threatened. If some children feel fearful, even if it is an unwarranted fear, we are not accomplishing our enjoyment goal. We may sometimes become exasperated at those who will not venture something and show reasonable courage and resolve, but we should never force or coerce a child to do something he/she is truly afraid to do. Their fear could make participation counter-productive and maybe even physically dangerous. Our task should be more one of gently and persistently leading and assuring them.

A word of caution is in order here. We must be careful in assessing the stresses our games place upon the children. It is not uncommon for students to vociferously exclaim that they want to play "Dodgeball" or some rough game akin to it. But can you really be sure that the sentiments of the most skilled and vocal reflect those of everyone? Can you expect a boy or girl who might be apprehensive about this game to stand up and admittedly announce that he/she is frightened? I don't think so. Many may accede to the cries of the majority, and even lend their votes and voices of support to a game they fear. We need to be sensitive to these kinds of social dynamics and pressures.

On-Task Activity

One of the best and easiest ways to evaluate a game is to look at the quantity of activity it produces. High participation rates are needed to best develop fitness, motor, and affective skills. In the most enjoyable and educational games everyone plays an important part and will be actively involved throughout. Little time will be spent waiting for turns and no one is eliminated from participation. Many of the traditional games you learned in school may not meet this criterion. Let us analyze a few old stand-by games and see if they can be altered for the better. If we learn to critically analyze these games we should be able apply this skill to improve many others which we know or will encounter.

Do you remember "Duck, Duck, Goose?" That is a game in which the children are seated in a circle, facing inward. One child walks around the outside of the circle tapping everyone on the head and saying "Duck." When the tapper taps someone and says "Goose!" the chase is on. The person who has been tapped tries to catch the person before he/she makes it around the circle and into the vacated spot. Children have long enjoyed this game, probably because of the suspense as to whether or not they will be picked. However, it is not difficult to see that the amount of activity is low. Only one or two children are physically active at a time and the others wait and wait. If we measured the percentage of time any one child was active during the course of the game we would probably find it to be something like 5 percent or less. Some children might not get picked at all. What could be done to increase activity? In games like this one, in which many students are standing or sitting as they await their turn, it often is possible to have them *Actively Waiting.* In "Duck, Duck, Goose", everyone could be jogging in place or walking counterclockwise as the chooser walked in the opposite direction. Think how much healthful walking the children would experience throughout the game. Another basic means of increasing activity levels is to see if the format of the game can be changed from one single game to numerous, simultaneously played *Mini-Games*. I know a teacher who played "Duck, Duck, Goose" in a format in which the students formed two lines down the center of the area. Everyone was paired with a partner, one line of partners faced away from the others. Each pair played their own mini-game. They took turns being the tapper and chased or fled to one line or the other based on whether or not they were pronounced a duck or goose. The amount of activity the children got in five minutes far exceeded that of what would have been produced in a half-hour under the traditional organization. As an example of wise *Anticipatory Set* usage, this teacher said that even the upper elementary children enjoyed this high activity version of "Duck, Duck, Goose" when the name had been changed to "I'm it! You're it!"

"Steal-the-Bacon" is a game that has been played across the country for many generations. I recall playing it when I was in school and I taught it many years in my early teaching career. The normal set-up is one in which two teams of students are aligned at opposing ends of the court. Each team was numbered one through whatever the number of players. Then, for instance, when the number 10 was called the number 10s from each side would run out and attempt to get the bacon, usually a knotted towel, and carry it back across his/her goal line without being tagged by the other player. Here again we find a game with a lot of exciting anticipation but with little total activity. Notice how we might again use the concepts of *Active Waiting* and *Mini-Game* formats to increase the activity. We could create *Active Waiting* by everyone walking or jogging in a circle. When a number is called, those two individuals rush into the center for the bacon and attempt an exit in any direction to the perimeter. All the rest of the children keep right on walking or jogging. Figure 9.1 depicts a sample mini-game format with three players per team. The teacher's call of one, two or three would initiate a number of games. All the ones, twos, or threes would go at the same time resulting in a third of the class members being involved at any one time. If you did not want children always playing against the same opponent, everyone could be moved one position clockwise by a simple rotation system. Also, to add some variety, variations of the games could be offered at the different sites. Stealing and dribbling basketballs or soccer balls could be done in one game while hockey sticks and pucks were used at another.

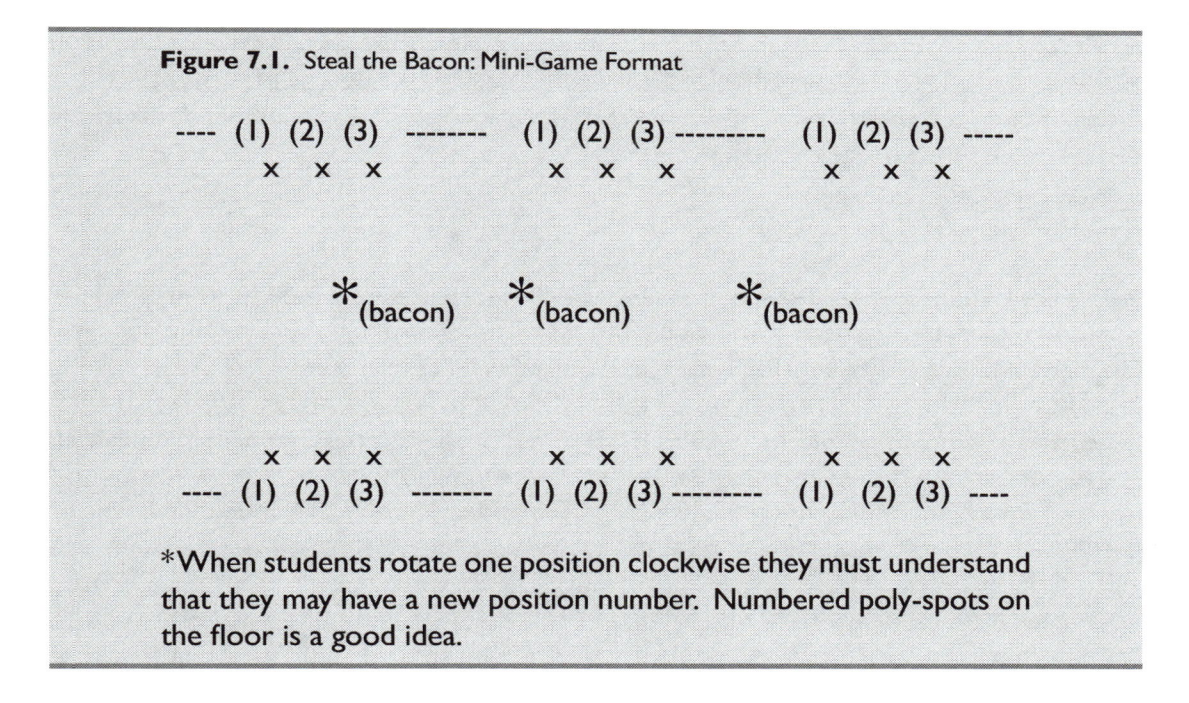

Figure 7.1. Steal the Bacon: Mini-Game Format

```
---- (1) (2) (3) -------- (1) (2) (3) --------- (1) (2) (3) -----
      x   x   x              x   x   x              x   x   x


       *(bacon)              *(bacon)              *(bacon)


      x   x   x              x   x   x              x   x   x
---- (1) (2) (3) -------- (1) (2) (3) --------- (1) (2) (3) ----
```

*When students rotate one position clockwise they must understand that they may have a new position number. Numbered poly-spots on the floor is a good idea.

Another simple way to insure more activity is to Eliminate the Elimination in elimination games. "Musical Chairs", as traditionally played, is a classic example of an elimination game. Everyone is circling around a double line of chairs which numbers one less than the number of children. When the music stops or the command is given everyone attempts to sit on a chair. The person left out is removed to spectator status. The game continues with one less chair each time until one winner remains. This game, and variants of it, can be great fun and still be played. Rather than eliminating those not finding a chair, why not simply assign them a point and allow all to continue. The excitement of the game will be still there as everyone strives to avoid points. I have played many successful variants of musical chairs where the children ran or dribbled basketballs and soccer balls around an area to music. When the music stopped everyone scrambled to get inside a hula-hoop or on a poly-spot. I found that having two or three less hoops or spots worked well because then no one was singled out as the sole person caught.

Making Games & Sports Fun & Educational

Finally, because many instructors commonly use relay games, a few words had best be said specifically about them. Activity rates in line relays will necessarily be low if the lines of children are long and only one team member at a time performs. The most obvious remedy, many times inexplicably overlooked, is to keep the lines short, four or less would seem wise. Another possibility is that of having more than one person going at a time. Could pairs of children be doing the activity together? Or what about the entire squads performing together in a cooperative manner? I have had children put hands on the waist or shoulders of the person in front of them and race train fashion, or join hand in a circle with a team member inside so as to transport them in a "circle of friends" fashion (or maybe it was a spaceship to ride in). Not only do these types of cooperative relays promote greater activity, cooperation is demanded and the races tend to be closely contested.

Successful

If you have been able to devise games where everyone is safely moving, that's terrific. But don't forget the second S in SOS. Is everyone generally experiencing success? Children will not enjoy a game if they are not experiencing success.

There are three different types of game structures: *individual, cooperative* and *competitive*. In *individual activities* the children are personally attempting to accomplish an activity according to a criterion. The key to ensuring high success rates in these individual games is the employment of the Long-Slanty Rope Principle introduced in Chapter 8. The children are either given different criteria suited to their abilities or they are given different versions of the task. For example, if we were going to have the children do as many skiers' jumps back and forth across a line in one minute, we might wish to set different criterion levels. We could say that if you can do 145 you are "Simmering!" Doing 175 equals " Cooking!" and at 185 you are "Hot Stuff!" Or we could encourage them to set their own personal targets, maybe to exceed the previous days achievement. Different versions of this particular task could entail one-legged performance, wider lines, or even a slightly raised obstacle to clear. An example of yet another skill would be to give the children a number of jump rope skills and then have them select those they think they may be able to accomplish in a given time.

In *cooperative activities* the children are attempting to accomplish a task either individually, in partners, small groups, or as an entire class. I think this approach to game organization can be especially conducive to feelings of success. This occurs because everyone tends to receive encouragement and help from his or her peers; everyone is on your side. Also, since the children are not being encouraged to compare their level of performance against other groups, they will be tending to work towards criteria appropriate for them. Of course, in cooperative games as with individual games, some thought may need to be given to making game variations to suit personal needs.

It is in *competitive activities* and games where we need to be especially vigilant about some students feeling unsuccessful. Competitive games can be great fun but competition can also be a set-up for failure; and a little failure can go a long way. If a child's skills are much below the skills of others, the competitive environment can become stressful and embarrassing. Suppose a relay race is being played in which the children are to crab walk down to a line and back. Imagine the feeling of children who cannot perform the skill well and flounder. Their ineptitude is displayed to all and their team is losing because of them. Because of this inherent problem in competitive games it is essential that we are sure that children possess the perquisite skill before we place them into these pressure, high profile game situations. In the following section we will address this issue of adjusting games to the children's skill levels and matching competitors.

MAKING SPORTS FUN & EDUCATIONAL

Some people are critical of including competitive games and sports in the regular school curriculum. They remember physical education class as placing too much emphasis on competition, especially competitive team sports. They believe that we should rather be offering cooperative experiences and life-long recreational activities. Such activities would be less stressful and, instead of focusing attention on comparing abilities and attempting to surpass others, the children would learn how to be satisfied with their own performances and how to get along with others. Some educators also feel that the larger than ever heterogeneity of today's classes are especially unsuited for the competitive approach; some children have had extensive training in youth sports while others have had precious little movement experiences; some children are gifted with many athletic abilities while others are not; the maturational levels of some children are far ahead or behind the age norms; and most classes typically include students with a range of disabilities. All these factors are thought to result in a sports experience in which the haves will dominate and the have-nots will be overrun or pushed to the sidelines. The less gifted, who might most benefit from learning to enjoy physical activity, are at risk of encountering failure and hence at risk to being turned off to the active lifestyle.

The above are legitimate concerns. I recognize the potential hazards of competitive sports and do not think they should dominate the physical experiences of children. All children would benefit from learning that movement experiences could be fun without competition. However, having said that, I do not agree that we should view competition as an evil to be always discouraged. Competition between sports performers can yield great excitement and joy. Your children will be beseeching you to play games and keep score. Many of us have had unforgettable, thrilling memories of competitive games and youthful sports involvement. If there are potential problems with competitive sports, as we have already established, the solution is to mend it, don't end it. Competitive games and sports can be a valuable part of children's education. They can be designed so that children of all ability levels and backgrounds can be successful and experience the fun and excitement of participation. They can be designed so they are an effective laboratory for teaching important affective skills such as: striving to do one's best, persevering, cooperating with teammates, respecting opponents, abiding by rules, winning gracefully, accepting defeat. In the following sections are ideas of how that might be achieved.

Changing the Rules

The rules of sports are generally written with the intent of establishing which of two skilled teams or players are the best, and worthy of being declared the winner. They are not written so as to accommodate players of lower abilities, nor are they written to maximize the activity levels and educational experiences of the participants.

Probably the most significant rule change we can make is the number of members on team sports. Activity is far from being maximized in ten-on-ten softball or kickball, eleven on eleven soccer or football, and six-on-six volleyball. And even less activity is present when you divide your class of 30 students into two teams and play fifteen-on-fifteen. When the ball-to-student ratio is low the amount of physical activity and skill development is low. Also, the better skilled of those groups will tend to monopolize a large share of the activity and the lesser skilled will be relatively inactive. In a typical mass-on-mass kickball game, each child will average only two or three kicks throughout a 40-minute game, average fielding experiences will be naturally low and they will be unequally distributed; the key positions of pitcher and shortstop will be more active at the expense of outfielders. It is obvious that such a set up will not come anywhere near our *Fifty-Percent Minimum Activity Standard.*

A *Mini-Game* format is educationally sound remedy. It should not be difficult to organize a number of simultaneous mini-games. A number of smaller hockey fields could be marked out by cones, basketball games could be run at each of the baskets, with a long net or rope strung across the gym or playing field multiple volleyball games could occur. A *Team-Size Rule of Thumb* is to keep the number of players on a team equivalent to or less than the grade level: first graders play one-on-one, second graders go two-on-two, third graders go three-on-three. The thinking here is that the younger children are not ready to understand the increased complexity that working with partners and teammates demands. For the older children it is still recommended that teams not normally increase beyond three per side. In three per side most strategy implications of the game remain intact, and activity levels are many times higher than normal.

In order to play mini-games other rule changes are necessary. Boundaries must be miniaturized. One goal, rather than two, might be used, and sizes of those goals might be reduced. Here are a couple of examples. A two-on-two volleyball game could be played in a small court space, the smaller the court space the more successful and longer the rallies would tend to be. The net or rope height might be adjusted. If the children could not consistently get their serve in and hence it was discouraging and holding up play, it could be dispensed with. Rather, an underhand throw-in or "courtesy toss" might work. Continuing to serve from a spot closer to the net will sometimes be effective.

For a game such as softball some major rule changes will be required. How, you are asking, can you play softball with only 2 or 3 per side? Instead of official softball I visualize playing games like "Over-the-line Softball" or "Bonkerball" (see Figure 9.2). In these kinds of mini-games certain aspects of the official game may be lost ("Over-the line Softball" does not require throwing or base running), but the skills of batting and catching are hugely increased. "Bonkerball" is a similar game but it does contain some throwing, catching, and base running elements. After the ball is batted the player must run around the cones before the fielders retrieve the ball and throw it to the cones.

Another useful rule change is to miniaturize the length of the games. Shorter games tend to be more exciting and less lopsided. Five or ten minutes might be sufficient.

Figure 9.2. Over-The Line Softball (the batters attempt to hit the ball over the line and the fielders attempt to catch it)

0	0	0
(fielders) 0	(fielders) 0	(fielders)
0	0	00
X (friendly pitcher)	X (friendly pitcher)	X (friendly pitcher)
X (batter)	X (batter)	X (batter)
X (on-deck player)	X (on-deck player)	(on-deck player)

Matching Competitors

One factor in helping to make competition enjoyable for all is the matching of competitors. Regardless of our degree of ability, competition can be an enjoyable experience when we are paired with and against people of our own level. Go to the tennis courts, golf courses or softball fields and observe some games in progress. You may notice that the courts and fields in which the people are unskillful are enjoying their contest just as much or more than the experienced performers. Excitement resides where reasonable challenges exist for all. However, when mis-matches exist, competition can easily become frustrating and threatening, boring or even physically dangerous.

There are a variety of ways individuals or teams can be ability matched. One is to allow the children to self-select: they can choose to play in the beginner's league, the experienced league, or the advanced league. I know one teacher who allows his volleyball students to choose between a "blood and guts" and a "hit and giggle" version. Or you might assign the children to teams. You could do this based on your estimates or perhaps on some try-out skill test. Another assignment method is to have student captains help equate the teams. I am not here advocating the *Slave-Market Approach* warned against in Chapter 7. Instead, a few skilled students privately help you divide the class into equal groups. They are not selecting people for their own squad but once that task is fulfilled you might assign them to a captain position.

Changing the Equipment and Facilities

Regulation sized equipment and facilities are not generally conducive to children's skill development or enjoyment. When confined to using official sized equipment and facilities, some weaker and less skilled students will learn incorrect techniques and will have frustratingly low success rates. I can still remember the initial dissatisfaction I held for basketball because of the size and weight of the ball and the height of the imposingly high rim. With some consideration given for equipment and facilities, virtually any child should be able to be successful. If a child cannot hit a pitched ball, a lighter, larger diameter bat may solve the problem; if that does not do it get a bigger ball; if not yet, a yet bigger ball or even beach ball; if not then, a batting tee could be used. A variety of equipment and facility modification ideas are offered in Figure 9.3.

Figure 9.3. Equipment Modifications

Softball
  Fat jumbo plastic bats:
  Flat bats (one side is flat):
  Larger and softer balls:
  Batting tees (large cones can serve this purpose well, if you cones are not large enough they can be raised by being placed on cardboard box)

Volleyball
  Balloons: They can be used in the beginning to learn the basic skill of setting, bumping and digging (some people are leery of using balloons because of the danger of children putting them in their mouths and choking; check your school's policy and be vigilant if you use them).

> *Beach balls or other large lightweight plastic balls:* They are not expensive and are easy to successfully play with. Another important benefit is that it does not hurt to hit or be hit by them (preventing these kinds of things early in the learning process can make the difference as to whether or not a child likes or dislikes the sport).
> *Trainer volleyballs:* These are bigger and lighter than regulation balls. They make a great progression between beach type balls and official volleyballs.
> *Ropes:* When strung down the length of the gym (from basketball rim to rim works) they become a serviceable net. The height can be adjusted to suit the needs of the different teams. Usually having them fairly high works best because then the ball must be projected high and permits the opposite side a better chance to get into receiving position. Of course, the rope is too high if some are having difficulty getting the ball up and over it.
>
> Basketball
> *Mini-basketballs:*
> *Waste cans:* These can serve as targets when set of chairs or other things
> Soccer
> *Soccer balls:* Sometimes they are easier to dribble when slightly deflated. I have even had younger children dribbling crushed milk containers around (they do not bounce and fly as out of control).
> Racquet Sports
> *Short handled wooden or plastic paddles:* These are a must for most elementary children, because speed and control can be much more easily regulated.
> *Coat hangers with nylon stretched over them:* This is a simple construction project to make a functional implement.
> *Shuttlecocks:* These work well in the early stages of learning because of their slower flight characteristics.

To gain access to equipment or other such learning aids I would first suggest that classroom teachers notify the physical education specialist in your area. Most specialists would love to see your interest and would find a means of getting you what is needed. If that fails, many items can be readily found in local toy stores. Others can, with a little construction ingenuity, be made. Three of the largest physical education equipment catalogs are WOLVERINE, SPORTIME, and THINGS FROM BELL. By googling them you will see the immense possibilities of cool things for purchase.

Perhaps the best of all possible sources of sports equipment might be gotten by getting on the web and contacting the various specific sports organizations. Whether it is the U.S. Soccer Association, U.S. Skiing Association, U.S. Gymnastic Association, U.S. Track and Field or most any sport association you can think of, they will likely have something to help you. All these organizations are desirous of promoting their sport and would love to have it introduced in the schools. Most have specific materials and programs developed for school grades K through 12. For example, if you contact the U.S. Tennis Association (USTA), PO Box 5046, White Plains, NY 10602-5046, (914) 696-700,

Making Games & Sports Fun & Educational

//www.usta.com/theusta /program.html#3 or the U.S. Handball Association, 2333 N. Tucson Blvd., Tucson, Arizona 85716, 1-800-345-2048, http://ushandball.org you would discover that they have excellent lesson and curriculum plans specifically designed for elementary schools and teachers like you. If you like, they will send representatives in to give demonstrations and/or in-service training. They will provide rackets and balls for all your students to keep. Everything is free.

UNITED STATES HANDBALL ASSOCIATION
1-800-345-2048
http://ushandball.org

Forget having to write up lesson plans! We will provide them for you at No cost. The USHA has developed teaching guides with 15 unit lesson plans for (1) Elementary students (separate lesson plans for grades K and 1, grades 2 and 3, and grades 4 and 5) (2) Junior and Senior High students, and (3) the 4-wall version of handball played in colleges and universities.

Just give us a little notice, and we will provide a handball workshop for teachers in your school district at No charge. All we will need is some wall space and a guarantee that you will put a handball unit into your curriculum.

With the invention of the new "white ace handball" a few years ago, handball has become a sport for everyone. This ball is slightly softer than the regulation handball and does not hurt the hands.

Adjusting the Contextual Aspects of Sports

What is meant by the *contextual aspects of sports*? Here is a list of six primary features integral to sports. (1) Seasons: sports usually last for an extended period of time, perhaps a few months. (2) Affiliation: sports see a number of teammates working together throughout the season. Close, long-term friendships are often formed. (3) Formal competition: practice times, league play and tournaments are scheduled prior to the season so that teams and individuals can anticipate and prepare appropriately. (4) Record keeping: as competition occurs, records of all kinds are kept on individual and team performances. (5) Festivity: sport is replete with banners, announcers, cheerleaders, publicists, bands, team names, uniforms, etc. (6) Culminating events: sports tournaments and post-season events with trophies, speeches and awards are a common practice.

To make sports enjoyable and educational, what approach should we take toward these contextual aspects? Should we view them as irrelevant detractors from the educational process? Do they create excessive stress and *hyper-competition*? If so, we should eliminate or reduce these aspects. On the other hand, should we view these contextual aspects as desirable additions to the sports experience which give it more meaning and fun? If so, we might want to incorporate and foster their presence. Based upon the philosophy I have advanced in the previous chapters you might correctly assume that I would subscribe to the more commonly excepted first point of view; that downplaying these contextual aspects is normally a sound practice. The reasoning is that it might be fun and educational to give children some competitive sports experiences, but we do not want to excessively heighten the importance of winning. Why not have team memberships frequently rotated so that cliques do not form and so everyone learns to play with everyone else? Why keep score? When a game is completed and the children ask who won the best response might be, "Did you have a good time? Did you get some good exercise and learn some skills? If so, then you won; we all won." We do not need league schedules, records, and culminating tournaments. The idea is to teach the young people to focus on their own performance and to not worry about how they compare to others; winning per se is not important

But does my above stance mean that you might be wise to always diminish the *contextual aspects of sports*? Perhaps not. Maybe an effective approach for some teachers and classes would be to do the opposite and take advantage of the contextual aspects to increase interest and commitment to the sport. For example, let's say that you have, at one time or another, richly enjoyed participating on a basketball team. You feel confident that you know the sport well, that you learned many valuable skills and lessons from the experience, and that you would like to provide that beneficial experience to your 5th graders. So here is what you did. You divided the class into 3 teams equally matched according to skills in this sport (maybe you used the private captain selection process previously described). Let us say that you had 24 students and hence three teams of 8 players. You explained to them that following some pre-season practices, they were going to have a basketball season with a schedule of contests. You encouraged team *esprit de corps* by having them practice as units and come up with team names and some sort of uniforms. Then, on the first day of the league play, team one played team two. The games were of the two-on-two *mini-game* format. This meant that team one had 4, two-person teams, and so would team 2. The squads had ranked themselves in A, B, C, and D levels. The games lasted 10 minutes, with the As playing the As, the Bs playing the Bs, and so on. Time permitted another round to be played that period, with the As playing the Bs and the Cs playing the Ds. Throughout the games, the role of the third, non-playing team, was that of fulfilling a variety of sport contextual roles. For instance, four of them served as officials and the others as record keepers, managers and publicists. When the next day of competition arrived, the teams were rotated so that team 3 became one of the playing teams while either team 1 or 2 assumed the roles of officials, scorekeepers, etc. At the end of the season a special round-robin tournament was scheduled in which some significant people were invited to attend. Awards and recognition of various kinds where made.

Some of you might be thinking that trying to incorporate all these contextual elements would be difficult and more than what you might be willing or able to do.

However, some of you might be emphatically saying "Yes! I see how I could organize something like this. I might not be able to do everything the first time, but I could start small and perhaps build off it in future years." And you might be thinking that the children could really get excited and motivated in such an environment. It contains many of the things you liked so much about sports. Furthermore, having the students playing the diverse roles of officiating, record keeping, and announcing, would be good learning experiences. The children would be learning to work together, take more responsibility for their own games, and might learn to better empathize with the work and difficulties of these jobs. Also, you might be able to integrate some of these duties into other academic areas: reporting and journalistic skills, record keeping and calculation skills, and more.

For a compete argument for the inclusion of the contextual aspects of sports, I would refer you to the text *Sports Education,* by Daryl Siedentop. The book is not long but provides many excellent ideas and implemented examples for teaching a variety of sports at a variety of grade levels. Siedentop's sport education philosophy is that competition is the essence of sports. Competition is fun and exciting and can be a great learning experience under our tutelage. We should make sports developmentally appropriate by matching the competition and modifying the rules, but let us not take the fun out of sports. Teaching children to fully compete and strive to win is not to be avoided but encouraged.

Traditional vs. Games Approach to Teaching Sport Skills

If classroom teachers would simply provide the opportunity and encouragement for their students to participate in some sports, either during recesses or physical education sessions, they would be helping the children improve their fitness, motor, and social skills. This small amount of helpful initiation from you could make a difference as to whether or not some children will engage in any active play throughout the day. Research shows that, if unprompted, approximately 35 percent of the children will remain inactive during free playtime. Many of the less fit children will be engaged in rather passive games or will simply sit and talk with friends. Data also shows that girls will on average be less active than the boys.

Although your fulfillment of the above recreational-supervisory role would be helpful, sports has the potential of teaching a great deal more if you are motivated enough to take a more active instructional role. Incorporating the ideas presented in the above sections (modifying rules and equipment, matching competitors, etc.) will better protect against some of the skilled students dominating play and the less adept being left out and feeling unsuccessful. However, there is another aspect that needs to be addressed if success is to be fully maximized. That aspect is skill instruction. Even with rule and equipment modifications many children will not possess adequate skills. They will adopt incorrect techniques and the games may sometimes break down because they cannot catch, throw, strike and so forth. Chapter 8 offered information of how to teach skills. What is covered in the following paragraphs is the question of whether sport skills are best taught in drills separate from the game, this being called the *Traditional Approach to Teaching Sports* (sometimes called the Technical Approach), or whether sport skills are more enjoyably and effectively taught within the context of the game, this is known as the *Games Approach to Teaching Sports* (sometimes called the *Tactical Approach*).

The *Traditional Approach to Teaching Sports* skills is to have the students participate in drills isolated from the game situation. In volleyball that would mean that we would have partners, or small circles of players, setting or bumping a ball to each other. They might also be divided up to serve the balls back and forth to each other; or they might be tossing or setting a ball for another to spike. The philosophy of the traditional approach is that many of the children will not have the prerequisite serving, setting, and bumping skills to successfully play the game unless the skills are first learned outside of the game. They reason that if those fundamental skills are not learned prior to the game, they will not be acquired in the game because the stress of competition is too great and the already skilled students will dominate.

In recent years many authorities have advanced the *Games Approach to Teaching Sports Skills*. I have included a good book on it in the Annotated References at the back of this book. Also, you could google either "Games Approach" or "Tactical Approach" for many other good sources. Proponents of this approach feel that the traditional approach has not been wholly effective for a couple of basic reasons. The first concern is that many students are not content with doing drills. They want to play the game and motivational levels are low until they can. The second concern is that students do not learn how to apply skills to the game when those skills have been practiced separate from it. They might get better at setting the balls around a circle but that does not mean they will correctly use that skill in the stress of specific game circumstances. The proper techniques acquired in practice may yield discouragingly little *transfer* to the game. I certainly can attest to having witnessed this phenomenon. In practice everyone is masterfully getting into good position to set the ball around the circle or properly underhand-passing the ball with their forearms, but when the same opportunity presents itself in the game, those positioning skills are not to be seen and the balls are almost invariably struck with open hands in an illegal fashion.

According to the *Games Approach*, it is best to allow the children to immediately begin playing and have them learn the techniques and strategies within the context in which the skills will be performed. But they are not advocating that we just throw out the ball and hope for the best. Rather, they see the learning key to lie in the progressive structuring of the games. Let us use the volleyball example again. The earliest introduction of children to volleyball, or any net sport, might consist of a one-on-one game in which each child has a very small area to guard. They throw the ball back and forth over a net or rope and attempt to have it land in their opponent's court.

The other player attempts to defend his/her area by catching the ball. All the children have the skills necessary to play this simple game and they are learning the beginning strategies and scoring rules that will form the foundation of future volleyball or other net sport games. The next progression is where the ball is hit over the net. Now the skills of setting and maybe underhand-passing are required. For the children who use improper techniques, some on-the-spot tips and instructions are given and the game is permitted to continue. Instruction introduced in this way hopefully has great relevancy and can be immediately applied. Eventually games with expanded court sizes will be organized and serving or other more advanced skills will be integrated. When two-on-two games are introduced, passing and other cooperative strategies are required. Now timely instructions on passing strategies will be given as the need arises. Overall, the concept of the *Games Approach* is that the children will understand and appreciate the role and need for skills as they play, and they will therefore be more eager to gain them. All the while, they of course will be enjoying playing the sport. You can see how *the Games Approach* dovetails well with the concept introduced in the previous chapter in which it was recommended that you strongly encourage children to practice individual sport skills outside of class time. By doing so they might be more ready for the in-class games.

It is hoped that the outlining of the arguments of the above two approaches will help you formulate a philosophy that will serve you. Rather than taking sides on the issue I would conclude by saying that your decision does not need to be one of either or. Drills do not need to be abandoned, but with wise progressions, some games could be initiated early in the learning process. Probably a useful concept to draw from this discussion would be that if we do use drills, we should make at least some of them as game-like as possible; by so doing, the children will better recognize how the skills tactically integrate into the game. For instance, instead of only having the students set and bump a ball around a circle, a task that is not done in a game, it would be more realistic to organize a drill where the ball comes from over the net and the performer's task is to pass it to a front line position.

Beyond Traditional Sports

I have previously made the point that there are advantages to having children learn a variety of games and sports. Children will have greatly different interests and aptitudes (remember the *Specificity of Motor Ability Hypothesis*). I also believe that if each year we continue to follow the pattern of repeatedly exposing children to the same limited range of traditional team sports experiences, we risk turning many of them off to adopting an active lifestyle. I call this the curriculum of *Overexposure*. It means that each year we reintroduce the same few sports for a week or two of rather superficial coverage. This is conducive to lowering interest and results in little in-depth learning.

Consider our most common traditional sports of football, softball, basketball, soccer and volleyball. They have much in common in that they favor a quite similar set of motor abilities. Those students who are bigger and who can sprint faster have a decided advantage. Also, all those sports favor similar psychological make-ups. If you like working in large social groups you will probably like them. But if you do not particularly care for the team atmosphere you could very well be unhappy. In Figure 9.4 I have provided a categorization of sports. Some of the placements are somewhat arbitrary but I think that they identify significant differences among the sports. In general the "invasion sports" have many similarities in games strategies, required physiological and motor abilities, and psychological propensities. Likewise, the other sports categories have their own unique set of basic strategies, ability requirements, and psychological demands.

Figure 9.4. Categorization of sports

Wall/Net Games
Strategies are very similar: making opponent move, attacking net to get angles, trying to find opponent weakness, returning to home base, clear to buy time, bisecting angle for best position, etc.
Techniques are moderately similar: striking and serving
Motor/physiological abilities very similar: quickness and fast reactions are essential
Psychological skills are similar: Except for volleyball, individual or partner

    Badminton
    Tennis
    Racquetball
    Volleyball
    Squash
    Handball
    Table Tennis

Invasion Games
Strategies are very similar: move with ball, give and go, feinting, move without ball, move to open space, signal, screen, fill lane to attack, stay between attacker, mark a man, mark a zone, use boundary lines, etc.
Techniques are only moderately similar: expect for Field Hockey and Ice Hockey and Rugby and Football
Motor/physiological abilities very similar: size and running speed, fast reactions
Psychological skills are very similar: body contact, aggressiveness, teamwork

    Basketball
    Soccer
    Rugby
    Football
    Field Hockey

       Ice Hockey
       Lacrosse

Striking/Fielding Games
Strategies are very similar: make contact, place ball in open spaces, learn when to hit long, short, positioning, fielding/where to throw, preventing, etc.
Techniques are very similar: most skills are almost identical (batting, throwing, fielding)
Motor/physiological abilities very similar: hand-eye coordination (tracking and catching)
Psychological skills are very similar: slower pace, suspenseful, strategic planning, teamwork
       Baseball
       Softball
       Rounders
       Cricket
       Kickball

Outdoor Recreational Activities
Strategies only moderately similar: careful planning and maintenance of equipment
Techniques not necessarily similar:
Motor/physiological abilities moderately similar: many athletic abilities not necessary, endurance and stamina, climbing and canoeing require strength
Psychological skills are very similar: enjoyment of nature, separating from crowds and engines, self-paced, reflective
       Hiking
       Camping
       Climbing
       Canoeing
       Sailing

Racing Events
Strategies moderately similar: pacing and achieving maximal effort
Techniques moderately similar: of course the running events are very similar
Motor/physiological abilities are very similar: muscular and cardiovascular endurance
Psychological skills are very similar: more individual, disciplined training
       Bicycling
       Track
       Swimming
       Duathloning/Triathloning
       Orienteering
       Adventure Racing

Form Sports
Strategies are very similar: learning routines, mental focusing
Techniques are very similar: take-offs, spins, rotations, landings, balances
Motor/physiological abilities are very similar: muscular strength and flexibility, balance, body and spatial awareness, small size not a disadvantage
Psychological skills are very similar: appreciation of the aesthetic aspects of movement, courage to learn and perform dangerous movements, individual
- Gymnastics
- Dance
- Diving

Target Sports
Strategies are very similar: focused concentration, control of anxiety and emotions
Techniques are not very similar:
Motor/physiological abilities are similar: fine motor control, hand steadiness
Psychological skills are very similar: individual, self-paced
- Bowling
- Golf
- Archery

Skiing/Skating/Balancing
Strategies are not very similar: this depends of whether the focus is on stunts or racing and leisure performance
Techniques are very similar: weight control, carving turns
Motor/physiological abilities are very similar: leg strength, dynamic balance
Psychological skills are very similar: courage to learn and perform dangerous movements, individual
- Water-skiing
- Snow Skiing
- Snow Boarding
- Skateboarding
- Ice Skating
- Inline Skating
- Endo boarding

An alternative to the *Overexposure* curriculum model would be a model in which, over the students' tenure in school, they would have a quality experience in an assortment of the sports categories. For example, third graders would have a unit of instruction in an "invasion sport" such as soccer. It would be rather thorough instruction replete with all the contextual elements of the *Sport Education Model*. The fourth graders might have an in-depth unit in a "net/wall sport" such as tennis. The fifth grade season might be devoted to a "form sport" such as gymnastics, and so on. You can see that the purpose of such a curriculum would be to provide the students with thorough training in some very different sports that would tap into a variety of different motor/physiological abilities and psychological interests. Those children who did not have the make-up to be very successful at soccer might discover that tennis or gymnastics was what they were better suited for. My preference would be that somewhere down the line, certainly by the high school grades, students could be given electives. The young people would be able to draw on their earlier experiences and select those kinds of activities they most preferred.

Of course, all this macro curriculum planning falls more under the purview of the physical education specialist than that of the classroom teacher. Nevertheless, I think it is important for the classroom teachers to recognize that your students will have different interest/abilities and you could play a part in introducing an activity that they may not be encountering in their physical education program or anywhere else. In wrapping up this chapter I offer some activities and unit plans for two sports that might not be normally covered. Whether or not you ever decide to use these specific lessons they should provide you some ideas for equipment modifications and lesson/unit planning.

TRACK & FIELD UNIT

Preface: the culminating activity of this unit is an *in-class track meet*. Every event is taught and practiced before the class track meet is held. Emphasize to the children that everyone's effort contributes to their team's performance so each child must do the best he/she can. If they encourage everyone on their team they improve their team's chances of doing the best they are capable of. No put downs are allowed. Only positive encouragement used.

Skills taught:
    1. Look Pass: distance relay
    2. Shuttle Pass: shuttle relay
    3. Hurdle form – i.e. lead leg & trail leg
    4. High jump form:
        a) scissors method
        b) Fosbury flop method
    5. Shot put form (intermediate grades only)
    6. Team cooperation toward healthy team competition

EVENT # 1: SHUTTLE RELAY
Points of emphasis:
    * use right hand only to pass and receive baton.

* hold baton like a candle (i.e. at the bottom with the flame on the top).
* receive at the top of the baton (i.e. the candle flame).
* "Punch" the baton against the body to slide the hand down to the bottom of the baton.
* always run past the next runner to the left of them (i.e. never cross the baton across your body).
* declare the number of passes you want the teams to make and then have the team members count them out loud as they make the passes.
* first team to have everyone sitting in line gets 4 pts, next gets 3 pts, etc... the last gets 1 pt.

***** _____ *****
             the four teams are split with half the team on each end of the gym
***** _____ *****

***** _____ *****

***** _____ *****

EVENT # 2: DISTANCE RELAY
Points of emphasis:
* *Look pass:*

    Outgoing runner
    * face shoulders toward inside of track and put left foot back
    * put inside hand (i.e. left) back with palm facing up.
    * look over inside (i.e. left) shoulder.
    * start to jog slowly when "incoming" runner crosses the warning line.
    * when incoming runner has placed the baton into you hand immediately transfer the baton into your right hand as you pick up speed.

    Incoming runner
    * baton should be in your right hand.
    * place baton into outgoing runner's left hand

General considerations:
* outgoing runner is the key because he/she is the freshest.
* outgoing runner must judge the speed of the incoming runner and not take-off too fast/
* outgoing runner must never run backward even though they look back.
* intermediate grades run from 5-7 laps.
* primary grades run from 3-5 laps each.
* have next runner up and in the outgoing runner position immediately after preceding runner has started his/her last lap.
* first team to be seated and in line gets 4 pts, next gets 3 pts and so on.

Making Games & Sports Fun & Educational

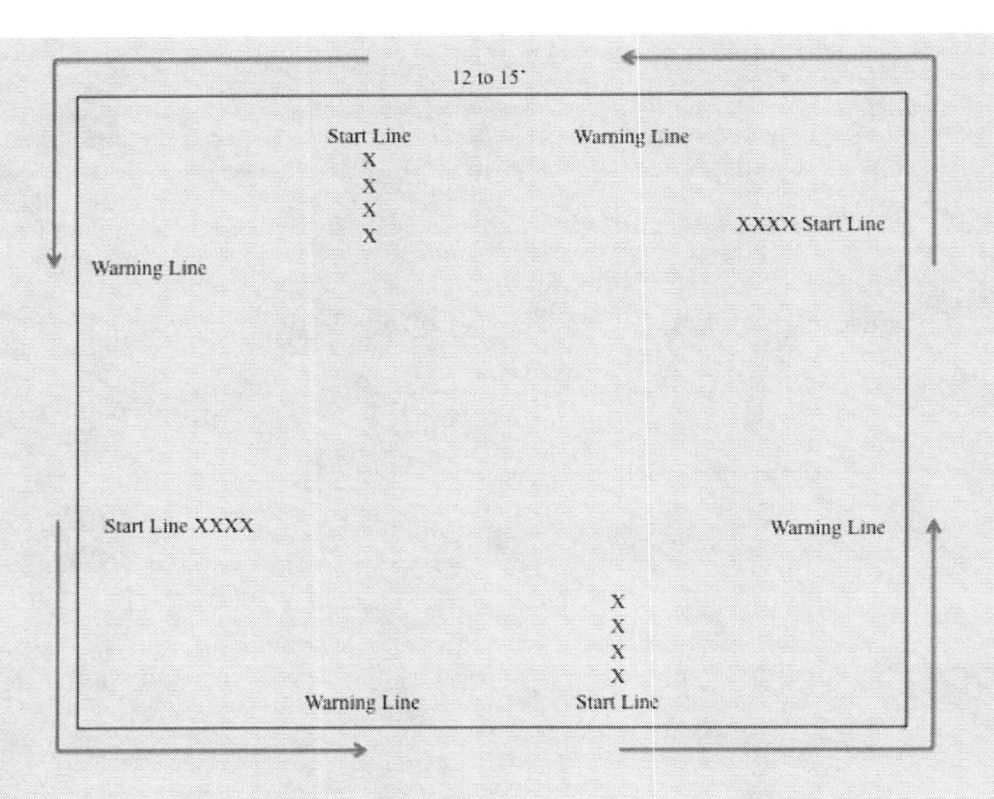

```
                    12 to 15'
         Start Line          Warning Line
             X
             X
             X                        XXXX Start Line
             X
   Warning Line




   Start Line XXXX                    Warning Line

                              X
                              X
                              X
                              X
         Warning Line     Start Line
```

EVENT #3: HURDLES

Points of emphasis:
- * "lead" leg is straight as possible.
- * "trail" leg is bent and toe is out to the side.
- * try to run over the hurdles and not to high jump over each one.
- * do the "layout" position hurdle stretch and imagine you are on top of the hurdle.

General considerations:
- * the hurdles (foam) can't hurt you.
- * don't slow down if you knock the hurdle over.
- * have two flights of hurdles going – one flight a bit higher than the other to allow for a challenge to those able to do it.
- * students must be able to go over the lower flight of hurdles without knocking over any of them before they are allowed to go over the higher flight.
- * adjust the heights according to the grade level and by the legs being used in an upright or flat position.
- * have three hurdles in each flight and have a mat at the end to run into.
- * allow kids to time practice runs.
- * always come back to the start along the outside of the hurdles and never between the hurdles.

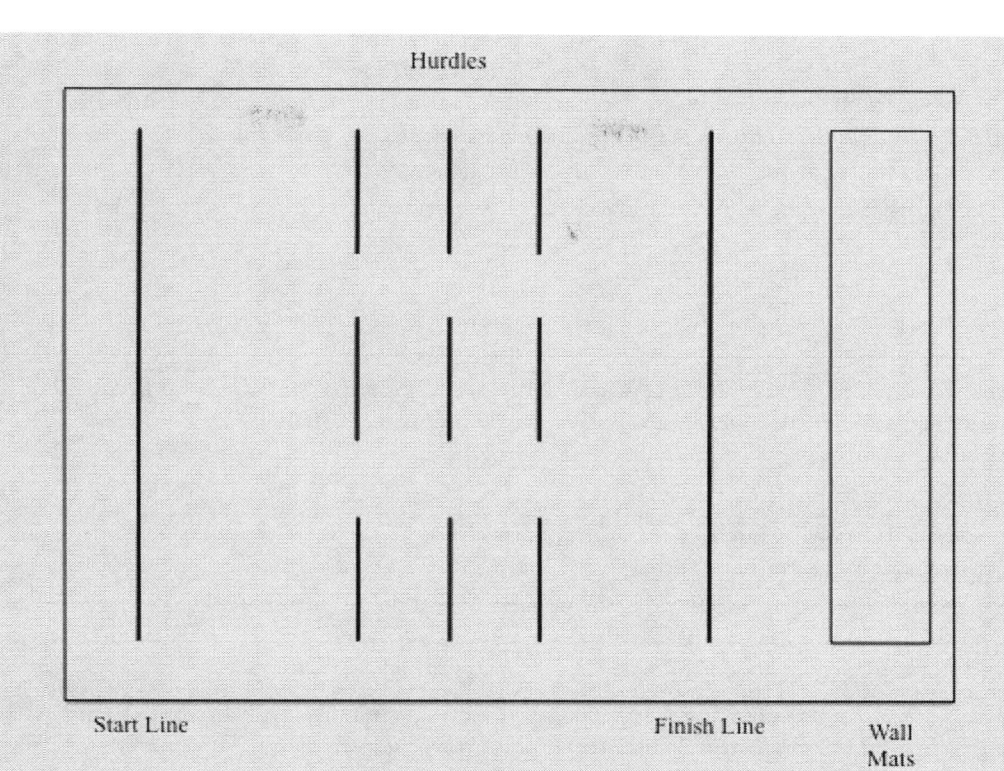

Diagram: Hurdles course with Start Line on left, Finish Line, and Wall Mats on right. Three rows of hurdles are shown between the start and finish lines.

EVENT # 4: HIGH JUMP

Points of emphasis for scissors style:
- start with scissors jump.
- emphasize straight legs.
- "near" leg goes up and over first.
- land on feet.
- try from both sides of bar to see which side is most comfortable to get the near leg up first.

Transition to Fosbury flop:
- same near leg as scissors but it is bent.
- instead of legs going over bar first, turn your back toward the bar and have your seat go over first.
- land on your seat.
- gradually try making your shoulders go over bar first by arching your back and landing on your back.

General considerations:
- let everyone get over a low height.
- give everyone a second chance at the lowest height to ensure a clearance and a team contribution.

* have one team at a time line up at the start cone of their choice (having already been determined in practice sessions).
* once a person has missed in the competition they may go and practice over the hurdles while others are still participating in the high jump.
* emphasize landing in the middle of the landing mat.
* some can't help but do the straddle where the stomach faces the bar and the outside leg goes over the bar first.
* during practice jumping the jumper may indicate to the event workers how high bar should be. This allows for appropriate comfort levels.
* make sure the side safety mats are always up against the side of the landing mat.

EVENT #5: SHOT PUT (FOR 4TH, 5TH, AND 6TH GRADES ONLY
Points of emphasis:
* THIS IS A PUT – NOT A THROW!!! This means that the shot must always precede the elbow in the direction of the put.
* start with the right foot facing the opposite direction of the put and the shot tucked under the right side of the chin. (these directions are for a right-handed putter so reverse the hands and feet directions for a left hander)
* the left hand is pointing down toward the back of the putting area so that the putter is leaning over at the waist with the body weight over his/her right foot.
* the shot is held in the fingers of the hand and not down in the palm.
* the putter then rapidly and forcefully scribes an arc with his/her left hand upward at about a 45 degree angle as he/she shifts the body weight to the left foot. During this motion the shoulders are rotating toward the front of the putting area and the shot is put off the shoulder in the direction of the putting area. The shot must precede the elbow in order to save damage to the elbow joint.
* EXTREME CARE MUST BE FOLLOWED SO THAT NO STUDENT IS IN THE PUTTING AREA WHEN THE SHOTS ARE BEING PUT!!!
* four putters can put at the same time but they may not be released to go get their shot until the teachers says "Retrieve your shot". This will ensure that no student gets hit with a shot.
* all other putters on the team are behind a line that is behind the putting area.
* make sure all four putters are in the starting position at the same time so that they are ready to put at the same time.
* the teacher's commands are: ("Putters ready" "Put" "Retrieve your shot")
* taped lines at 10, 15, 20, 25, and 30 feet are put on the floor and if the shot hits the line or beyond it the putter gets credit for that distance.

```
30'_____  30'_____  30'_____

25'_____  25'_____  25'_____

20'_____  20'_____  20'_____

15'_____  15'_____  15'_____

10'_____  10'_____  10'_____

Putting _____      _____    _____     _____
Line      X         X          X          X
_____
Safety line
```

HANDBALL UNIT (K-1)

LESSON 1 (GRADES K-1)
Activity: Eye/Hand Coordination Drills
Objective: (1) Develop eye/hand coordination. (2) Develop one-handed striking skills of smaller objects.
Equipment: Balloons, large Nerf (foam) balls
Facility: Any controlled area. Indoor area is better.
Drills: (1) Student taps (strikes) balloon 3 times with right hand. Same with left. (2) Student taps balloon once with right hand and once with left hand. (3) "See how many times you can tap with your right hand." Same with left. (4) RELAYS: Groups of 2 or 4. Student does tapping activity then passes balloon to next person. (5) "Tap the balloon to yourself with your right hand, then tap to your partner." (6) "How many times can you tap with your right hand in 10 seconds?" Same with left. (7) Student taps balloon within a limited space, such as a hula-hoop. As tapping in a controlled space is mastered, movement may be even more limited by having student kneel or sit within the hoop.

LESSON 2 (GRADES K-1)
Activity: Eye/Hand Coordination Drills
Objective: (1) Develop eye/hand coordination. (2) Develop catching skills.
Equipment: Bean bags
Facility: Any controlled area
Drills: (1) Student tosses bean bag up (no more than 3 feet) with right hand and catches with right hand. Repeat several times. Same with left hand. (2) Student tosses bean bag up with right hand and catches with left hand. Repeat several times. Same, only left to right. "How many times can you toss and catch in 15 second?" (3) With partner about 6 feet away, student tosses to partner with right hand. Partner catches with right hand and tosses back. Repeat several times. Same with left. (4) Student performs previous drills within a limited space, such as a hula-hoop.

LESSON 3 (GRADES K-1)
Activity: Eye/Hand Coordination Drills
Objective: (1) Develop eye/hand coordination. (2) Develop one-handed striking skills of smaller objects.
Equipment: Smaller Nerf balls, sponge balls or yarn balls
Facility: any controlled area. Indoor area is better.
Drills: Same as in Lesson 1
Comments: The same drills may be used, but, if possible, make them more challenging (more repetitions or for a longer time, or in a more limited space). Emphasize "Watch the ball," or "Watch your hand make contact with the ball."

LESSON 4 (GRADES K-1)
Activity: Drop and "Push"
Objective: (1) Develop eye/hand coordination. (2) Develop striking skills

Equipment: 10-inch playground ball

Facility: Any area that is flat, wall space

Drills: (1) Student holds ball at waist (with two hands), drops and catches (with two hands). (2) Student is positioned approximately 5 feet from wall. Student drops and "pushed" the ball to wall and catches on rebound after first bounce. (3) Student continues same drill with increasing repetitions. (4) Repeat with one or two hands.

Comment: (1) Emphasize "watching" the ball. (2) Students who are able to perform drills with one hand should be encouraged to do so.

LESSON 5 (GRADES K-1)

Activity 2 Square (modified)

Objective: (1) Understand the concept of striking. (2) Participate in a partner activity.

Equipment: 10-inch playground ball

Facility: Any area that is flat and can be marked with line

Drills: (1) Partner A drops ball and hits to his/her partner (one or two hands). Partner B catches and repeats. This game is similar to Newcomb volleyball. (2) Student performs previous drill while hitting with dominant hand only. (3) Student performs previous drill while hitting with non-dominant hand.

Comments: (1) Regulation 2 Square size (6' x 12' or 9' x 18') will work, although a smaller size will probably work better. (2) Bouncing or dribbling is a good warm-up or lead-up. "Watch your hand hit the ball." (3) Make this a cooperative activity by having partners work together to see how many repetitions they can complete before the ball bounces twice or gets away. (4) Emphasize "watching the ball."

LESSON 6 (GRADES K-1)

Activity: 2 Square (one hand without catch). This is regular 2 Square, but contact with the ball can be made with one hand at a time.

Objective: (1) Understand the concept of striking. (2) Participate in a partner activity.

Equipment: 10-inch playground ball

Facility: Any area that is flat and can be marked with line

Drills: (1) Partner A drops ball and hits (one hand) to his/her partner. Continue. (2) Student performs previous drill with specified hand.

Comments: (1) Emphasize cooperative theme. "You want your partner to hit the ball." (2) If the ball does not bounce in the correct area (on partner's die of line), student should catch the ball and start again.

LESSON 7 (GRADES K-1)

Activity: 2 Square (one hand). This is regular 2 Square, but contact with the ball can be made with only one hand at a time.

Objective: (1) Develop one-hand striking ability. (2) Participate in a partner activity.
Equipment: 8 or 10-inch playground ball
Facility: Any area that is flat and can be marked with line
Drills: (1) Same as previous lesson. (2) Student performs previous drill while alternating hand (depending on the side of the body to which the ball rebounds).
Comments: (1) Some students may be able to work with 8-inch balls while others may need 10 inch balls. (2) Emphasize cooperative theme to avoid students striking the ball too hard. This can be done by using "time trials" (15 seconds – 1 minute). Have students count how many times they and their partners make contact with one hand. (3) Begin to emphasize use of non-dominant hand. "If the ball goes to your left side, use your left hand."

LESSON 8 (GRADES K-1)
Activity: Rebound Activities
Objective: (1) Understand the angles of rebound. (2) Intercept a rolled or thrown ball rebounding from a wall.
Equipment: 8-inch playground ball
Facility: Level area, wall space
Drills: (1) Student rolls ball to wall and retrieves ball on rebound. (2) Partner A rolls ball to wall, Partner B retrieves. Alternate. (3) Student tosses ball to wall and catches after first bounce. (4) Partner A tosses ball to wall, Partner B catches after first bounce. Alternate.
Comments: (1) Tosses to wall should be tow-handed underhand or easy chest passes. (2) If possible, a line drawn on the wall about 2 feet from the ground will indicate how high tosses need to be. Emphasize cooperative theme. "You are working WITH your partner." (4) If possible, students need to start 5 feet away from wall. If students are extremely successful, you may want to back them further from the wall. (5) Students could work in groups of 4. Two partners would participate (for time or completion of a task) while the other two partners act as retrievers about 10 feet back. Alternate pairs.

LESSON 9 (GRADES K-1)
Activity: Striking Drills (dominant hand)
Objective: (1) Develop striking skills. (2) Participate in partner or small group activity.
Equipment: 8-inch playground ball
Facility: Level area, wall space
Drills: (1) Warm up with Lesson 8 drills. (2) Student stands behind line 5 feet from wall and drop ball to floor. As ball bounce up, student hits it to wall. Student then catches rebounding ball after first bounce. (3) Partner A drops and hits ball to wall. Partner B catches after first bounce. Alternate. (Alternate pairs or rotate). (4) Relay activities – Use same drill as (3). Instead of 'partner', use 'next person'.
Comments: (1) Emphasize cooperative theme. "You want your partner to be successful." (2) A hit ball should rebound from the wall and make contact with the ground in front of the 5-foot line. "If the

ball bounces behind the 5 foot line, it is out of bounds." (3) Ideally, students should contact the ball about waist high. (4) Individual drills can be done singularly, or in small groups while taking turns. Partner drills work best with 4 students.

LESSON 10 (GRADES K-1)
Activity: Striking Skills (non-dominant hand)
Objective: (1) Develop striking skills. (2) Participate in partner or small group activity.
Equipment: 8-inch playground ball
Facility: Level area, wall space
Drills: Same as previous lesson except done with non-dominant hand

LESSON 11 (GRADES K-1)
Activity: Striking Skills (dominant hand)
Objective: (1) Develop striking skills. (2) Participate in partner or small group activity.
Equipment: 8-inch playground ball
Facility: Level area, wall space
Drills: (1) Warm-up with previous drills. (2) Student tosses ball to wall and strikes rebounding ball after first bounce. Partner acts as retriever about 10 feet back. Alternate. (3) Partner A tosses ball to wall. Partner B hits rebounding ball after first bounce. Alternate. Another pair acts as retrievers. Alternate pairs or rotate.
Comments: (1) Retrievers (partner or other pair) need to be about 10 feet back. (2) Begin to introduce "position." Ideally, student should have side to the wall when striking the ball (as in baseball), especially when striking the ball from a shoulder high or lower position. "Face the front wall more when striking from higher than shoulder high."

LESSON 12 (GRADE K-1)
Activity: Striking Skills (non-dominant hand)
Objective: (1) Develop striking skills. (2) Participate in partner or small group activity.
Equipment: 8-inch playground ball
Facility: Level area, wall space
Drills: Same as previous lesson except done with non-dominant hand

LESSONS 13, 14, 15 (GRADES K-1)
Activity: One-Wall Handball
Objective: (1) Develop striking skills. (2) Develop eye/hand coordination. (3) Participate in partner activity. (4) Participate in a "lifetime sport." (5) Understand the concept of rebound.
Equipment: 8-inch playground ball, 6-inch playground ball for the more skilled students
Facility: Level area, wall space
Comments: Partner A starts rally from behind the 5-foot line. Partner B returns the ball, and partners attempt to rally (hit the ball to the wall before the ball bounces twice on the floor). Ball must rebound

from wall and bounce in front of the 5-foot line or it is considered out. This game should be played in a cooperative way. "Try to hit the ball so your partner can hit it." Have students count how many times they can keep the ball in play. Alternate pairs or rotate. Retrievers should be encouraged to go after ball as quickly as possible.

HANDBALL UNIT (2-5)

LESSON 1 (GRADES 2-5)
Activity: 2 Square (1 handed). Students play regular 2 Square, but contact must be made with one hand.
Objective: (1) Understand the basic concept of striking. (2) Participate in a partner activity.
Equipment: 8 inch playground ball (Grades 2,3), 6 inch playground ball (Grades 4,5)
Facility: Any area that is flat and can be marked with lines
Comments: (1) Emphasize "watching the ball." (2) Encourage students to use non-dominant hand, as well as dominant hand. (3) Make this a cooperative activity. Have partners work together to see how long they can keep the ball in play. "You want to make your partner successful"

LESSON 2 (GRADES 2-5)
Activity: same as previous less
Objectives: Same as previous lesson
Equipment: Same as previous lesson
Facility: same as previous lesson
Comment: Especially with grades 4 and 5, challenge students to play with non-dominant hand only

LESSON 3 (GRADES 2-5)
Activity: Eye/Hand Coordination Drills
Objective: (1) Develop skill of one-handed striking of small objects. (2) Develop eye/hand coordination.
Equipment: Balloons, large Nerf balls
Facility: Any controlled area. Indoor area is better.
Drills: (1) Student hits balloon (or Nerf ball) 5 times in a row with right hand. Same with left. (2) "how many times can you hit the balloon with your right hand in 30 seconds?" (3) "How many times can you alternate hitting with your right, then your left, then right, and so on?" (4) "How many times in a row can you and your partner hit with your right hands only?" Same with left. (5) RELAY Activities – Divide students into small groups. Have student perform same drills, then pass balloon to next person.
Comments: (1) Number of completed tasks (i.e. five in a row) or time (i.e. 30 seconds) will vary according to grade level. (2) Bouncing or dribbling 6-inch balls or racquetballs (grades 4 and 5) is a good warm-up activity. "Watch the ball hit your hand."

LESSON 4 (GRADES 2-5)
Activity: Eye/Hand Coordination Drills
Objective: Same as previous lesson
Equipment: Yarn balls, balloons. Racquetballs (Grades 4 and 5).
Facility: Same as previous lesson
Drills: same as previous lesson

Comments: (1) Increase the number of times students need to hit in a row, or increase the time in which students attempt to make maximum successful contacts. (2) In grades 4 and 5, alternating hands while bouncing the racquetball is a good warm-up activity.

LESSON 5 (GRADE 2-5)
Activity: Throwing – Sidearm and overhand (dominant hand)
Objective: (1) Develop sidearm throw with proper reciprocation. (2) Develop the overhand throw with proper reciprocation.
Equipment: Racquetballs
Facility: Wall space, level area
Drills: (1) Student throws ball to wall with overhand stroke and catches after first bounce on rebound. (2) Partner A throws ball to wall with overhand stroke. Partner B catches on first bounce after rebound. Alternate. (3) Partner A throws ball with sidearm stroke. Partner B catches after first bounce on rebound. Alternate. (4) RELAY activities – Same drills as above except substitute 'next person' for 'partner'. Have students work in small groups.
Comments: If using racquetballs, have students (grade 2 and 3) start about 10 feet from wall when throwing ball. If 6-inch balls are used, the distance should be shorter. Grades 4 and 5 should start about 15 feet from wall when using racquetballs.

LESSON 6 (GRADES 2-5)
Activity: Throwing – Sidearm and Overhead (non-dominant hand)
Objective: (1) Develop sidearm throw with proper reciprocation. (2) Develop the overhand throw with proper reciprocation.
Equipment: Racquetballs
Facility: Wall space, level area
Drills: Same as previous lesson except done with non-dominant hand.
Comments: (10) Student should attempt to imitate the throwing motion of dominant hand. (2) Pay particular attention to the footwork. "Step toward the wall as you throw."

LESSON 7 (GRADE 2-5)
Activity: Drop and Hit (dominant hand)
Objective: (1) Develop striking skills. (2) Develop eye/hand coordination.
Equipment: 6-inch playground balls (grades 2,3), racquetballs (grades 4,5)
Facility: Wall space, level area
Drills: (1) Student drops the ball (bounces it) and hits it to the wall with a sidearm stroke. Student retrieves as next student moves to line to hit. This works well in groups of 4. Grades 2 and 3 should start about 8 feet from the wall and grades 4 and 5 should be about 15 feet from the wall. ALL grades should start with 6-inch playground balls. Grades 4 and 5 should progress to racquetballs. (2) Partner A drops and hits ball to wall with sidearm stroke. Partner B attempts to catch ball after first bounce.
Comments: (1) Remember, the hitting stroke should imitate the throwing stroke. (2) When students begin to hit the racquetball, encourage them to "cup your hands and relax your arms." (3) Students

can work in groups of 4 in a rotation. The 3 back may serve as retrievers and boundaries (far enough back so that they are not in the way and they can prevent the ball from going past them). Students rotate one position counterclockwise after completed task.

LESSON 8 (GRADES 2-5)
Activity: Drop and Hit (non-dominant hand)
Objective: (1) Develop striking skills. (2) Develop eye/hand coordination.
Equipment: 6-inch playground balls (grade 2,3), racquetballs (grades 4,5)
Facility: Wall space, level area
Drills: Same as previous lesson except done with non-dominant hand.
Comments: Make sure students drop ball far enough away from their body so that their elbow is slightly bent as the hand contacts the ball.

LESSON 9 (GRADES 2-5)
Activity: Move and Hit (dominant hand)
Objective: Develop striking skill when contacting a thrown ball rebounding from a wall.
Equipment: 6-inch playground balls (grades 2,3), racquetballs (grades 4,5)
Facility: Wall space, level area
Drills: (1) Student stands behind line and tosses ball to wall so that it rebounds in front of line. Student attempts to hit ball to wall before ball bounces twice on floor. Grades 2 and 3 start 8 feet from the wall. Grades 4 and 5 start 15 feet from the wall. Student retrieves own hit as next student moves to line to toss (or 3 back can retrieve). (2) Partner A tosses ball to wall. Partner B moves and hits rebounding ball to wall. Other pair of partners may retrieve. Alternate. Alternate pairs or rotate.
Comments: (1) Always emphasize cooperative theme. Keep score (number of successful hits) of partners – NOT individuals. "You want to make your partner successful." (2) If a partner throws the ball to the wall, and it rebounds back toward himself, he/she should quickly move out of the way so as not to interfere with the partner's hit.

LESSON 10 (GRADES 2-5)
Activity: Move and Hit (non-dominant hand)
Objective: Develop striking skill when contacting a thrown ball rebounding from a wall.
Equipment: 6-inch playground balls (grades 2,3), racquetballs (grades 4,5)
Facility: Wall space, level area
Drills: Same as previous lesson except drills done with non-dominant hand
Comments: Throws that begin drills should be with dominant hand.

LESSON 11 (GRADE 2-5)
Activity: Rally
Objective: (1) Develop striking skills. (2) Participate in a partner activity.
Equipment: 6-inch playground balls (grades 2,3), racquetballs (grade 4,5)
Facility: Wall space, level area

Drills: (1) Student stands behind line (8 or 15 feet) and tosses ball to wall and attempts to hit the ball to the wall in succession as many times as possible. Ball must bounce in front of line after rebounding from wall. (2) Partner A stands behind line and tosses ball to wall. Partner B attempts to hit the ball back to the wall. Then Partner A attempts to return, and so on. Partner pairs alternate, or players rotate.

Comments: (1) If a continuous rally is too difficult, make the goal 2 hits or 3 hits. (2) Emphasize use of non-dominant hand. Perhaps require rally to start with a hit by non-dominant hand. (3) Player who hits ball must make every effort to get out of the way of the other player attempting to hit. Students must understand that this is a rule.

LESSONS 12, 13, 14, 15 (GRADES 2-5)

Activity: One-Wall Handball

Objective (1) Participate in a partner activity. (2) Develop eye/hand coordination. (3) Develop striking skills with both hands. (4) Learn and participate in a "lifetime sport" activity.

Equipment: Wall space, level area

Comments: (1) Students begin rally by hitting ball to wall from behind line. Rally continues as long as: (a) Ball rebounds off wall in front of line. (b) Students return ball to wall before it bounces twice (rebounding ball does not have to bounce; it can be hit "on a fly"). (c) Ball goes directly to wall after leaving student's hand. (2) Instead of the winner of the rally serving the next ball, have one player serve for 3-5 rallies, and then the next player. (3) This is a good activity for the 4-person rotation set-up. The ball will get away many times, and the 3 back players may serve as retrievers.

CHAPTER COMPREHENSION CHECK

The concept of *anticipatory set* is re-introduced. What is it?
What is the author's *Three-Rule Rule* and *The Expansion Principle*?
My *SOS Principle* is re-introduced. What is it?
What is the legal standard we are held to regarding the safety of our students?
What are at least three commonly played games what are considered unacceptably dangerous by the legal profession?
What is the concept of *Actively Waiting*?
What is the *Mini-Games* concept?
What is the concept of *Eliminate the Elimination*?
What are the three different types of game structures? What are the particular strengths of each?
Why do some teachers and schools disapprove of offering competitive games and sport during the school day? How might others argue otherwise?
The *Fifty-Percent Minimum Activity Standard* is re-introduced. What is it?
What is the *Team-Size Rule of Thumb*?
What are the basic rules of *Over-the-Line Softball* and *Bonkerball*? What would be some of the advantages of playing these games over an "official" softball game?
The concept of the *Slave-Market Approach* was warned against in Chapter 7. What is it?
What was the author's stance on playing for official rules and using official size bats, ball, clubs, etc.?
What were the author's ideas for matching competitors ability-wise, and what were his arguments for doing so?
What is meant by the *contextual aspects of sports*?
What is the concept of *hyper-competition*?
What is the philosophy of *Sports Education*?
Approximately what percent of children remain inactive during free play periods?
What are the basics of the *Traditional (Technical)* and the *Games Approach (Tactical)* to teaching sport skills?
What are considered the two major drawbacks of the *Traditional Approach*?
What is the *Overexposure* concept?
Sports can be placed into categories containing common tactical strategies? What are those categories and how might they be useful to a curriculum planner?

Making Games & Sports Fun & Educational

[CHAPTER 10]

ASSESSMENT OF THE PSYCHOMOTOR DOMAIN

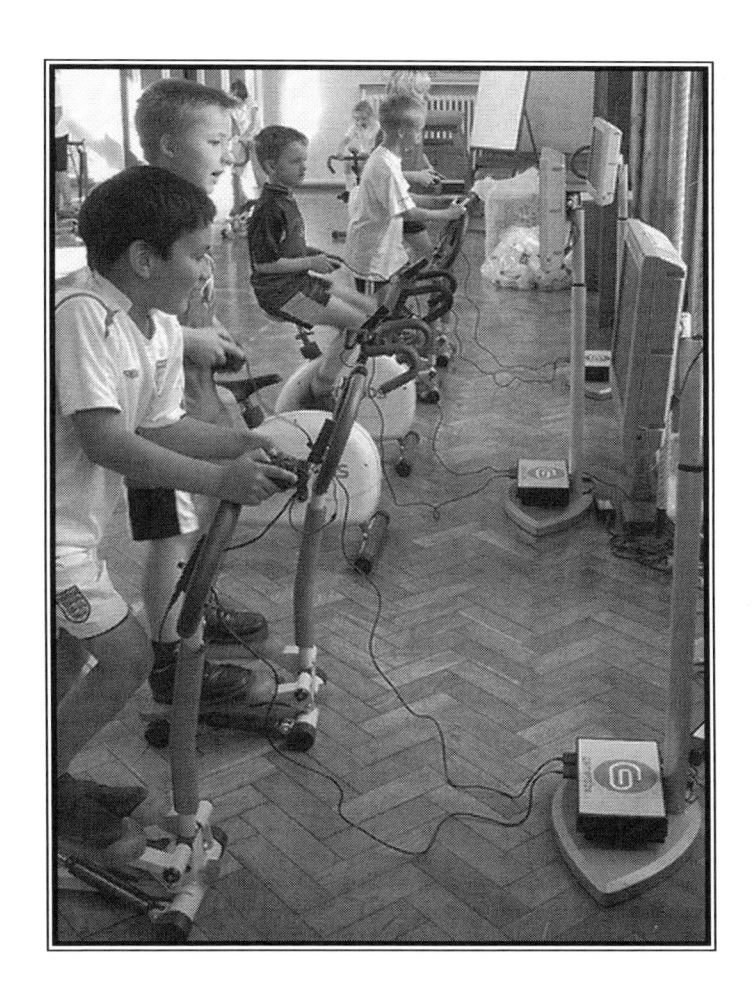

EVALUATION OF PHYSICAL ACTIVITY

Physical Activity Assessment Instruments
Self-Report Logs
Pedometers
Heart-Rate Monitors

EVALUATION OF PHYSICAL FITNESS

What Does a Physical Fitness Test Tell?
Three Approaches to Physical Fitness Testing
The Traditional Approach
The Personal Approach
The Challenge Approach
Selecting a Physical Fitness Test
The President's Challenge
Fitnessgram

EVALUATION OF MOTOR SKILLS

Formal vs. Informal Evaluation
Process vs. Product Evaluation
Authentic Evaluation
Holistic Evaluation

REPORTING & GRADING OF THE PSCHOMOTOR DOMAIN

Reporting
Grading

CHAPTER COMPREHENSION CHECK

> *"That which gets measured gets done."*
> ~ Ralph Waldo Emerson

> *"Increasing a child's aerobic capacity or maximal strength should be a by-product of games and activity not the primary goal"*
> ~ Charles Corbin

This is the age of educational assessment. Over my forty some years of teaching I have never experienced such a monomaniacal emphasis on testing. School administrators and teachers are all feeling the pressure to measure and document the achievement of ever expanding national, state and/or district standards. Physical education specialists are being expected to produce objective data in the health and fitness domain. They are asked to verify what cognitive, affective, and pyschomotor skills have been acquired or will be acquired on some scheduled date. And if the school has not been able to afford adequate physical education staffing, those assessment responsibilities necessarily devolve upon the classroom teachers.

Beyond being well versed in measurement techniques to meet these weighty administrative demands, having good evaluation procedures serves a number of practical, helping functions. They can provide you with more personal accountability of your instruction and offer insights regarding teaching methods that work and those that need reconsideration. But by far the most important role it can have is that of lifting the motivation of you and your students. What can be more rewarding than clear evidence that you indeed are having a positive effect on the knowledge and behavior of the children? No matter how hard your work may be, or how marginal your financial gains, teaching is a joy when you know that you have made an impact. However, without this assuring verification, doubt, weariness and burnout can threaten. Also, like teachers, the children's enthusiasm can easily wane when there are no noticeable improvements. This discouragement can be countered when you provide them with data verifying that they are doing more sit-ups then earlier in the year or that they are making measurable improvements in their throwing skills. Learning is often a painfully slow process and we must miss no opportunities to help children appreciate learning whenever it occurs. Telling yourself or the children that progress is being made might be sufficient, but sometimes more tangible evidence is needed.

In this chapter you will be introduced to a variety of ideas concerning how you might evaluate your students' practices and skills in the psychomotor domain. We will separately look at assessing physical activity, physical fitness and motor skills.

EVALUATION OF PHYSICAL ACTIVITY

If you will recall from Chapter 2, a primary goal is to move children into an active lifestyle. More specifically we ideally want children to adhere to *The Activity Pyramid*. At the basic level young people should be establishing lifestyle behaviors that that will result in at least 60 minutes of light/moderate activity everyday (*The Lifetime Physical Activity Model*). And hopefully, in addition to that, they will be participating in both vigorous aerobic activities at least three times per week and muscular strength/dynamic flexibility activities three or four times per week.

With this being a worthy, agreed upon goal, it is most strange to me that so little evaluation of physical activity has been done in the schools. I believe it should be the responsibility of all physical educators to assess each class they teach to determine whether or not what they did that day was likely to increase the probability that their students would be physically active tomorrow and in the future. A suggestion is to base program success on an average school increase in physical activity. What could be more important for health and wellness than increasing the amount of activity that children accumulate on a daily basis? Most parents would be delighted if their children were taught to live an active lifestyle. That could be one of the best legacies a physical education program could leave students.

The evaluation of movement could easily be begun in a simple informal manner. It would not have to be any more complex than asking for responses or a show of hands. You could ask how many felt like they got some good exercise in class. You might use *The Perceived Exertion Scale* to help them judge the intensity of their performance. Or you might get estimates of the physical activity engaged in outside of class, "Over the weekend, how many participated in at least 60 minutes of physical activity?" "How many remembered to do their sit-ups yesterday?" Research confirms that self-reports are reasonably reliable with children over age 10. I know from experience that it can be hugely rewarding to get an indication that some students are being influenced by my instruction. And if I happen to receive an indication that many were not following through as I had hoped, that too was good for me to know.

To take the above informal assessment one small step further you might easily and profitably begin to record and track their movement behaviors. "Let's put up on the board the number of us who were able to get an hour of activity the previous day and we will see if we can do even better the rest of the week." Maybe you could begin recording the number of children participating in a walking program or the level of activity of some formerly inactive students during recess. Another idea is to have the children begin tracking their own behaviors. Simple log keeping could be a good skill for them to learn and it could be made a part of their portfolios. Checking those logs could be a useful way to verify the effect of your instruction.

Physical Activity Assessment Instruments

In recent years, three technological instruments have begun to be used in schools to measure physical activity: Self-Report Logs, Pedometers, and Heart-Rate Monitors.

Self-Report Logs

Recently, a variety of reliable and valid physical activity assessments tools have been developed specifically for children. While most have been developed primarily for research purposes, here are two that would be easy to use in your classroom with your intermediate grade students. The simplest would be the *Centers for Disease Control (CDC) Activity Calendar*. If you have your students google CDC BAM (Body and Mind), and then click on the *Activity Calendar*, they will find a simple calendar for planning and recording their weekly activities. The other useful self-report log is the ACTIVITYGRAM developed by the Cooper Institute for Aerobics Research. It works by having the children log in three days worth of activities and then gives them a print out of reinforcements and recommendations (Figure 10.1).

Having students use and maintain logs of these kind could be an excellent assignment for the students. They would provide great information for class discussions and could be used for reinforcing and grading purposes. Even though promoting out-of-school physical activity is the stated goal of physical education teachers, a recent study found that less than 5 percent of their lesson actually prompted or rewarded the students for out-of-school participation. Regular referencing to these calendars could help remedy this omission.

Figure 10.1. ACTIVITYGRAM

Previous Day Physical Activity Recall

Name _____ Teacher _____ Grade _____ Date _____

Think back to yesterday after you finished school. For each of the 30-minute periods, select a primary activity that you performed and put the number in the Activity Number box. For each activity, then check how hard the activity was in terms of physical effort. Use the terms 'Very Light¹, 'Light', 'Medium' or 'Hard' to estimate the intensity. Light is like slow walking, medium is like fast walking and hard is like fast running.

		ActivityNumber	Very Light	Light	Medium	Hard
Afternoon	3:00					
	3:30					
	4:00					
	4:30					
Supper	5:00					
	5:30					
	6:00					
	630					
Evening	700					
	7:30					
	8:00					
	8:30					
	9:00					
Night	930					
	10:00					
	10:30					
	11:00					

Health AND *Fitness* An Elementary Teacher's Guide

Activity Numbers

Eating	Work/School	16.	25. Use skateboard
1. Meal/Snack	8. Homework	17.	26. Play organized sport
Sleep/Bathing	9. House chores	**Physical Activities**	27. Did Individual exercise
2. Sleeping	**Spare Time**	18. Walk	28. Did active game outside
3. Resting	10. Watch TV	19. Jog/run	29. Other (list) _____
4. Shower/bath	11. Go to movies/concert	20. Dance (for fun)	
Transportation	12. Listen to music	21. Swim (for fun)	
5. Ride in car, bus	13. Talk on phone	22. Swim laps	
6. Travel by walking	14.	23. Ride Bicycle	
7. Travel by bike	15.	24. Lift weights	

Pedometers

Pedometers are small devises worn on the belt and rather accurately measure how many steps a person takes. They function by means of detecting the simple pendulum action of each stride, whether it be walking or running. They cost between $11 and $22 apiece, depending on the type, so the outlay for a class of 36 would be between $400 and $800. In many cases, parent-teacher associations have agreed to fund pedometers after learning about their value form a presentation made to the group. Most models will translate steps taken into miles covered and calories burned. Some brands also track the amount of time moving, a feature that is useful if you have an activity-time goal.

Pedometers can teach students about accumulating activity not just during the school day but outside of class as well. They are effective at showing kids that everyday *lifestyle activities* can make a valuable contribution to health. A visit to google will discover endless ways to use pedometers creatively.

Classroom teachers and students can wear pedometers during the school day. At the end of the day, students check the number of steps they have accumulated. Physical activity goals are then discussed and set, and students try to meet their personal goal for two consecutive days. Students can be asked to monitor their parents or another significant adult for one day. To be considered to have an active lifestyle and derive significant health benefits a commonly set daily goal for adults is The 10,000 Steps Criteria. Depending on stride length, 10,000 steps translate into around 5 miles. The purpose of this assignment is to familiarize parents with the need for daily activity and to make them aware of their own and their children's activity levels. A brisk 30-minute walk usually requires approximately 3,800 to 4,000 steps. Research shows that the average classroom teacher takes around 3,000 to 7000 steps per day.

Rather than "a one standard fits all" approach, I favor using a baseline and goal-setting technique. This method requires that each individual identify his or her average daily activity (baseline) level. For elementary school students, this requires four days of monitoring pedometer step counts (or activity time). For adolescents and adults, it requires eight days of activity monitoring (because their days are much more variable). After the baseline level of activity has been established, each individual has a reference point for setting a personal goal. The personal goal is established by taking the baseline activity level and adding 10 percent more steps to that level. For example, assume someone has a baseline of 6,000 steps plus 600 (10 percent) more steps for a total of 6,600 steps. This will be the personal goal for the next two weeks. If the goal is reached for a majority of the days during this two-week period, another 10 percent (600) is added to the goal and the process is repeated. For most people, a top goal of 4,000 to 6,000 steps above their baseline level is a reasonable expectation. Using the example of 6,000 baseline steps here, a goal of 10,000 to 12,000 steps would be the ultimate activity level.

Pedometers can be used to evaluate the baseline activity levels of students at or near the start of the school year and then used to monitor their activity a number of times throughout the school year. School administrators might accept a two percent increase in physical activity accumulated as a school-wide goal over an 18-week period. Activity levels both in and out of schools could be used as separate outcomes. Out-of-school activity can be regarded as physical education homework.

A good way to increases enthusiasm for pedometer use is with a school-wide steps contest. The step counts of all students in each class, including the teacher, are added and then divided by the number of students. Finding the average number of steps for the entire class makes this a group competition and avoids putting down students who are less active. A gentle reminder here is that students should not have to reveal their step count unless they choose to do so. A sensitive approach is to have the students place their step counts anonymously on a tally sheet.

PEDOMETER CHALLENGE
CALCULATING STRIDE LENGTH

CHALLENGE NO. 1: Estimate the number of steps that you think it would take you to walk a mile.
CHALLENGE NO. 2: Walk one mile (4 laps around a 440 yard track) wearing a pedometer. Walk with normal, regular strides. Record the number of steps that it took to cover the mile distance.
CHALLENGE NO. 3: How many feet are in a mile. Figure your stride length with the information you have gathered (5,280 feet divided by number of steps).

Heart-Rate Monitors

Heart-rate monitors consist of a chest belt that detects a person's heart rate and a wristwatch that picks up that information for display. They can be used to inform the student and teacher of exercise intensity and whether or not the performer is in his or her aerobic training zone. The devises are as of yet rather expensive and thus it is difficult to use them in large classes or for outside of class assignments. Nevertheless some teachers like to have students take turns wearing them and then discussing the findings with the rest of the class.

Although elementary students can be taught to use heart-rate monitors, I have not found them to be particularly accurate in monitoring and interpreting their readings. I believe that the time it takes to teach and use the procedures could probably be better spent engaging children in activity. More global and less time-consuming indicators of intensity, such as sweating, breathing hard, and the *Perceived Exertion Scale* are likely more useful in elementary schools. And of course there is the question of what types of activity you are prioritizing. Heart-rate Monitors place all the emphasis upon the vigorousness of activity and remaining in a determined target heart rate zone. Elsewhere in this text I have made it clear that children are inherently interval trainers, preferring short bouts of activity interspersed with rest. Expecting them to enjoy adult like, steady-state, high-intensity exercise is unrealistic for most of them.

EVALUATION OF PHYSICAL FITNESS

What about physical fitness testing? What does it tell us? How should we use them? Which test should we use?

What Does a Physical Fitness Test Tell?

There are four basic factors that determine how well a child will do on a physical fitness test. Before referring to Figure 10.2, ask yourself what you think these factors may be and select which of those might have the most pronounced effect. Have you done so? Okay. The amount of "physical activity" the child is engaging in might have been the most obvious one and the first to come to your mind. After all, the more one is exercising the better they will be prepared for the test. The "lifestyle" factor is referring to things like sleep, nutrition, stress, and medical care. Inadequacies in any of these areas, singly or particularly in concert, can potentially impair vigorous performance. The "heredity" factor is simply the recognition that each individual is born with unique capabilities in the various components of physical fitness. Some people are going to be inherently many times stronger than others, while others may be far more flexible, or leaner, or have greater aerobic capacities. These large genetic variations are often known as The *Principle of Individual Differences*. Finally, "maturation" is recognition that children develop at different rates. I hope you did not forget this one. A child may naturally mature a year or even two years earlier or later than the norm of his/her age group. This means that even if your class contains children of all the same chronological age, it can be expected, due to early and later maturing, there will exist a developmental range potentially as large as four years. Obviously, those children who develop earlier will have a decided advantage on many components of fitness.

Figure 10.2. Factors Contributing to Fitness Test Scores

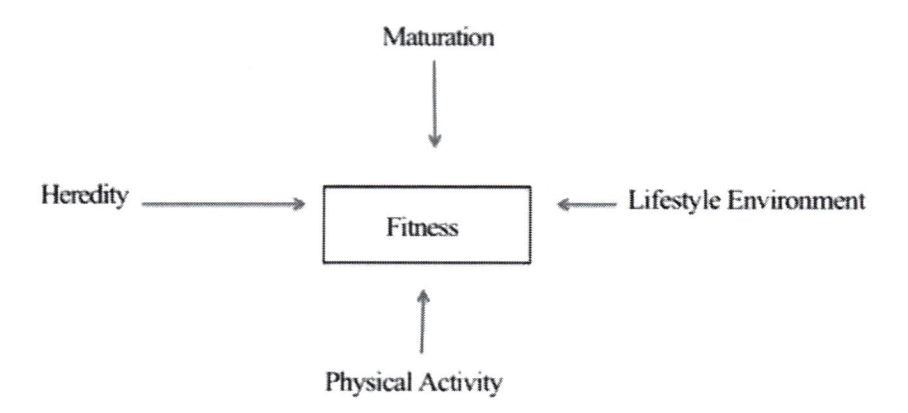

Of the above four factors, it is important to understand that the combination of the latter two, heredity and maturation, have much the dominant impact on children's fitness test scores. It is estimated that genetic abilities alone account for well over half the variances in performance. This is true for both children and adults. Also, the typical four-year spread in maturational levels can mightily impinge upon performance. Allow me to give an example of some research that dramatically accents this point. A number of years ago some physiological data was collected on ballplayers participating in the "Little League World Series" held in Williamsport, Pennsylvania. Teams were drawn from all across the United States and from many other nations. The young players were eleven and twelve years old. Measurements of bone density and pubic hair growth confirmed that the most dominant players (the clean-up hitters, pitchers) had an average maturational age comparable to fourteen-year-olds. Clearly early maturation was playing a major role in their successful performance.

We need also understand that exercise and lifestyle do not affect children's physical fitness scores nearly as much as they do for adults. This is true because pre-pubescent children are not as *trainable* (remember this term from Chapter 3) as are adults. They simply do not yet have all the hormones that needed to physiologically adapt to exercise. Nor have the environmental factors of inactivity and poor lifestyle choices had years to accumulate and degrade fitness. How well adults do on a physical fitness test much better reflects lifestyle choices than tests of children, and as adults age this becomes even more the case. In youth we can abuse our bodies with much less immediate consequences than we can later on. This reminds me of a pertinent poetic passage, *"Oh for boyhood's painless play, / Sleep that wakes in laughing day, / Health that mocks the doctor's rules, / Knowledge never learned in school, ... / Oh that thou couldst know thy joy, / Ere it passes, barefoot boy!"*

Now that we know what a physical fitness test might or, more to the point might not tell us the teacher, what may the results be telling the child? To them, what could be the implication of a low correlation existing between their fitness test performances and their health practices? Consider these two scenarios. Child A has been dutiful and conscientiously following your exercise and nutritional prescriptions throughout the year. But because he is maturing slower than most of the other children, and because he is not particularly genetically gifted or *trainable* in a number of fitness components, he still makes only modest gains and sees that his fitness test performance is far below most of his peers. Quite naturally that child may be despondent and discouraged. His conclusion could be "What's the use? Why try?" Clearly such a reaction would be a demonstration of *learned helplessness*. Research data has confirmed that poor performance on a fitness test has a tendency to reduce a child's motivation to engage in further physical activities.

In our second scenario, Child B has not been so carefully adhering to advisable exercise or eating practices; in fact, she may be wallowing in a foul sink of sloth and nutritional debauchery. But, because she happens to be maturing early and is relatively physically gifted, she scores near the top of the class on the fitness test. What does she think? She might erroneously feel reassured that her habits are just fine, even though they are leading her down the primrose road to some future health problems.

Okay, where does all this leave us? Are physical fitness tests archaic, not worthwhile or even counter productive? Should they be abandoned? Not necessarily. The manner in which we do the testing could determine whether the motivational effects are good or bad. Let us judge the merits of three possible approaches.

Three Approaches to Physical Fitness Testing

Traditional Approach

The *traditional approach* is where everyone is required to take the test. Test performance and scores are carefully evaluated and counted by judges to ensure accuracy. Also, the test results are distributed to everyone, with the better performers typically receiving special recognition in the form of patches, certificates or public displays of names. Some of these tests are *norm referenced* because a child's performance is compared to other children either within the school, the school district, or nationwide. To earn the special recognition of having passed the test, a percentile score of something like 50 or 80 percent must be achieved on all the test items. *Criterion reference* tests are those in which a cut-off level has been set for each component of fitness. The level is an arbitrary one, but it is hoped to represent a minimal level of fitness below which none of the children should fall. Under this system it is of course theoretically possible that everyone could be recognized for passing.

Possibly there is something to be gained from the schools accurately tracking the physical fitness status of its students. It may identify areas of strengths or weaknesses and might detect significant group trends. However, to fulfill this institutional role it is doubtful that yearly instructional and administrative time is justifiable. Perhaps a few spot checks throughout the school years would be sufficient (maybe once in the upper- elementary, middle school, and high school years). Whatever the schedule, because testing for these purposes is large scale and needs to be very accurately done to ensure reliability and validity, it should normally fall under the province of the physical education specialist.

Traditional testing is also justified on motivational grounds; namely, the existence of the tests will serve to make the children more diligent about their fitness. We need to be careful here. As discussed earlier, even if all the children do view it as an incentive to work determinedly on their fitness, some likely will still fail to perform well on the test because of maturational, genetic and trainability factors. These people could be very deflated by the results, particularly if they are normative evaluations. I would say that another danger is that many of the lower fitness students will not be motivated to do well on the test because they already know that it would be futile for them to try. They perceive they are low in fitness, and the approach of the testing process is only something to dread. They fear their ineptitude will be displayed in a highly public forum. Physical skills are highly valued in children; can you not empathize with the feelings of a child struggling, and failing to do a pull-up in front of a waiting line of peers? Or chugging along with a red face as other students are lapping you? The net effect seems to be one in which those possessing above average fitness abilities are likely being motivated (although some of the very fittest may not be because the cut-off levels are too easy for them) while those of low fitness, who are most at risk and in need of encouragement, are being ill served.

Personal Approach

The essence of the *personal approach* has the children less formally self-testing themselves and then setting individual goals. Suppose you thought it important for the children to do regular sit-ups so as to have firm abdominal muscles. Besides having them do sit-ups in class and encouraging them to continue outside of class, you add an evaluation component. Shortly after introducing the concepts of how and why to do abdominal exercises you say, "Let's all give ourselves a test to see where we are. Following these procedures do as many sit-ups as you possibly can." After they have completed the task, you tell them to remember how they did and to be prepared for the same test latter in the term. You also encourage each to set a reasonable personal improvement goal.

To my mind, this personal approach to testing has some real pluses. Although the students' self-scoring may not be as accurate as under the traditional instructor scored system, it should tend to be motivational to all the students. Everyone should be capable of making some improvement toward his/her *self-performance goal*. The potential for embarrassment is minimal because everyone is simultaneously working and not likely to be standing about watching others. Also, their results and goals are private, maybe known only to themselves, the teacher, or to those friends with whom they wish to share.

The personal testing approach could take on more elaborate forms if you so chose. A battery of test items could be administered where the children either scored or worked with a partner. The goal setting process could involve you sitting down with each child and helping them set and write challenging, but reasonable goals. Practice plans and schedules could be designed. Short-term enabling objectives could be established and monitored. Incentives and recognition could be developed for all those who achieve their goals. Everything could be made a part of their portfolios. This sort of personal *self-performance goal* setting process could be a valuable learning experience for teaching perseverance.

Challenge Approach

Some of you might give credence to the potential problems of the traditional testing approach, and yet you are not comfortable in evaluating only on improvements and totally dispensing with fitness standards. Surely you are thinking, there can be some goodness in establishing a desirable fitness standard and recognizing those who can attain it. The *challenge approach* to physical fitness testing is the same as the *traditional approach* but with the exception that participation is voluntary. Using this system we might announce a physical fitness "challenge" test to be administered near the end of the term or year. It is to be an extra-class event scheduled during a lunch hour or after school. You explain what the test consists of and what standards must be achieved to pass the test. You make clear that passing the test may not be possible for everyone and that those planning on participating will need to be seriously training for it. A few special training practices may even be planned.

The *challenge approach* is much like that with which we take in sports and in many other disciplines. If a child shows good aptitude in the track or gymnastic activities introduced in class, we quite appropriately would encourage them to go out for a school or club team and thus maximize their talents. If a child were good in music or math we would attempt to integrate him/her into any programs, clubs or contests which might exist in these fields.

Selecting a Physical Fitness Test

A good first step in deciding what to evaluate is to ask yourself what it is you believe in most strongly and what kind of instruction and experiences have you been giving the children. It makes little sense to give a physical fitness test, or any test for that matter, if you have not been assiduously teaching for improvement. If you have been encouraging the students to engage in aerobic activities than you want to use a test that assesses that component of fitness. If you have devoted attention to diet and calorie burning then assessment of body fat is in order. My view is that those components of physical fitness which are most related to long-term health are of central concern. In Chapter 3 it was pointed out that all the components of fitness can relate, in one way or another, to both our athletic performance and our long-term health. However, we saw that some components play a more significant role in health than others. Aerobic cardiovascular fitness and body fat control would certainly need to be listed as such because of their relationship to common disabilities. Tests that focus on these aspects of health are classified as *health related physical fitness tests.* Anaerobic fitness and muscular power play a big part in many sports activities but much less of a central one for long-term health. Tests that include assessment of these aspects of fitness are classified as *performance related physical fitness tests*. Example items they would be testing would be a sprinting shuttle run, standing broad or vertical jump, or softball throw for distance. It can be seen that coaches in many different sports might be interested in testing some of these.

There are many different physical fitness tests from which you can select and possibly your school district may already have a policy for using one. The two most widely used national physical fitness tests are *The President's Challenge* developed by the President's Council on Physical Fitness and Sports and *FITNESSGRAM* developed by The Cooper Institute for Aerobics Research. The basics of each are described below. You should be able to discern that the FITNESSGRAM fits my philosophy better in that it focuses somewhat more on the health-related components of fitness, and sets healthy criterion levels for them.

The President's Challenge

The primary purpose of *The President's Challenge* has been to motivate children and youth age 6-17 to begin and continue an active lifestyle by providing awards for reaching appropriate fitness levels and engagement in an active lifestyle. Different attractive patches are awarded for each of the five awards. Suggested guidelines are included for accommodating special needs students.

The Presidential Active Lifestyle Award rewards an active lifestyle. Students who are active for 60 minutes per day, five days per week, for six weeks are eligible for this award. They are encouraged to repeat their participation throughout the year, earning a series of stickers placed on the certificate indicating the number of times the award has been won.

The Presidential Physical Fitness Award recognizes an outstanding level of physical fitness. Boys and girls who score at or above the 85th percentile on all five items of *The President's Challenge*: (sit-ups or partial sit-ups, shuttle run, endurance run/walk 1/4 mile – 6-7 year old, 1/2 mile – 8-9 year old, 1 mile – 10-17 year old, pull-ups or right angle push-ups, v-sit reach or sit and reach) are eligible to receive the award. Emblems are numbered to correspond with the total number of times the award is earned.

The National Physical Fitness Award recognizes the achievement of a basic yet challenging level of physical fitness. Boys and girls scoring at or above the 50th percentile on all five items on *The President's Challenge* are eligible to receive this award.

The Participant Physical Fitness Award recognizes boys and girls who attempt all five test items on *The President's Challenge* but whose scores fall below the 50th percentile on one or more of them.

The Health Fitness Award recognizes students who achieve a healthy level of fitness. As with the physical fitness award, the HFA is given based on the results of a five-item assessment: (partial sit-ups, one mile run/walk: 1/4 mile 6-7 year old, 1.2 mile 8-9 year old, 1 mile 10-17 year old, V-sit: sit and reach, right angle push-ups or pull-ups and a measurement of body mass index). Body Mass Index is an easy way, based on height and weight, to estimate body composition without actually measuring body fat.

Assessment of the Psychomotor Domain

Fitnessgram

FITNESSGRAM is a comprehensive health-related fitness and activity assessment and computerized reporting system. All elements within *FITNESSGRAM* are designed to assist teachers in accomplishing the primary objective of youth fitness programs, which is to help students establish physical activity as a part of their daily lives. Criterion-referenced standards are used to evaluate fitness performance. These standards have been established to represent a level of fitness that offers some degree of protection against diseases that result from sedentary living. Performance is classified in two general areas: "Needs Improvement" and "Healthy Fitness Zone" (HFZ). In Figure 10.3 are the test items. All students are expected to strive to achieve a score that places them inside the HFZ. *FITNESSGRAM* acknowledges performance above the HFZ but does not recommend this level of performance as an appropriate goal level for all students.

Figure 10.3. FITNESSGRAM Test Items

Aerobic Capacity
Teachers select one of the following:
  * The PACER
  One-mile run
  The walk test (secondary students)

Body Composition
Teachers select one of the following:
  * Skinfold measurements
  Body mass index

Abdominal Strength & Endurance
Teachers must select this:
  * Sit-up

Trunk Extensor Strength & Flexibility
Teachers must select this:
  * Trunk lift

Upper Body Strength
Teachers select one of the following:
  * Push-up
  Modified pull-up
  Pull-up
  Flexed arm hang

Flexibility
Teachers select one of the following:
  Back-saver sit and reach
  Shoulder stretch

* Recommended test.

Research findings were used as the basis for establishing the *FITNESSGRAM* health fitness standards. With regard to aerobic fitness level, studies have shown that a significant decrease in risk of mortality results from getting out of the lower 20% of the population. Aerobic capacity standards for the HFZ have been established so that the lower end of the zone corresponds to getting out of the lower 20 percent of the population. The upper end of the Healthy Fitness Zone corresponds to a fitness level that would include up to 60 percent of the population.

The higher end of the body composition HFZ corresponds with 25 percent body fat for boys and 32 percent for girls. This is based on research showing that boys and girls with body composition readings above these figures are much more likely to have elevated cholesterol levels and hypertension. The lower end of the HFZ corresponds with 8 percent body fat for boys and 13 percent for girls. Some students may be healthy at lower levels of percent body fat but it is good to detect those that are this lean so that they know that they could encounter health problems. Also, it could be a tip-off of those who might be suffering from an eating disorder. It is important to understand that the interpretation of body composition from both skinfold measurements and the body mass index (BMI) are only estimates. Even if you have good experience using skinfold methods measurement error of 3 to 5 percent are expected. The body mass index, because it is based on height and weight measures, also has a degree of inaccuracy in that it tends to overestimate the amount of body fat in the heavier boned and muscular students, and underestimate the amount of body fat in the smaller boned and less muscular.

There are four other positive aspects of the *FITNESSGRAM* that deserve mention. The first is the *ACTIVITYGRAM*, which was discussed, in the first part of this chapter. It is very useful in reliably measuring physical activity and of course can be used in conjunction with or separately from the fitness test. It is designed to fit nicely in with *The Activity Pyramid* guidelines.

The *PACER* test is the recommended test of aerobic performance. The students are paced by music as they run back and forth between cones that are placed 20 meters apart. The music gradually becomes faster and the children try to keep up with it as long as they can. Their score is based on how many laps they are able to do. It is easy to administer, valid and reliable, and kids generally like it much better than a mile run test. Kindergarten through third-graders enjoy doing the *PACER* test but it is not recommended that any scores be recorded at this stage. Just let them do it as long as they are having fun. It usually will only take a few minutes before they are tired.

Third, a strong feature of the *FITNESSGRAM* is its software. It is easy to use and the outcome printouts are very complete. The data is easy to enter and best of all, it is possible for the students to do the entering themselves. They can enter both their test scores and also their physical activity logs for the *ACTIVITYGRAM*. As the students enter data there are useful helping prompts.

Finally, there are some useful testing items and procedures for students with special needs.

Assessment of the Psychomotor Domain

EVALUATION OF MOTOR SKILLS

In Chapter 2, my overriding goals were to get children active and eating healthily. I did not give the acquisition of motor skills primary goal status. Some authorities feel otherwise. They believe that developing strong movement skills should be the central purpose of physical education experiences. Teaching and evaluating them should be a core part of the program. They see the possession of good motor skills as critically important to the ultimate adoption of active lifestyles. Without good skills participation options are greatly limited and we do not normally choose to pursue endeavors for which we feel inept.

I do not disagree that the learning of motor skills is something we wish to accomplish. The only reason I did not give it primary priority is that research has failed to show a strong relationship between physical skill competency in students, and their health and activity levels in adulthood. The correlation between the two is a positive one, but a very weak positive one. I personally have known many people who were not particularly physically active in school but who subsequently integrated regular exercise, sports or recreational activities into their adult routines. Conversely, I have known many ex-scholastic and collegiate athletes who now are very much sedentary. Be this as it may, helping children acquire good movement skills surely is a good thing, we should be teaching them as much as we can, and assessing there acquisition whenever possible.

Motor skills can be broken into two kinds: *fundamental* and *sport specific*. *Fundamental motor skills* are skills can be broken into *locomotor fundamental motor skills* such as walking, running, skipping, jumping, leaping, sliding, and galloping. *Object control fundamental motor skills* are throwing (underhand and overhand), catching, kicking, and striking. There are two reasons it is hoped that children will acquire these skills during the primary grades. Firstly, these skills form the underlying basis of all future sports performance. Possession of these basic movement skills is said to have a positive *transfer* effect on the learning of sport skills. For instance, if a child has never learned the step-hop sequence involved in skipping, it likely will be difficult for him/her to later learn to perform a sport specific basketball lay-up which involves this skipping action. If he/she has not first learned to make a lateral slide step, later difficulties will be encountered when having to move quickly to the side when guarding a soccer player or covering a tennis court. It is obvious how the fundamental skills of running, throwing, catching and striking are prerequisite to sports that demand specific versions of those movements.

The second reason it is desirable for young children to master these fundamental skills is the terrific significance they have at this developmental stage. These motor skills tend to be valued more highly than all other aspects of a child's life. If a child cannot run or catch nearly as well as his/her peer group, it can be a bitter dose to a young and forming self-concept. We adults, who have come to place greater value on many other intellectual and affective aspects of our lives, sometimes forget the once paramount significance of showing parents and playmates that you were good at jumping rope, hitting a ball, or that we at least could keep up with others and participate in the common cultural games.

Of course, it is ultimately desirable that children learn not only the *fundamental motor skills* but that they also then apply those skills to achieving some more advanced skills in specific sports. The larger one's repertoire of *specific sport skills* the greater the likelihood of adoption of an active lifestyle. Those who own these movement tools will be more successful at an expanded array of activities and will be less prone to injuries.

Before beginning to discuss the particulars of evaluating fundamental and sport specific skills, permit me to make a couple more points concerning the need of these skills being taught in the schools. Many people mistakenly assume that *fundamental skills* are acquired as a natural part of the maturation process. Although these skills are basic movement patterns, they are by no means instinctual and must therefore be practiced just as is any other skill. Granting that basic motor skills must be learned, others will say that young children are inherently active and learn these skills as a result of their own volition; witness them racing about, you literally cannot stop them from exuberant running, hopping, and bouncing. While there is truth in granting high energy levels to young children, we need understand that in today's society not all children are getting a wealth of movement experiences. In my introductory chapter I mentioned a number of environmental factors which were causing less activity in young people: the multifarious media attractions, reduction of safe play areas, greater reliance on motorized transportation, more unsupervised latch-key situations, etc. Not only does less activity mean demonstrably lower physical fitness levels, it also brings lower movement skills. Because of the more movement-restricting environment that many of today's children face, we are seeing a greater share of children exhibiting deficient fundamental skills. Also, it is worth noting that the early grades are considered a *critical period* for learning these skills; this is when most children are gaining these skills and if a child falls behind, it is generally the case that they will fall further behind rather than catch-up in later grades. Remedial programs for adults are commonly not effective because of the stigma of spending time working on skills which have long ago been mastered by our peers. Also, some recent research suggests that learning skills during these formative years has an affect on the structural formation of the brain. Skills not learned during this period may never be learned to a high level.

Finally, a point needs to be made about teaching sport specific skills during the school day. There is growing evidence that more and more school-aged children are deficient in a variety of sport skills. Why is this the case? Although many young people participate in youth sports programs, there still are those who are not involved, and many more that do so for only a limited length of time. A majority drops out of sports programs as early as elementary and junior high school ages and the trend towards earlier dropout has been occurring. Furthermore, even the more athletically advanced children who remain in youth sports are tending to acquire a narrower range of sport specific skills. This is because of a dramatic trend toward earlier and earlier specialization in single sports. A sports arms race to have the best team has been developing at the university and high school levels. This pressure is reverberating all the way to the youth sports level. The competition is tough and the coaches, parents and children are affected by it. The less talented are weeded out sooner and the more talented are channeled into year round devotion to one sport. This sports specialization undoubtedly results in higher skill attainment in the selected sport, but it also means they may be less prepared to diversify and enjoy other sporting activities later in life. If all one has done is focus on basketball, football, or soccer throughout school, will he/she not have missed out on some other athletic experiences? Will he/she easily be able to join a softball team, a master's swim club, a tennis league?

Formal vs. Informal Evaluation

Suppose you are convinced of the importance of motor skills and would like all your students to have adequate levels of them. But you foresee a couple of problems. For one thing, you may not have had an athletic background and hence do not feel sufficiently qualified to teach and evaluate in this area. The second problem is that even though you may have enjoyed sports and feel competent, you are afraid that evaluation of your student's motor skills will necessitate the addition of too great a burden on your other already heavy teaching responsibilities; as much as you might wish to, you simply cannot visualize yourself having time to be judging and recording everyone's performances.

Both of these doubts about sufficient knowledge and feasibility are legitimate practical concerns in need of being addressed. In response to competency concerns I would only say this, if your background skills are not great, you obviously must bow to your limitations and not expect to instruct and evaluate many skills. That is okay. However, surely you have knowledge of some basic movement patterns and can recognize major flaws. This might be particularly true with regards to the most fundamental elements of walking, running, or hopping, etc. As for your fear that motor skill evaluation will be too time demanding let me begin by giving you two examples of motor skills being assessed. Teacher A will represent a very complete and formal approach to evaluation, teacher B will be highly informal.

Teacher A desires that all her third graders have good fundamental motor skills. Early in the year she teaches her students a circuit training system in which they move from station to station while being paced by music. Twice each week she positions herself at one of the stations. Armed with a list of fundamental motor skills test (Figure 10.4) and a checklist, she evaluates groups of four or five children as they rotate by. On the first day she might be able to assess the entire class on the criteria associated with each of the skills of running, skipping, and sliding (each criterion is scored as mastered, partially mastered, un-met). The next day, as she has the children throwing and catching balls, she measures the criteria related to those skills. After approximately four or five testing sessions everyone has been evaluated. The test results are then used in a variety of ways: she uses them as a guide to insure that she provides instructional help where deficiency have been identified, she files the results for future accountability sessions with administrators, and she has the outcomes sent home to the children's homes with a cover letter. The letter informs the parent(s) why it is important for their child to be mastering these basic skills at this developmental time. It also solicits their helping at home and tells them to anticipate another set of test results towards the end of the year.

Figure 10.4. Fundamental Motor Skills Test

FUNDAMENTAL LOCOMOTOR SKILLS:
   RUN
      1. Brief period in which both feet are off the ground
      2. Arms in opposition to legs, elbows bent
      3. Foot placement near or on line (not flat footed)
      4. Non-support leg bent approximately 90 degrees (close to buttocks)
   GALLOP
      1. A step forward with the lead foot followed by a step with the trailing foot to a position adjacent to or behind the lead foot
      2. A brief period in which both feet are off the ground
      3. Arms bent and lifted to waist level
      4. Able to lead with the right and left foot
   HOP
      1. Foot of the nonsupport leg is bent and carried in back of body
      2. Nonsupport leg swings in pendulum fashion to produce force
      3. Arms bent at elbows and swing forward on take-off
      4. Able to hop on the right and left foot
   LEAP
      1. Take off on one foot and land on the opposite foot
      2. A period in which both feet are off the ground (longer than running)
      3. Forward reach with arm opposite the lead foot
   HORIZONTAL JUMP
      1. Preparatory movement includes flexing of both knees with the arms extended behind the body
      2. Arms extend forcefully forward and upward reaching full extension above the head

3. Take off and land on both feet simultaneously
4. Arms are brought downward during landing

    SKIP
1. A rhythmical repetition of the step-hop on alternate feet
2. Foot of nonsupport leg carried near surface during hop phase
3. Arms alternately moving in opposition to legs at about waist level

    SLIDE
1. Body turned sideways to desired direction of travel
2. A step sideways followed by a slide of the trailing foot to a point next to the lead foot
3. A short period in which both feet are off the floor
4. able to slide to the right and to the left

FUNDAMENTAL OBJECT CONTROL SKILLS

    TWO-HAND STRIKE
1. Dominant hand grips the bat above non-dominant hand
2. Non-dominant side of body faces an imaginary tosser (feet parallel to the batting tee)
3. Hip and spine rotation
4. Weight is transferred by stepping forward with the front foot

    STATIONARY BOUNCE
1. Contact ball with one hand at about hip height
2. Push ball with fingers (not a slap)
3. Ball contacts floor in front of (or outside of) foot the side of hand being used

    CATCH
1. Preparation phase in which elbows are flexed and hands are in front of the body
2. Arms extended in preparation for ball contact
3. Ball is caught and controlled by hands only
4. Elbows bent to absorb force

    KICK
1. A rapid continuous approach to the ball
2. The trunks is inclined backward during ball contact
3. Forward swing of the arm opposite the kicking foot
4. Follow-through by hopping on the non-kicking foot

    OVERHAND THROW
1. A downward arc of the throwing arm initiates the windup
2. Rotation of hip and spine to a point at which the non dominant side faces an imaginary target
3. Weight is transferred by stepping with the foot opposite the throwing hand
4. Follow-through beyond ball release diagonally across body toward side opposite the throwing hand

Teacher B also is aware that it is beneficial for children to have sound motor skills. He does not have an extensive background in sports but he has played softball and can recognize a fundamentally good throw from a bad one. He knows for instance that it is essential to step forward with the foot opposite the throwing hand and that a good follow-through is one in which the arm finishes down across the body. One day he takes his second grade class out to play a game called "messy backyard." The game's arrangement has the class divided so that half the children are on one side of the play space and the others on the other. These areas are known as their "backyards." A number of yarn and nerf-balls have been equally distributed to both areas. When he shouts, "go," both sides are to clean up their yard as quickly as possible by throwing the cluttering balls from their yard to the other sides. Constant throwing ensues by everyone until the stop command is given. While the game is in progress our teacher B monitors the action and also looks to see if there is anyone throwing with poor technique. If anyone is noticed, he makes a mental note of finding an opportunity to give him/her a corrective tip or two.

It is apparent that Teachers A and B are at opposite ends of a formality in evaluation continuum. Teacher A's formal system is to be admired and it likely would yield more thorough results than teacher B. However, the methods used by Teacher A are much more demanding of time and preparation, maybe more demanding than can be generally expected of most classroom teachers and even physical education specialists. Certainly, in this dawning age of outcome based education, all physical education specialists will be required to implement this sort of in-depth evaluation. Instead of making independent decisions about which if any skills to assess, they will be held accountable for specific learning standards developed by state or professional organizations. And of course, if a school does not have a physical education specialist, or only minimal access to one, the mandated standards will still need to be met, and guess who might be ultimately asked to see that it is done – the classroom teachers?

To give you an idea of the kinds of skills children may be expected to demonstrate, refer to Figures 10.5. The Figure gives grade-specific benchmarks (K-4) established by The National Association for Sport and Physical Education (NASPE). Those states mandating outcome-based education will probably be developing their guidelines around a template much like these.

Figure 10.5. Fundamental Skill Benchmarks

KINDERGARTEN
The student is able to:
____ Travel in different ways, in a large group without bumping into others or falling.
    ____ Walk   ____ Skip   ____ Slide   ____ Gallop
    ____ Run   ____ Hop   ____ Jump
____ Travel in a forward and sideways direction, and change direction quickly in response to a signal.
    ____ Forwards
    ____ Sideways
    ____ Change direction in response to a signal
____ Distinguish between straight, curved, and zig-zag pathways while traveling in various ways.
    ____ Straight
        ____ Walk   ____ Skip   ____ Slide   ____ Gallop
        ____ Run   ____ Hop   ____ Jump
    ____ Curved
        ____ Walk   ____ Skip   ____ Slide   ____ Gallop
        ____ Run   ____ Hop   ____ Jump
    ____ Zig-zag
        ____ Walk   ____ Skip   ____ Slide   ____ Gallop
        ____ Run   ____ Hop   ____ Jump
____ Make both small and large body shapes while traveling.
    ____ Small shapes while traveling
    ____ Large shapes while traveling
____ Travel demonstrating a variety of relationships with objects.
    ____ Under while moving
    ____ Over while moving
    ____ Behind while moving
    ____ Alongside while moving
    ____ Through while moving
____ Without falling, walk forward and sideways the length of a bench.
    ____ Forward the length of a bench
    ____ Sideways the length of a bench
____ Roll sideways (right and left) without hesitating or stopping.
    ____ Roll sideways to the right
    ____ Roll sideways to the left
____ Toss a ball and catch it before it bounces.
____ Demonstrate the difference between an overhand and underhand throw.
    ____ Overhand
    ____ Underhand

Health AND **Fitness** An Elementary Teacher's Guide

_____ Kick a stationary ball using a running approach without hesitating or stopping.
_____ Continuously jump a swinging rope held by others.
_____ Form wide, narrow, or twisted bodies alone and with a partner.
    _____ Wide
        _____ *Alone*
        _____ *With a partner*
    _____ Narrow
        _____ *Alone*
        _____ *With a partner*
    _____ Twisted
        _____ *Alone*
        _____ *With a partner*
_____ Sustain moderate physical activity.

FIRST AND SECOND GRADERS

The student is able to:

_____ Travel in a backward direction and change direction quickly and safely without falls.
    _____ Travel backward
    _____ Change direction quickly
    _____ Does not fall
_____ Change speed and direction in response to various rhythms.
    _____ Change speeds: slow-fast, fast-slow
    _____ Change directions
        _____ Forward-backward
        _____ Backward-forward
        _____ Backward-sideways
        _____ Sideways-forward
        _____ Sideways-backward
    _____ Use a variety of rhythms
        _____ Four-counts
        _____ Eight-counts
_____ Combine traveling patterns in time to music
    _____ Walk with music
    _____ Run with music
    _____ Skip with music
    _____ Hop with music
    _____ Slide with music
    _____ Jump with music
_____ Jump and land using a combination of one and two foot take-offs and landings.
    _____ One foot take-off
    _____ One foot landing

   _____ Two foot take-off
   _____ Two foot landing
_____ Demonstrate skills of chasing, fleeing, and dodging to avoid or catch others.
   _____ Chases
   _____ Flees
   _____ Dodges
   _____ Avoids or catches others
_____ Roll smoothly in a forward direction without hesitating or stopping.
_____ Balance: Demonstrate momentary stillness in symmetrical and asymmetrical shapes on different body parts.
   _____ Right foot
   _____ Left foot
   _____ Both feet
   _____ Right knee
   _____ Left knee
   _____ Both knees
_____ Move the feet in a high level by placing weight on hands and landing in control.
   _____ Handstand against wall
_____ Use the inside of the foot or instep of the foot to kick a slowly rolling ball into the air or along the ground.
   _____ Uses the inside of the foot to kick a slow rolling ball.
   _____ Kicks ball into the air
   _____ Kicks the ball along the ground
_____ Throw a ball hard while demonstrating a correct throwing technique.
_____ Catch using properly positioned hands.
   _____ Fingers pointed up for ball caught above waist
   _____ Fingers pointed down for ball caught below waist
_____ Consistently dribble a ball using hands without losing control.
_____ Use at least three different body parts to strike a ball.
   _____ Hand to strike a ball to a target
   _____ Foot to strike a ball to a target
   _____ Forearm to strike a ball to a target
_____ Continuously dribble the ball using feet without losing control.
_____ Strike a ball repeatedly with a paddle to a wall or partner.
_____ Repeatedly jump a self-turned rope.
_____ Consistently strike a ball with a bat from a tee or cone, using the correct grip and side to target.
   _____ Can consistently strike a ball with a bat from a tee.
   _____ Uses correct grip
   _____ Side is facing target

_____ Skip, hop, gallop, and slide using age level motor skill.
    _____ Skip
    _____ Hop
    _____ Gallop
    _____ Slide
_____ Demonstrate safety when participating in physical activity.
_____ Identify appropriate behaviors when playing with others.

THIRD AND FOURTH GRADERS
The student is able to:
_____ While traveling, avoid or catch an individual or object.
    _____ Avoids individuals
    _____ Avoids objects
    _____ Catches individuals
    _____ Catches objects
_____ Leap, leading with either foot.
    _____ Right foot
    _____ Left foot
_____ Jump and land for height or jump and land for distance, using correct motor pattern.
    _____ Jump and land for height
    _____ Jump and land for distance
_____ Roll in a backward direction without hesitating or stopping.
_____ Transfer weight from feet to hands at fast and slow speeds, using large group extensions.
    _____ Transfers weight from feet to hands
    _____ Transfers fast from feet to hands
    _____ Transfers slow from feet to hands
_____ Hand dribble and foot dribble a ball
    _____ Hand dribble
    _____ Foot dribble
_____ Strike a softly thrown lightweight ball back to a partner using a variety of body parts and combinations of body parts.
    _____ Can strike a thrown lightweight ball with thigh (as in soccer) back to a partner.
    _____ Can strike a thrown lightweight ball with the forearms (like a bump in volleyball) back to a partner.
    _____ Can use a combination of body parts - forearm, foot, etc.
_____ Strike a softly thrown ball with a bat or paddle while demonstrating correct grip, side to target, and level swing.
    _____ Can strike a thrown ball with a bat or paddle
    _____ Can demonstrate correct grip

   _____ Side is to target
   _____ Swing is level
_____ Develop patterns and combination of movement into repeatable sequences. (Grapevine)
_____ Without hesitating, travel into and out of a rope turned by others.
   _____ Into
   _____ Out of
_____ Balance, with control, on a variety of moving objects.
   _____ Balance boards
_____ Throw, catch, and kick using correct motor patterns.
   _____ Can throw with correct motor patterns
   _____ Can catch with correct motor patterns
   _____ Can kick with correct motor patterns
_____ Demonstrate competence in basic swimming stroke and water survival skills.
   _____ Competence in basic swimming stroke
   _____ Competence in survival skills
     _____ In water
     _____ On water
     _____ Around water
_____ Maintain continuous aerobic activity for a specific time.
_____ Maintain proper body alignment during activity.
   _____ Can lift correctly
   _____ Can carry correctly
   _____ Can push correctly
   _____ Can pull correctly
_____ Can support, lift, and control body weight in a variety of activities.
   _____ Can support body weight
   _____ Can lift body weight
   _____ Can control body movement
_____ Regularly participate in physical activity for the purpose of improving skillful performance and physical fitness.
   _____ Regularly participate in physical activity
   _____ Purpose of activity is to improve skill
   _____ Purpose of activity is to improve fitness
_____ Analyze potential risks associated with physical activity.
_____ Identify activities that contribute to personal feeling of joy.
_____ Enjoy feelings resulting from involvement in physical activity.

Although the advent of greater documentation of student learning can seem worrisome and daunting to both physical education specialist and classroom teachers, I do not feel we should conclude that these are totally unrealistic expectations. Rather, we must face the facts and learn to do it; it can be done. I know a number of teachers who are now very successfully finding ways of regularly integrating evaluation into their lessons and who feel that their teaching has been enriched as a consequence. Computer technology has been a savior for some. A good example is the use of hand held computers (palm pilots) for entering student behaviors and skill criteria data. These allow information gathered in the field to be directly downloaded on to a computer for storage and organization.

To conclude this section, it is clear that you will have to weigh a number of factors in making your decisions regarding the degree of formality of your evaluation practices. Your unique situation might favor your following the less systematic model of Teacher B. Hopefully, as did he, you will be on the lookout for opportunities to help some children over rough spots in their attainment of motor skills. Opportune aid to one or two could be so important. And on the other hand, if circumstances permit, perhaps it will be possible for you to year by year meet the challenge of developing a more elaborate, but workable, system of motor skill evaluation. It would be no small thing indeed if along with what you were teaching the children in the classroom you could play a significant role in insuring all your children become effective movers.

Process vs. Product Evaluation

Earlier in this chapter you were encouraged to consider evaluating whether or not the students were in the process of being physically active. That is what is important for health in the long run, and it is a realizable goal for everyone. We saw that measuring physical fitness outcomes was not as much under the students' control. Genetics and maturation rates skewed fitness scores.

When evaluating motor skills it is also useful to consider the difference between process and product outcome evaluations. *Process evaluation* of motor skills is where the focus is on how much the skill is being practiced and/or on the technique being used by the performer. If you or the child keeps a record of how much batting practice is occurring over a few week's time, that is evaluating the process. If you are judging the goodness of your students' dribbling technique or their volleyball service technique, that is also evaluating the process. The motor development test in Figure 10.4 would be considered process oriented, as are the *NASPE fundamental skills benchmarks* of Figure 10.5. Although the dividing line between process and product evaluation is not always perfectly clear, *product evaluation* is when the emphasis is on the outcome rather than how the skill is done. It is a product test when the measurement pertains to how fast someone runs a given distance or how far he/she throws a ball.

The arguments in favor of using *process evaluation* as opposed to *product evaluation* of motor skills are similar to those presented for physical fitness. The product outcome level a child is able to achieve on a motor skill, as with physical fitness, is going to be effected by not only the amount of practice but also by genetics and maturational status. If you test running speed or batting distance outcomes, your results might not always tell you who has been practicing the most or even who has best developed the proper running or swinging technique which will best serve them in the long term. Someone could be batting cross-handed and not correctly transferring his/her weight forward into the swing and yet, because of more advanced inherent development, is still hitting the balls further than all others. Conversely, another child could be employing an essentially sound technique and still have less than mediocre outcome success.

> Assess the Process and the Product Will Follow
> Assess the Product and the Process is Hollow

Because a child's motor outcomes are determined in large part by genetics and maturation, outcome achievements are to only a minor degree under the students' control; this is not true regarding the process of doing the skills. With the exception of some children with physical disabilities, everyone will have sufficient physical capabilities to permit the use of proper technique in all the fundamental and sport specific skills. As a consequence it follows that, given sound instruction, you should generally be able to successfully develop, in a relatively short period of time, measurable improvements in everybody's technique.

In conclusion, although our ultimate motor development wish is to help our students produce good motor outcomes, i.e. running faster and batting balls farther, it would appear that our instructional goal is best directed at the acquisition of proper technique. Accordingly we should be generally selecting or developing motor skill assessments of process. If we can help the children to perform correctly and avoid developing initially bad movement habits, and we should be able to readily accomplish this, we have done what is most important for the long run. Once we have them on the right technique track, we can be assured that they will then be in a position to achieve their full potential. The final realization of that potential will be a function of their genetics and how much they continue to practice.

Figure 10.6 is an example of a test of a tennis groundstroke. Obviously you will not normally be this detailed in your evaluation of a sport specific skill, but the test is a good example of *process evaluation*. With much practice I have learned to quickly evaluate these criteria; seeing two or three swings is usually sufficient. If you were going to assess your students on this skill, you could simplify your task by paring the criteria to one or two aspects that you thought to be most important. There is no reason you could not establish your own *rubrics* for other sport skills with which you are familiar.

Figure: 10.6. Process Evaluation of a Tennis Ground Stroke

5 - *Excellent*	Proper grip, good balance, footwork, and near perfect form. Consistently demonstrates correct stroke mechanics. Shots are hit with power and consistently placed appropriately.
4 - *Good*	Proper grip, good balance, adequate footwork, and acceptable, but not perfect form. Demonstrates above average consistency of of stroke mechanics. Moderate power and consistent placement within court area.
3 - *Satisfactory*	Proper grip, acceptable balance, but footwork is poor. Form is somewhat erratic and inefficient, resulting in inconsistent shot placement. Style of stroke is more defensive in nature, but can sustain a short rally.
2 - *Fair*	Uses improper grip at times, poor footwork and basically incorrect form. Inconsistent stroke mechanics. Defensive style of play, merely trying to get the ball over the net. Unable to sustain a rally.
1 - *Poor*	Incorrect grip, off-balance, with poor footwork. Form is very poor and erratic. Virtually no control of ball placement. Experiences difficulty in getting ball over net.

Authentic Evaluation

Your evaluating of motor skills can be done in drill situations isolated from the game or while the student is actually participating in game competition. The advantage of evaluating during drills is that you can organize the environment to get a good look at every person's skill under the exact same conditions. For example, you could have a circuit training situation set up so that you would be sure to have a good minute or two for each student to demonstrate his/her ability to execute an underhand volleyball pass or tennis groundstroke under controlled conditions. They might have the ball tossed to them or could be hitting off of a wall. I have done a good deal of testing like this to see if the students can demonstrate the correct technique.

Evaluating skills while they are being performed in a game situation is called *authentic evaluation*. There are two advantages of this type of evaluation. One is that it can be easily done while the children enjoy playing the game. No special circuit training or testing stations is required. The other advantage is that how the skill is applied in the game situation is the real test of whether or not the student has learned to use the skill; that is why it is called *authentic evaluation*. I mentioned in an earlier chapter that it is not unusual to see a deterioration of skill technique when the transition must be made from practice drills to the game. According to the exponents of *authentic evaluation* it makes sense for us to be judging the real thing, the ultimate objective.

One point needs to be made if *authentic evaluation* is going to be feasible. It is essential that the *mini-games* concept is being employed. Otherwise, it will be a long time before you will see players perform the game skills you are wishing to assess. As they wait and wait for a turn, you will also wait. But get them involved in games where they are on their own or with a partner or two and you will know what they can do very quickly.

Holistic Evaluation

In the Figures and examples provided thus far we have been zeroing in on evaluating specific process skills used within a sport. Is their groundstroke form correct? Is their underhand passing technique as it should be? In *holistic evaluation* you are making a more general assessment of the student's performance. You are not just evaluating a person's specific serving technique but are making a more generic assessment of all his/her overall tennis techniques, strategies and knowledge of rules and etiquette. Figure 10.7 provides an example of *holistic evaluation*. Notice that we are lumping all their techniques together to make a general judgment of goodness of technique, and that we do the same with their strategic decisions, knowledge of the game rules and affective behaviors.

With little or no adaptation you could easily apply the Figure 10.7 rubric to most any team sport. Holistic evaluation is only an estimate of sorts but it does give the instructor some objective guidelines. When small-sides games are in progress it is possible to completely evaluate everyone in a period or two. And certainly *holistic assessment* has the virtue of being authentic.

Figure: 10.7. Holistic Assessment of Sport Skills

5 - Excellent	Demonstrates mastery of sport specific skills and ability to consistently perform with little or no conscious effort resulting in few errors. Extensive knowledge base and understanding of sport or activity. Employs effective strategy specific to the tasks or situation.
4 - Good	Demonstrates competency and ability to perform basic skills without making many errors. Complete understanding of rules and strategies of the specific sport or activity. Usually selects appropriate strategy and skill for situations and generally displays consistent performance.
3 - Satisfactory	Displays basic knowledge of sport or activity and ability to perform fundamental skills adequately to be able to play game. Performance is frequently inconsistent, resulting in numerous errors being made. Understands basic strategies, but lacks ability to effectively employ.
2 - Fair	Demonstrate inability to perform more than the basic skills. Has difficulty in executing even the basic skills, making frequent errors, some critical, during performance. Generally inconsistent performance with only a minimal understanding of strategies and rules.
1 - Poor	Rarely, if ever, performs skills well enough to be able to play a meaningful game. Demonstrates little understanding of sport or activity and inability to execute skills without making significant and frequent errors. Makes little attempt to adjust performance.

REPORTING & GRADING OF THE PSYCHOMOTOR DOMAIN

Reporting

Throughout this book I have advocated regular communication with the parents. We should do the best we can to keep them informed of our goals, practices, and of course, how their children are learning and performing. We should be thoroughly assessing in the cognitive domain to determine the extent of learning about nutrition, exercise and other health practices. And those results should be conveyed to the homes to demonstrate what has been taught and learned. In the psychomotor realm we need to have the parents and guardians tied in with process of the motor skill homework assignments and the logging of physical activity and exercise both in and out of school. Summary reports should give the big picture to document the active lifestyle that the school is promoting, and how faithfully the child has been achieving it. We need always remember that above all else, we are promoting the enjoyment of an active lifestyle.

I also believe that two or three times per year it would be useful to provide a comprehensive report on each child's health status. This would consist of any physical fitness scores that had been collected. If the program stressed aerobic fitness it may have used a test such as the PACER, and/or a walking test. Interpretation of those test scores in terms of their relationship to VO2 measures and mile-run estimates would be helpful. If strength testing had been done, such as sit-up, push-up, or pull-up testing, they too should be relayed to the homes. Rather then explaining any of the tests in normative terms (percentile rankings), it would be better to focus more on how the scores relate to healthy criteria levels. The point should not be on pointing out how a parent's child did relative to classmates or nationally. What needs to be understood is whether or not the child has what is generally considered to have a healthy level of fitness in each tested fitness component, and what are the potential health consequences and remedial actions if necessary.

I definitely believe that Body Mass Index (BMI) Scores should be reported. Body fat estimates are simply too vital a health issue to be treated as a taboo subject. Dealing with the real problem of overweight and obesity is undeniably a major responsibility of health and fitness instructors. Avoiding doing so because it is a sensitive topic cannot be justified. Doing so would be as irresponsible as biology teachers failing to address evolution, historians downplaying the holocaust, or geologists overlooking global warming, Some states and individual school districts are now requiring that each student's BMI be calculated and the result sent home to parents. The point of this practice is to share with parents the status of their child's weight, as many parents fail to perceive the fact that their children are overweight. For instance, in a survey from the University of Michigan of more than 2,000 parents, more than 40 percent appeared unaware of their child's obesity, instead reporting that their child was "about the right weight."

The easiest way to determine a child's BMI is to use the CDC's Calculator for Teens and Children. The calculator requires a child's date of birth, date of measurement, sex, height without shoes, and weight. The calculator outputs the BMI, the BMI-for-age percentile, and the child's weight status category (Figure 10.8). The CDC BMI-for-age charts offer a visual tool for showing parents how their child's BMI score compares to other students the same age. These growth charts can be used to communicate to parents what are considered to be healthy weight percentiles or to suggest they may want to consult their healthcare provider if their child falls into the other categories. As a teacher, it is important to remember that the BMI is an *estimate* of levels of body fat that is reliable for most, but not all, children. The child's healthcare provider will do further analysis and use different methods to determine whether there are any issues that need to be addressed. Thus, the main reason school districts share children's BMI with parents is not to intervene, but simply to alert parents to potential issues so that they can make an informed decision about consulting their healthcare provider.

Figure 10.8. Body Mass Index Weight Status Categories

Weight Status	Percentile
Underweight	Less than the 5th percentile
Healthy Weight	5th percentile to less than the 85th percentile
At Risk of Overweight	85th to less than the 95th percentile
Overweight	Equal to or greater than the 95th percentile

Finally, there exist many other vital health statistics that large percentages of our population do not, but should, know about themselves. Monitoring of many of these markers could easily be begun as early as the intermediate grades. I am referring to things like resting pulse rates, blood pressure, cholesterol readings, and hearing and sight test scores. The teachers could administer some such measures and others gathered from the school nurse. Including this kind of information might serve as a lesson for the children, making them aware that these are important indicators of health that everyone should be tracking.

Grading

In mathematics we grade on how well the students can do on math test, not how long and hard they studied. Likewise in all the other academic subjects the students' grades are based not on effort but on the content knowledge they ultimately display on examinations. Consistency may lead therefore to the conclusion that physical education grades should reflect performance on physical fitness and movement/sport skills tests. After all, the purpose of the academic disciplines is to make students competent in math, science, literature, etc. Is not the purpose then, of health and physical education, to make students physically fit and skillful in various movement/sport skills. I say no, at least not directly. Let me explain.

In the introductory chapters I never stated physical fitness or achievement of masterful motor skills as a program goal. Doing so would be setting both the children and the teachers up for failure. We know that how well young people do on a fitness test is largely not under their control. Hereditary factors and maturation are the primary determinants, and their prepubescent bodies are not especially *trainable*. And we have learned of the colossal hours required to develop most complex movement/sport skills. If we base grades on physical fitness and motor performance skills tests it very possibly would convey discouraging information to some students (remember *learned helplessness*), and furthermore, it would not necessarily tell us much about how active the children are.

As for the teachers, does either a physical education specialist or classroom teacher ever have enough activity time with his/her students to reasonably produce and document a rise in fitness scores or to make low skilled students into good ballplayers? Remember how many miles it takes to burn up one pound of body fat; how many weeks of regular, target zone exercise it takes to improve aerobic fitness; how many thousands of hours of shooting baskets and dribbling balls to start to become competent at just those aspects of basketball. A teacher is in an untenable situation if he/she is to be held accountable for these kinds of improvements across the school year. Students will likely demonstrate somewhat higher scores at the end of the year because they have matured for nearly a year, but real increases in fitness and skills due to the teacher's training interdictions are bound to be marginal and necessarily limited to a small set of fitness components and motor skills.

The chief psychomotor goal I enunciated in Chapter 2 was to help the children enjoy an active lifestyle. I further clarified that goal by defining exercise in terms of *The Physical Activity Pyramid*. Priority was placed on trying to get all the children adhering to the 60 minutes of daily lifestyle activities which forms the base of the pyramid, and then, as much as possible, promoting more vigorous aerobic participation and muscular strength/dynamic flexibility activities. That being my purpose, it follows that I should as accurately and thoroughly as possible assess and grade the students' compliance. Doing so would entail regularly tracking how well the students were completing their activity homework assignments and faithfully organizing and logging their weekly activity plans. I would also feel justified in factoring in examination scores which demonstrated their cognitive understanding of the psychomotor principles necessary for knowing how and why to take care of one's body. Obviously these self-reports will never perfectly reflect what was actually done, but if good communication channels are established with parents and guardians, their help in monitoring and signing off on assignments should be achievable.

If motor skill assessment scores have been collected they too might be factored into the student's grade. However, I would do so only for the process-oriented skills tests advocated earlier in the chapter. Demonstrating the processes of employing the correct techniques, applying knowledge of the rules and strategies, and exhibiting self-responsible-caring affective behaviors are all largely under the control of the student regardless o entry skill levels. Displaying these kinds of psychomotor skills is all we can rightfully expect of the children, and if they do not display them, a lower grade would be justifiable. This places the grade not on athleticism but on what it should be, technique/strategies, effort and attitudes.

CHAPTER COMPREHENSION CHECK

Beyond assessing to meet administrative demands, what are two reasons assessment is important to the teacher?

Has it been common for schools to be assessing the physical activity levels of students?

Has it been found that intermediate level elementary students can reliably self-report their physical activity levels?

What are two self-report tools that can be used to formally assess the physical activity levels of elementary students? What are the characteristics of each?

What are pedometers? How do they work? Are they considered a reasonably accurate measurement of physical activity?

The *10,000 Step Criteria* translates into approximately how many miles of walking?

What is the average number of steps elementary classroom teachers normally take each day?

What alternative does the author offer in place of the *10,000 Step Criteria*? Why?

What size of increase in accumulated steps might a school accept as achieving a yearly goal of increasing physical activity?

What are heart-rate monitors? How do they work? What are the author's views and arguments regarding their use with elementary aged children?

What are the four major factors that determine an elementary student's score on a physical fitness test? Which two of the four are considered to be most potent?

What is meant by saying that pre-pubescent children are not particularly *trainable*?

What typically happens to a child's level of physical activity following a low performance score on a fitness test?

The term *learned helplessness* is re-introduced. How does it relate to the use of physical fitness testing?
What is the difference between *norm referenced* and *criterion* fitness tests?
What are the three basic approaches of administering physical fitness tests? What are the characteristics of each?
Which of the three approaches to fitness testing is more directly related to the setting of *self-performance goals*?
What factors should you consider when selecting a physical fitness test?
What is the difference between a *health related physical fitness test* and a *performance related physical fitness test*?
When are the two most common physical fitness tests? What are the basic differences between them?
On what basis are the aerobic and body composition "Healthy Fitness Zone" criteria established?
What is the ACTIVITYGRAM?
What is the PACER?
What is the relationship between having good motor skills and adult activity levels?
What is the difference between *fundamental* and *sport specific* motor skills?
Why is it good for children to acquire *fundamental motor skills* during the elementary school years?
What is the concept of *critical periods*?
What is the *sports arms race* concept? What implications does it have?
What is the distinction between the *process evaluation* and *product evaluation* of motor skills? Which does the author view as more appropriate and why?
What is *authentic evaluation*? What is its advantage compared to un-authentic evaluation?
What is *holistic assessment*?
What kinds of things does the author recommend being reported to parents? Why?
How good have parents been found to estimate their children's BMI status relative to other children?
What is the justification for grading physical education in a fundamentally different manner than other academic subjects?
What kinds of things does the author feel should be graded, and what kinds of things not graded? Why?

[CHAPTER 11]

OFTEN ASKED QUESTIONS

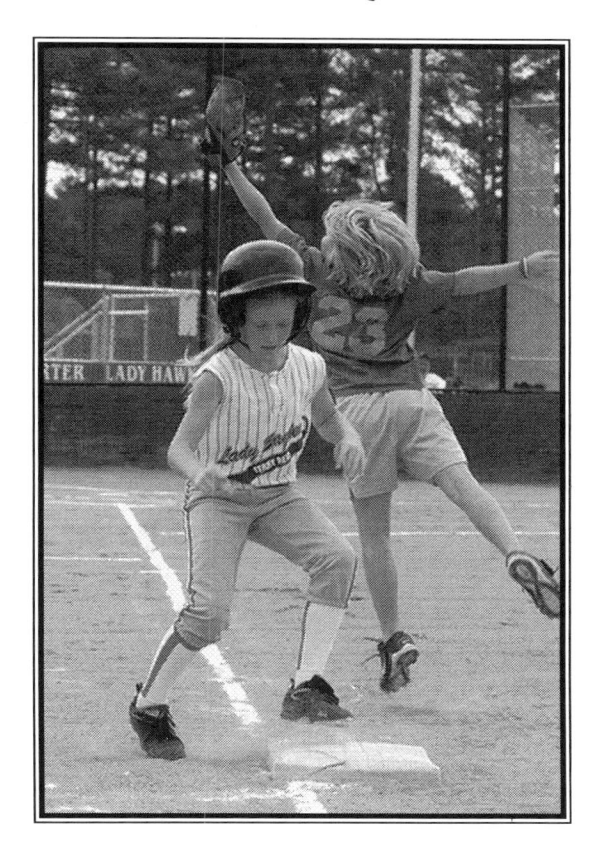

WHAT IS AND ISN'T APPROPRIATE TOUCHING IN THE ACTIVITY ENVIRONMENT?

HOW CAN I ACCOMMODATE STUDENTS WITH SPECIAL NEEDS?

HOW CAN I TEACH MOVEMENT ACTIVITIES IN THE CLASSROOM?

WHAT ARE MY SAFETY & LEGAL RESPONSIBILITIES?

WHAT EQUIPMENT WILL I NEED & HOW MIGHT I ACQUIRE IT?

WHEN SHOULD & SHOULDN'T BOYS & GIRLS PLAY TOGETHER?

I HAVE BEEN URGENTLY ASKED TO COACH YOUTH SPORTS. WHAT DO I DO?

WHAT ARE APPROPRIATE PHYSICAL ACTIVITIES & TEACHING METHODS FOR THE PRE-SCHOOL CHILD?

CHAPTER COMPREHENSION CHECK

> *"I had six honest serving men —They taught me all I knew: Their names were Where and What and When — and Why and How and Who"*
> ~ Rudyard Kipling

> *"It is a shameful thing to be weary of inquiry when what we search for is excellent."*
> ~ Cicero

WHAT IS AND ISN'T APPROPRIATE TOUCHING IN THE ACTIVITY ENVIRONMENT?

If all questions are good, this qualifies as an good good question. When teaching physical activities, many situations arise in which touching might occur either between the teacher and the student or among the students. Teacher-student contact might happen for a variety of reasons. Firstly, when physical skills are being learned it may be appropriate for the instructor to want to provide manual guidance. As related in Chapter 8, when children still do not perform a skill properly following instructor verbalizations and repeated demonstrations, manual guiding might be in order. For instance, you might tell a child to swipe his leg and keep his toe more pointed when making a soccer kick. If that does not satisfactorily convey the message you might then demonstrate it a number of times. If the student continues to lack an understanding, it may be time to provide the proprioceptive sensation of the movement by actually grasping the lower leg and foot and moving him/her through the desired pattern. The hope is to give the idea of what the skill should feel like when done properly.

A second situation that calls for teacher/student contact is that of spotting. This is where the teacher gives physical assistance to help in actual completion of a task. An example might be where a child is tentative about trying a forward roll. Both performance success and safety could be contingent on the teacher laying on hands to give some uplifting support under the shoulders and a bit of rotation impetus to the legs.

The sexual harassment authorities and guidelines I have consulted unanimously felt that it was appropriate for teachers to provide physical guidance and spotting for skills like those described above. However, they all were agreed that such help should not be applied if it would make the student feel uncomfortable. They recommended that rather than immediately jumping in and providing unsolicited physical assistance, it would be better to preface your action with a statement such as... "May I physically assist you through this?" or "Is it okay if I help you?" In most cases there will not be a problem and you may come to know where there is no possibility of any difficulty. But in that rare event when a child might have reason to not wish to be touched, we would know to refrain.

Besides lending guidance and spotting assistance, teachers are also frequently touching students to console, congratulate and minister to injuries. Here again contact may be inappropriate if it is perceived discomforting to the student. Probably the action of congratulating with handshakes, high 10's, and pats on the back will be acceptable to all. But what about embracing, arms around the shoulders, and pats on the butt? No, today's society considers these more intimate behaviors as potentially dangerous and therefore inappropriate between teacher and student. As for treating injuries, certainly it is our duty to attempt to respond to them with application of appropriate first aid. But for the everyday bruises and scrapes, we are being asked to exhibit some restraint in our handling and condolences, to wipe the tears away without hugs and kisses.

I know that there are you who will feel some resistance to adopting this level of aloofness, I do. I fondly remember having three or four first graders hanging on each of my legs because they are glad to see me; and I remember hugging crying children who had failed at a task or hurt themselves. But I think we cannot blithely dismiss these new restrictions as totally uncaring foolishness and legal absurdities. We must remind ourselves that everyone, young and old, has a right to a degree of personal space and privacy, and that there are always going to be a few people, in every profession, who will either knowingly or unknowingly overstep those borders. I would imagine that most of us, at some point in our lives, have experienced such a violation, great or small. If we do not accept any limitations to close contacts with children, some children will be abused who would not be otherwise. Surely we can compromise a little, we do not have to have completely unfettered liberties to still show warmly sincere, affectionate behaviors.

What about the physical contacts among the children? Physical contact is an integral part of many games and activities: bumping, pushing, pulling, holding, supporting, guiding, lifting, etc. Generally, I think it is a good experience for children to work closely together in these ways. It can break down barriers and produce an accepting, inclusive environment. Also, if we expect students to display caring behaviors, they will sometimes need to model your physically assisting, spotting, praising and consoling of others. Having said this, we must be cognizant of the potential for bad touches as well as good. Perhaps a first step to reduce problems is to educate all children that they have a right to some personal space. If they feel uncomfortable with any too-close contact with another student, they should be able to say so. And we should teach everyone to be respectful of the privacy rights of others.

We, as teachers, can show our sensitivity to privacy rights by making it known that anyone can opt out of an activity that would be threatening to personal space. As much as we might believe a game to be beneficial, and as much as we might be disappointed by non-participation, forced involvement will likely be counter-productive. Perhaps a more fruitful approach in dealing with such problems is to consider modifications that would decrease the frightening features of an activity without eliminating the cooperative spirit. Instead of holding hands, arms around shoulders, or closed dance positions, maybe elbow touching or simple back-of-hand contact would sometimes be serviceable substitutes. Or in some instances equipment can be used to provide a level of separation. An example that comes to my mind here is a levitation activity I once had the children play. The children lay down in a circle with their heads close together. They then put their arms up to support a child which I laid backwards onto the surface of hands. This done they then were to rotate the rigid suspendee. While this was a good and enjoyable game I did find that some did not wish to have this many hands up and down their backside, and there were one or two situations in which I sensed bad touches might be occurring. A solution to the game was found in having the levitated person rest of a small tumbling mat.

HOW CAN I ACCOMMODATE STUDENTS WITH SPECIAL NEEDS?

It is so important we design our physical activities to enable successful participation of those children with mental and physical disabilities. They have the same desires, interests, and expectations to belong and achieve as their peers. With good encouragement and instruction, children with mental impairments can sometimes find more success and enjoyment in physical activities than what may be found in more intellectually demanding realms. And children with physical limitations are frequently in greatest need of establishing active lifestyle patterns because restricted movement opportunities are often leading them down a road to pathologically low fitness levels. It is wrong to think a physical disability precludes a lifestyle rich in exercise and sports (see Figure 11.1). Finally, it is critical that the children without disabilities participate with those who do; such experiences can teach them how to accept the strengths and limitations of everyone.

Figure 11.1. Activities for Those with Impairments

Physical impairments need not consign people to a life of inactivity. Listed below are some sports and recreational pursuits which would require no, or minimal adaptations. Can you think of a few more?

Major impairment of the visual system:
    Step aerobics
    Bicycling (exercise bicycle, tandem and "Spinning" classes)
    Swimming (lane lines and a gutter beeper might be needed)
    Water aerobics
    Stair steppers

> Running (treadmills and partner running – using the elbow as a guide)
> Walking
> Weight training, lifting and bodybuilding
> Stretching and Yoga
> Wrestling
> Track (throwing events)
> Dance
>
> Major impairment to the lower musculoskeletal system:
> Archery
> Darts
> Horseshoes
> Swimming
> Wheelchair racing
> Wheelchair sports (basketball, tennis, etc.)
> Weight training and lifting
> Kayaking, canoeing and sailing
>
> Major impairment to the upper musculoskeletal system:
> Walking and hiking
> Running
> Soccer
> Dance
> Step Aerobics
> Stair steppers
> Bicycling (exercise bicycle, tandem and "Spinning" classes)

The first idea I would offer regarding the inclusion of special needs students is that you consider the three types of activity structures that were presented in Chapter 9: *individual, cooperative, and competitive*. In that chapter the point was made that it is easier to accommodate differences in ability when activities are designed as individual or cooperative. In *individual activities* everyone is working independently and hence not holding up or being held up by others. For example, those with impairments can be happily working on simpler ball or movement skills while the more gifted, without conflict, can simultaneously be experimenting with more advance tasks. In *cooperative activities*, group goals generally require everyone to help each other. The more advanced students will be forced not to disregard those who are slower, but rather to give them assistance. The cooperative structure will tend to elicit more caring behaviors. *Competitive activities* pose greater difficulties for inclusion of diverse abilities because mis-matches in abilities can result in the spotlighting of those differences. The performance of lesser-skilled individuals will be more evident if they are causing their team to fare poorly relative to others. This, of course, can result in embarrassment and frustration.

The point to be drawn from the above paragraph is that ways to achieve inclusion will be easier to find if all your activities are not socially competitive. However, it should not be concluded that competition cannot also be designed to yield successful performances for all, it just may require a bit more careful thought. Below are listed some elements of activities and games that can be altered regardless of the activity type. Throughout the text I have stressed the need to individualize tasks to match the disparate ability levels which exist in every class. Remember the *Long-Slanty Rope Principle*? Including children with disabilities simply means that we must extend the long-slanty rope a bit further. For getting a list of specific inclusion games and activities you are referred to the pecentral.com web site.

1. **Equipment:** Change the weight and size of objects and implements, target size, and ball resiliency. Bigger is usually better. Bigger balls are generally easier to bat and catch. Bigger and lighter bats are easier to use. Bigger targets are easier to hit. Softer, less resilient balls move slower and are easier to control; partially deflated soccer balls are easier to dribble, deader balls will rebound less erratically from rackets. Rigid paddles provide more controlled rebounds than tautly strung ones.

2. **Space:** Change the space involved in the activity, such as the distance from the target, the height of the target, or the number of yards between bases. Lower the nets and shrink the court sizes and areas to be defended.

3. **Time:** Vary the time it takes to complete an activity or the number of repetitions. Repeat dance steps before moving to the next.

4. **Environmental dynamics:** Motor skills can be classified as *environmentally closed* or *environmentally open*. *Environmentally closed* refers to situations in which the performer is dealing with fairly static surroundings. Hitting a ball from a batting tee is a more closed skill than contending with the dynamics of a thrown pitch. *Environmentally open* skills are those in which a performer must adjust to a quickly changing environment. A further example would be catching a ball while on a run or throwing to a moving teammate. It should be obvious that closed skills tend to place less processing demands on the performer and thus should be considered as a means

of adapting activities to lower skill levels. In ball sports, low skilled individuals may be able to more easily fill the roles of serving, foul attempts, throw-ins.

HOW DO I TEACH MOVEMENT ACTIVITIES IN THE CLASSROOM OR LIMITED SPACE?

It is important to continue activities even when the weather prohibits outdoor activities and when there is no available gym or large multipurpose room. Stretching and exercise breaks are good health practices to instill, and children need to learn that regular exercise is something you find time to do everyday, regardless of the weather or circumstance. You have taught them the Reversibility Principle, now you must take the even more important step of modeling behaviors to counter it.

It is hard to make particular activity recommendations without knowing the specifics of your facilities but there are a few general ideas that can be given. You can always make some space if your desks and chairs are moveable. Moving everything to one side of the room should provide a small space sufficient for many activities and games. A few small circuit training stations could be formed; poly-spot and carpet squares could be arranged so each child would have a personal space for individual exercises and stunts; games like "No Touch", "Daytona Speedway", or "Walking / Beanbag Tag" could be played. Moving furniture to the center of the room can result in a perimeter area adequate for various circle formation games and activities ("Creative circles", folk dancing, "Around-the-clock" games, "Astronaut drills", etc.). When the desks cannot be moved out of the way activity space is more constrained but there is still much that can be done. Students can do calisthenics, in-place jogging, stretches and isometric exercises beside their desks; they can do manipulative activities with lummi sticks, balls, and other objects; or they can follow each other up and down the aisles doing some of the same activities as those mentioned above.

When exercising in the classroom there is a need to keep the exuberance under control. Too much noise will frequently be disrupting to neighboring classrooms. Also, because the play space will be limited, extra care must be taken to avoid collisions with surrounding obstacles and each other. Rather than attempting to play with regular sports balls and bats, consider using less abrasive objects such as balloons, yard balls, beanbags, and foam balls.

For a large number of specific ideas refer to the "Classroom Activities" listed in Chapter 12.

WHAT DO I NEED TO KNOW ABOUT SAFETY & LEGAL LIABILITY?

More than 50 percent of all accidents in the school setting occur on the playground and in the gymnasium. It therefore is essential that you know how to make your activities as safe as possible. Also, it is important for you to understand a few basic facts regarding your legal obligations. Teachers must offer a standard of care that any *reasonable and prudent person* with similar training would apply under the given circumstances. They are expected to anticipate foreseeable dangers and take necessary precautions to prevent such problems. Below are three basic duties that must be met.

> 1. *Supervision:* Supervision can be classified as general or specific. *General supervision* means that the actions of all the children can be regularly monitored. The teacher is responsible for always maintaining this level of supervision. You should never leave your class unattended nor have some of your students participating in activity areas which you cannot watch. Even when dealing with emergency situations you must be able to maintain a degree of awareness of the rest of the class. For instance, if a child experienced a significant injury in class, the teacher should not leave to get help; rather, a student or two should be sent to get help or to find a responsible adult to monitor the class in your absence. *With-it-ness* is a term for the teaching skill of being able to attend to more than one thing at a time. Can you talk to someone or administer to a "boo boo" and still have an idea of the whereabouts and the behaviors of your class? With experience you will likely find your *with-it-ness* developing. One way to increase *with-it-ness* is to normally position yourself on the perimeter of the group so that your back will not be turned if a dangerous situation should arise (remember the *Back-to-the Wall Principle?*).
>
> *Specific supervision* is when the teacher is directly present at the site of an activity and can quickly regulate or stop the action if necessary. This level of supervision is required when a child is performing a dangerous movement. Obvious examples would be when a child was high up on the climbing ropes

or beginning to learn a gymnastic flip. Another kind of dangerous situation would exist if the students where in route to a playing field which required the crossing of a busy highway. To safely cross the street the teacher would have to be at the site of the crossing so as to be able to signal traffic and stop the children. It would not be sufficient for the teacher to have warned the children as to the proper manner of crossing the street and then to have trustfully followed at a distance while exercising general supervision.

2. *Safe Activities:* All the activities you introduce must be reasonably safe. If a prudent person could foresee the eventual likelihood of an injury, the activity should be stopped immediately and then modified or terminated. We should be able to see some activities as apparently dangerous. Football, "red-rover" and tag games in which tackling was occurring would be examples. "Dodgeball" games where playground and volleyballs are thrown at each other would be another. Having rules specifying that "Dodgeball" and kickball players must be hit below the waist would not satisfactorily solve the problem; we are still making children targets of potentially injurious balls and misdirected throws will inevitably occur.

The safety of most activities and games depends upon whether or not the children possess sufficient skill to handle the conditions demanded of them. If your class has not practiced rolling progressions, some of the students may not be fit or skilled enough to safely perform unassisted forward rolls. Even though the children may be able to execute a wheelbarrow walk, putting it into a relay race might exceed the ability of someone who could subsequently be pushed onto his/her face. It might be fine to match the children according to size and strength and progressively teach a skill like the fire person's carry, but piggyback relay races would make the activity much more hazardous. Broken teeth and noses have occurred in wheelbarrow races, and shattered kneecaps have resulted from piggyback relays. Even where the students have been size matched, the courts have ruled against teachers in such cases.

Skill levels become increasingly important to safety as the activities and sports involve more interaction and physical contact. For example, having low and high skilled students competing together in unmodified soccer, softball and basketball games could easily become unacceptably dangerous; those who are twice as big, and can move their bodies three times as fast as some other children, can pose a foreseeable risk to those students who are less mature and not ball savvy. Visualize yourself on the fields and courts of powerful professional athletes – would you be safe? The best suggestion I can give to reduce large skill miss-matches in sports is to utilize the *mini-game* format suggested in Chapter 9 and then equate the teams and pairings.

Any activity can also become unsafe if the rules of conduct are violated. It is your responsibility to make corrections as soon as you notice any potentially dangerous procedure violations. If misbehavior has been occurring for a period of time, and it leads to an injury, you would be held accountable. You should have had the supervision to be aware of it, and you should have remedied it. Only in rare situations would the elementary level teacher be absolved of responsibility due to the concept of *contributory negligence*. *Contributory negligence* is a legal term for situations where others may be held partially or totally accountable for their own actions. Take this as an example, a teacher gave clear warning to her sixth graders that swinging bats was dangerous and prohibited until everyone was spread out on the playing field. Then, out-of-the-blue, one of the students suddenly swung and injured somebody. If there was no good reason (past history or disability) to have suspected the child of this behavior, the teacher could hardly be thought neglectful; normal six-graders should be assumed to possess this much self-control. However, *contributory negligence* is not legally attributed to children less than seven years of age. This means that you should not feel confident that your warnings, no matter how clear they may be, will suffice to prevent inappropriate actions. Telling them not to swing the implements in their hands might be little more effective than telling them not to put peas up their noses (it might only give them the idea of doing so).

Often Asked Questions

3. *Safe Play Environment:* The teacher always has the duty to make activities as safe as possible. This means that the facilities and equipment must be made not just safe, but as safe as they reasonably can be. Always inspect the play space and look for things like wet spots on the floor, gravel on the pavement, or holes or sprinkler heads in the fields. Also, look for obstacles such as protruding bleachers, tables, chairs, or posts. Remove them if you can or establish boundaries to ensure adequate buffer zones. I am always amazed when the end lines and boundaries of relays, tag games and sports are immediately next to these all too too solid, harsh realities. Finally, take heed to keep the facility uncluttered after activity begins; don't leave your clipboard, papers or computer message pad lying about. Watch for clothing articles that the children have the habit of leaving lying about.

The selection of equipment can have a major impact on safety. Always consider whether or not softer, lighter weight balls can be used. Yarn and nerf-balls work great for many games. And it seems foolish to play softball with an official hard ball when softer ones are available which would be safer and probably much better suited to limited skills levels and play spaces.

The children's clothing has bearing on safety. Pendulous garments and jewelry should be removed. From my experience, improper footwear is the greatest dress hazard because slipping and turned ankles can often result. Flip-flops and large heeled "klomper-stomper" shoes are not acceptable. Denying activity is the surest course and probably conveys a good safety message. Allowing participation in bare feet might be acceptable for some few activities. Performing in socking feet should be more unacceptable.

A legal term that relates to the environment is *attractive nuisance*. Occurrences of *attractive nuisances* would be leaving climbing ropes hanging, a mini-trampoline set-up, or a javelin lying about. Such items would be enticing to many children and must never be left available for unsupervised use. Make sure these kinds of things are not available before you get to the activity area and that they are put away before you leave.

Finally, besides supervision, safe activities, and environmental factors, here are four other recommendations.

1. Have formulated in your mind a clear emergency care plan. It should include phone numbers, how the help of other school personal will be gained, and the basic first aid steps you should follow.

2. Do not force students to do activities they are afraid of. Make it clear that the choice of activity belongs to them. Although it can be frustrating when a child refuses to participate in a potentially beneficial activity, we should do no more than offer constant help and encouragement. Fear itself can make a task dangerous. Along the same line, we must honor all parental and doctor notes to be excused from participation.

3. Be cautious about having the children exercising when it is hot and/or humid. Children do not cope with heat stress nearly as well as do adults. Their sweating capacity is not as great and it is important to provide frequent activity breaks and regular fluid replacements. Overweight individuals have a larger problem with exercising in the heat because their surface area to mass ratios are smaller and hence heat dissipation is not as effective.

4. It is always our responsibility to warn participants of the *inherent risks* involved in activities. Make it a habit to tell or show the students what to watch out for and then check to see if they understood. Beyond that, courts are always pleased to see a *paper trail* that documents your lessons including this advice.

5. Remember the untenable position you put yourself in if you use exercise as a punishment procedure. This practice can be viewed as a form of corporal punishment and you could face suite if either physical or psychological injury was determined.

WHAT EQUIPMENT WILL I NEED & HOW MIGHT I ACQUIRE IT?

One of the themes of this text has been to maximize movement; this means a shift away from games and activities in which 30 students are playing with one ball or are impatiently lined up to await a turn on the tumbling mat or a shot at the basket. No, if high levels of activity and skills are to be attained it is requisite that we have play equipment for most every child in the class, ever as much as other academic subjects require books and writing paper. Nevertheless, the overall amount of equipment needed for a varied range of experiences does not have to be prohibitively great. First of all, there are many types of equipment for which it is not difficult to purchase or have enough made for each child. Examples would be bean-bags, nerf-balls, yarn-balls, jump-ropes, hula-hoops, Frisbees, carpet squares, poly spots, paddles, birdies. With these items alone, and some creativity, there are endless activity possibilities. I have known teachers who have had parents or school personnel inexpensively make the likes of yarn-balls, bean-bags, jump-ropes, hula-hoops and wooden paddles. Equipment procurement is one of the areas where a formation of a wellness team could produce some dividends.

If you wish to introduce the children to certain sports, you should have a large number of sports balls and implements, ideally enough for every class member or one for every two students. Although these items are more expensive to attain, good accumulations of them may be feasible. The physical education specialist and wellness team might be able to get donations from different sources. Remember that the sports equipment that might be most useful to you will not likely be "regulation" sized and weighted. I would like to have extra big, and soft, softballs; light weight fat bats, bigger and lighter volleyballs, junior size basketballs, soft-pliable hockey sticks, etc.

In addition to having the above for most everyone, I think you would find a good, easily portable sound system to be essential not just for dance type activities but also for general motivation and management purposes. A number of small cones would serve you well in delineating game and activity boundaries and target zones. Some type of jerseys are nice to lessen confusion in team games. A variety of longer length ropes make for a variety of group and Double-Dutch jumping challenges.

Finally, I would encourage you not to limit your equipment horizons. More expensive specialty equipment can sometimes be obtained through grants, civic organizations, and benefactors. Unicycles, rollerblading skates and accouterments, endo-boards, tumbling mats and crash pads, climbing walls, rope courses, hiking gear, pedometers, heart monitors, bicycles and helmets, and portable basketball hoops have all been gotten by other enterprising souls. Also, be aware that many school districts are now acquiring popular specialty equipment for shared use across schools. Have a look at the catalogs and web sites listed in the Annotated Resources section for other equipment and supply ideas.

WHEN SHOULD & SHOULDN'T BOYS & GIRLS PLAY TOGETHER?

My view is that throughout the elementary years, there should be no gender segregation in regular school physical activities. We should be attempting to convey the message that we are friendly caring people, we do not discriminate on the basis of disabilities, race, gender or anything else. We treat everyone with respect and uncomplainingly play with the nearest person. And we should not foster stereotypical roles by suggesting that certain activities are more for boys or girls. Nor should we allow to go unchallenged talk of "throwing like a girl" or girls being better at dance or rope jumping. Let us provide male and female models for all children and not unnecessary limit anyone's aspirations. I would not require the assumption of boy and girl roles in dance or gymnastic activities and I would not encourage an us against them mentality by having all boys' teams playing against girl's teams.

As was made clear in more than one chapter, ability matching is needful in competitive physical activities, without it safety, enjoyment and skill development is threatened. At the intermediate level you will be seeing that some boys in your class will be significantly excelling the girls in sports involving physical power and aggressive play behaviors. However, I do not believe this should lead to separate boys and girls games. Overlap will surely exist in which some girls will be competitive with the better boys and more advanced than many of the boys. Let everyone appreciate this reality by matching solely according to ability.

Before leaving this topic, something should be said about the controversial issue of co-educational, after-school sports. Some people feel that up through sixth grade the teams should continue to be co-educational. Their reasoning is much the same as that made above for common, regular physical education experiences. However, there is another school of thought, with which I concur, which believes that some fifth and sixth grade after-school sports teams are best separated. Basketball, soccer, softball and other sports with a premium on physical power will see many boys beginning to exhibit a decided advantage over the girls. Although there may still be some girls who are capable of competing with the boys at this higher level, it is not going to be as common as was the case in regular class play. The elective sports teams will be attracting a pool of the best boy performers and thus it should be expected that only a very select few of the girls will be able to keep up. The larger the student population the more likely this will be the result (Figure 11.2).

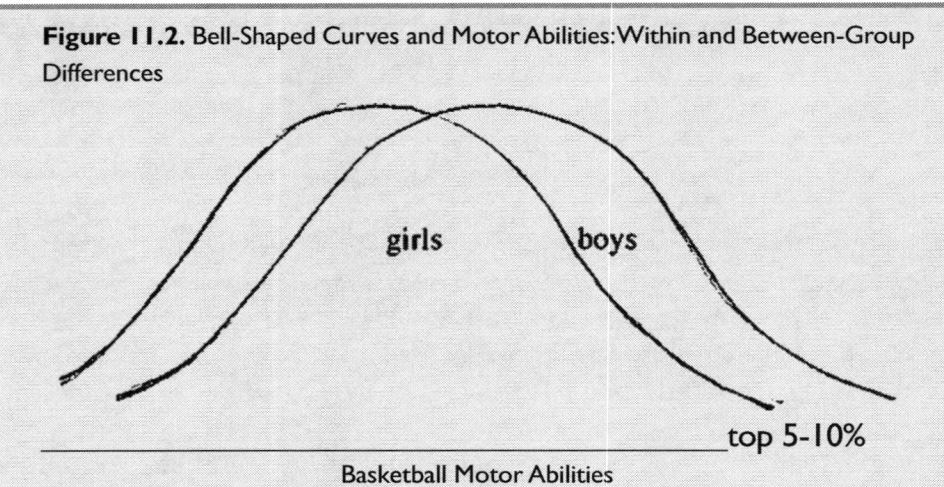

Figure 11.2. Bell-Shaped Curves and Motor Abilities: Within and Between-Group Differences

girls   boys

top 5-10%

Basketball Motor Abilities

Given a large population, the distribution of innate abilities will normally assume a bell-shaped curve. For example, if fifth and sixth grade boys had a small physiological power advantage for playing a sport such as basketball, we would expect the displacement of the bell-shaped curves as depicted above. Because the individual ability differences within the boy and girl populations would be greater than the between-group differences, many of the girls would be expected to be able to outperform a sizable segment of the boys. However, if only the top 5 or 10 percentage of the composite group were selected for a sports team, it could be expected that those elite performers would be all, or nearly all, boys.

The implication of this normal overlapping of motor ability curves would be that we can not reliably predict gender differences in a small group of children in a normal classroom. Other the other hand, we might expect the boy's or girls to predominate if they have a slight motor ability advantage and we are selecting only the very best performers from a very large group.

With boys and girls maturing much earlier than in past years, and most school sports programs drawing from larger populations, I would argue for having separate sports teams for the genders. I believe they afford more girls the opportunity to participate and be leaders. But if we do organize separate teams, we have the duty of making sure the teams are given equal prestige and rights. Schedules, equipment, coaches' pay, and our support deserves to be equably distributed.

I HAVE BEEN URGENTLY ASKED TO COACH YOUTH SPORTS. WHAT DO I DO?

Of course, your decision as to whether or not to coach a youth sports team depends upon you and your situation. But perhaps I can provide some information to weigh. Probably the two most common factors arguing against taking on a coaching duty are (1) not having the time and (2) insufficient knowledge. Time undoubtedly is a concern for all and doing a good job of coaching will require a significant commitment. If you elect to coach, will you still have adequate time for work, family, and personal intellectual/physical development? It will not be easy but with good time management skills it may be possible.

A number of points can be made regarding your knowledge to do a good job. Firstly, I would say that your Health and Fitness or Elementary Education studies are a solid foundation for dealing with young people in any context. Your training in educational philosophy, child development, and your close working with children will give you an advantage over many other coaches who lack this background. Also, the principles you have learned from this text should provide a sound theoretical basis from which to begin; you have learned about physiological training principles, effective demonstrating and feedback provision, how to go about modifying drills and games to promote greater activity and skill development, management techniques, discipline procedures, how to make activities enjoyable, and much more.

Although you might feel comfortable with your educational/pedagogical foundation skills, you may yet question whether or not you have enough knowledge in the X and O specifics of the sport. This is certainly a legitimate concern. It is not essential that you were an outstanding athlete or even that you played the sport, but you do need to know the fundamental techniques, strategies, and rules of the game. If you lack this kind of sport specific understanding it might be best to postpone your acceptance until you have upgraded these skills. There are a number of ways to acquire sports specific knowledge. A first step would be to talk to, observe, and if possible, assist an experienced master coach. Be aware too that there are many excellent texts and videos on the market for both beginning and experienced coaches. I would specifically recommend you visit the *Human Kinetics* web site. They are the largest publisher of books and videos for coaching all kinds of sports, at all levels. Finally, you might wish to take a step further and earn some coaching credentials by attending certifying workshops or completing a university degree program. Local universities may give coaching workshops and/or offer a coaching minor degree program. Various coaching organizations provide workshops and certification courses. The most widely used coaching certification is provided by *The American Sports Education Program* (ASEP). They offer well-developed programs for beginner and advance coaches.

A final point I would make is that coaching can be a tremendously rewarding position. Sports are a highly valued experience in young people's lives and it is not uncommon for a coach to be listed as the person of most influence. This is a weighty responsibility that deserves to be held by the best society can provide. Sadly, we do not always have the best of role models as coaches. There is a high turnover rate in coaching (approximately two years is the average tenure) and thus inexperience is a recurrent problem. Also, because of the excitement of sports and the impressive images of sometimes dubious professional coaching behaviors, some youth sport coaches can be led to over stress winning at the expense of fun and educational purposes. We need to have leaders who will remember that it is full striving to win, not winning *per se*, that is most important, and that the welfare of the young athletes is what must always take precedence over winning. If you could be such a person, please coach, we need you. This is doubly true for women coaches. Although the number of sports programs for girls have greatly increased in recent years, the number of women coaches is small, and has been significantly decreasing.

WHAT ARE APPROPRIATE PHYSICAL ACTIVITIES & TEACHING METHODS FOR THE PRE-SCHOOL CHILD?

You will find it enjoyable to teach physical activities to pre-schoolers. They are so full of energy and take such delight in games and moving. Frequent short bouts are good for their developing bodies and will make for more attentive students.

The very simplest of individual and partner activities will generally work best. Any games with more than one or two rules will not be understood; team play and competitions are too advanced for them. At this age it is good to have them experience all kinds of locomotor skills: walking, running, skipping, jumping, leaping, sliding, hoping, galloping. Doing these skills in different directions and patterns, and at different rates, will develop their motor schema of how to move and will serve as the foundation from which later sport specific skills can be built. Look back to Figure 10.5 for the NASPE Kindergarten Benchmarks.

Early childhood is also the time to begin learning the overlapping concepts of *body awareness, directionality* and *laterality*. *Body awareness* refers to the children knowing their body parts and how they move. *Directionality* refers to a comprehension of the orientation of one's body and body parts in space. *Laterality* is more specific and means knowing left from right and the relationships between them. In Figure 11.3 are some sample activities.

Health AND *Fitness* An Elementary Teacher's Guide

Figure 11.3. Preschool Body Awareness, Laterality and Directionality Activities

Body Awareness Activities

put elbows together	touch one elbow
touch both elbows	elbows to knees
knees together	knee to toe
hands on top of head	elbows on hips
back of hands together	touch one shoulder
touch heels together	hands on ears
raise your shoulders	curl your body, extend it
hold one foot	jingles (head, hips, back, heels)

Laterality & Directionality Activities

- stand in front of spot, back, left, right
- hold spot in front, back, right side, over
- stand on spot and face away, right side towards me
- move away from your spot, forwards it
- draw a square in air (triangle, etc.)
- clap twice behind back
- lie on your back, front, left, right
- raise right arm, foot, elbow, shoulder, hip, knee
- lean to left, right, forwards, backwards
- bend left, right, backwards, forwards, sidewards
- stand on left foot, toes, heel
- stand on left foot and swing the right foot forwards, backwards
- lift your right knee and left elbow
- circle arms out in front, side, behind
- turn knees towards each other, away, left, right

Preschoolers are especially fond of sing along activities, rhythmics and simple dances. They love to pretend and act-out things. Examples would be animals (chickens, horses, bunnies, elephant, ducks, frogs, cats, alligators); daily activities (waking up, getting dressed, washing body parts, brushing teeth, do exercises, running for the bus, carrying groceries); sports (skating, race walking, baseball, trampoline, swimming, dancing, soccer, basketball, volleyball); vehicles (airplane, bicycle, lawn mower, fire truck, row boat, unicycle). Manipulative games will also be enjoyable and beneficial for them; bean-bags, streamers, beach-balls, yarn-balls, nerf-balls and rhythm sticks work great. It would be good to have enough pieces of equipment for everyone so as to maximize skill development, but also keep in mind that they will tire quickly and will require frequent rest periods.

Often Asked Questions

For a more comprehensive coverage of preschool activities and method suggestions I would recommend acquisition of the following two texts: (1) McCall, R. M. & Craft, D. H. *Moving With A Purpose: Developing Programs for Preschoolers of All Abilities*. Human Kinetics, 2000 and (2) Hammett, C. T. *Movement Activities for Early Childhood*, Human Kinetics, 1992 (http://www.humankinetics.com/). The pecentral.org web site will also have a section devoted to preschool issues and activities.

CHAPTER COMPREHENSION CHECK

What are the situations in which touching between the teacher and student is called for?
What is considered inappropriate touching between the teacher and student?
What are some things that can be done to reduce the touching among the students as they participate in games?
How do the three types of activity structures (individual, cooperative, and competitive) relate to teaching students who have special needs?
What are the concepts of *environmentally open* and *environmentally closed* motor skills? How do they relate to the teaching of children with special needs?
What are the teacher's legal requirements regarding *general* and *specific supervision*?
What is the concept of *With-it-ness*? What is a technique to be used to increase *with-it-ness*?
From a legal perspective, is it important to match the children according to abilities when they will be competing in sports and games when physical contact is possible? Why?
What is the concept *contributory negligence*? At what age is it a legal factor?
What is and is not considered acceptable footwear for most physical activities?
What is the concept of *attractive nuisance*?
How well do children handle heat stress relative to adults? Why.
What is the concept of *inherent risk* and what is the teacher's responsibility relative to it?
What are the author's views regard boys and girls teams in gym class? In 5th and 6th grade sports teams?
What has normally been found regarding bell-shaped curves of motor abilities? are the differences usually greater within groups or between groups? What implications might that have for expectations of performance?
What skills are needed to coach and which skills not needed?
Why might you want to be aware of *Human Kinetic Publishers*?
What is the *American Sports Education Program (ASEP)*?
What are the concepts of *directionality*, *laterality*, and *body awareness*?

[CHAPTER 12]

ACTIVITIES TO HELP YOU START

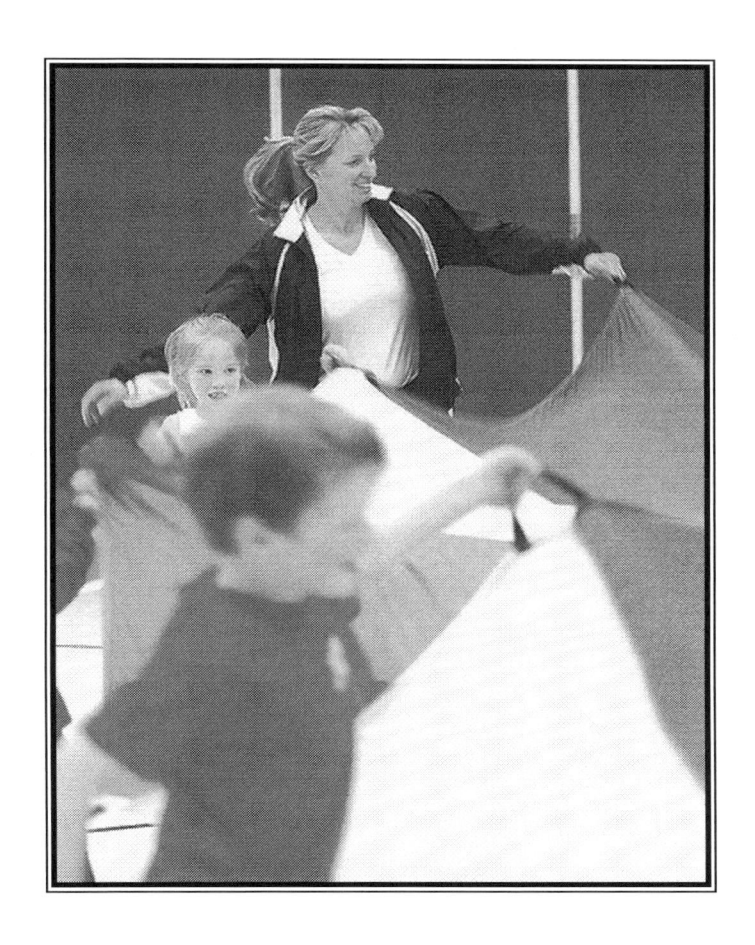

BEANBAG ACTIVITIES

CLASSROOM BASED ACTIVITIES

COOL-DOWNS

COOPERATIVE/NEW GAMES

DANCE
Golden Oldies
Folk Dance
Square Dance

GENERAL GAMES

HULA-HOOP ACTIVITIES

MUSIC ACTIVITIES

PARACHUTE ACTIVITIES

RELAYS

ROPE ACTIVITIES

TAG GAMES

STUNTS (INDIVIDUAL CHALLENGES)

STUNTS (PARTNER CHALLENGES)

WALK/RUN ACTIVITIES

WARM-UPS

"*I know of no more encouraging fact than this... If one advances confidently in the direction of his dreams, and endeavors to live the life he has imagined, he will meet with success unexpected in common hours.*"
~ H.D. Thoreau

"*Nothing great was ever accomplished without enthusiasm.*"
~ R.W. Emerson

Hopefully you have gotten numerous activity ideas throughout this text, and more importantly, you have developed an understanding of how to create and evaluate your own. In this final chapter I will add some of my favorite selections. All these activities have been effectively used by me or other teachers of elementary children. They have passed the *SOS Test*: they can (1) be played Safely, (2) keep everyone actively On-task, and (3) Successfully enjoyed by all the children regardless of their ability levels. However, I do not guarantee that any of these activities will work for you. Unless effective management procedures have been established, the most commendable of games can be torn apart by unruly students. Also, you will need to further vary and build off of these suggestions to suit the specific grade level, skills, temperaments and interests of your students. You may have to alter them in light of your unique environment and equipment possessions. And finally, as I hope you have realized from studying this book, there are many pedagogical skills that make for a good teacher (*anticipatory set, the three-rule rule, teacher movement, effective questioning, proximity control, with-it-ness, varied reinforcement,* etc.). These skills will require months and years of patient and purposeful practice before fully effective games and lessons can be implemented.

Permit me to conclude by saying that I hope these following activities will, in a small way, add to what you have learned in this text and help you to begin an enjoyable career of teaching of physical activities. The quotes at the beginning of this chapter have been an inspiration to me. I truly believe that if you are determined and enthusiastic, you can make yourself into a master teacher. No other goal could be worthier. Thank you for your patient reading.

"May the gods go with you. Upon your sword sit laurel victory and may smooth success be strewed before your feet." - W. Shakespeare

BEANBAG ACTIVITIES

I have suggested games with beanbags in other places of this text so I will introduce only a couple new ones here. I good home position for beanbags is balanced on top of heads. This certainly restricts fidgeting.

Quick hands: Partners are seated crossed legged facing each other. A beanbag is placed directly between. When the teacher calls "ready" students place their hands on their thighs. When the teacher calls "right," "left," or "both," the students react by grabbing for the bag with the appropriate hand or hands. Sundry starting conditions can be stipulated: hands on hips, over eyes, behind back, on head. Also, there are other possibilities besides the seated position: push-up and curl-up position.

Put & take: One person is in push-up position facing his/her seated partner. The seated person has a beanbag resting in each hand; palms up. On a signal the push up person reaches up and takes one bean bag and puts it on the floor, then reaches up with the opposite hand and removes the second beanbag. When both beanbags are on the floor, the push-up person reverses the procedure by sequentially moving the bags from the floor to the hands. The object is to see how many can be moved in a given time period.

CLASSROOM-BASED ACTIVITIES

If at least one or two classroom activities were done daily, it would add up to a significant amount of physical activity over the course of the year. Studies show that such breaks improve the students' attention/behaviors and do not impair academic performance (some show better performance).

Major Muscle Workout: These would be good exercises you or one of the students could initially lead everyone through together. However, later we might sometimes want to give the students a little flexibility as to activity pacing and selection. In this game you could list the following exercises on the board or on an overhead. Then you set a time of 4 or 5 minutes (cooking timers work good for this purpose). The students are told that they are to determine their own workout pace and see how many exercises they get done. Instead of listing the benefited muscle groups as I did here, you might leave blanks and then quiz them afterwards. I also tell them that if they want really strong muscles, they need to do these kinds of exercise until the muscles are really tired, and they need to do them two or three times per week. I do.

```
30 SEATED CRUNCHES …………..…ABDOMINALS
30 LARGE MARCHING STEPS………WARMING UP & CARDIO
30 RUNNING THIGH SLAPS………..WARMING UP & CARDIO
30 LEG LUNGES……………………......QUADRICEPS
30 CALF RAISES……………………...GASTROCNEMIUS
30 SQUATS…………………………....GLUTEUS & HAMSTRINGS
```

Health AND *Fitness* An Elementary Teacher's Guide

```
30 ARM CURLS (WITH BOOK)........BICEPS
30 DIPS USING CHAIR.................TRICEPS
30 PUSH-UP USING CHAIR............PECTORALS
```

Calisthenics: These can consist of stretches and more rigorous movements such as jumping jacks and jogging in place. The teacher might lead the activities but eventually can have student captains be at the front.

One Behind: The teacher begins an activity but the students only observe. When the teacher clearly switches to a different activity the students begin doing the prior one. This continues with the students staying one behind. For further variation the students might stay two behind, or parts of the class could be one behind while others were two or three behind. Of course student captains might be used as leaders.

Ski Boggying: This activity is done by side jumping back and forth as quickly as possible. A good challenge might be to go for a minute and see how many can be made (140 warm, 155 simmering, 170 cooking, 180 hot stuff). A break and heart rate check might be given and one or two more repetitions can be done. One leg versions are a challenge.

Power Walk: This is simply walking in place, raising the knees high and vigorously swinging the arms.

Calorie Count Walk: This is the same as the above but with an estimation of the calories burned. Having everyone take 25 big steps in place will burn up approximately 1 calorie (yard length steps for a 150# person). Thus, if we all took 100 big steps we would burn how many calories? One hundred big steps would of course be 4 calories, that is about how many calories are in an M&M. It might be fun and educational to have the children calculate and burn off some different foods such as a pad of butter, 5 potato chips or a half can of pop.

Sport Imaging: Sport skills can be practiced without the implements. Throwing balls and javelins; swinging rackets, bats and clubs; jumping hurdles and tacklers, refining martial arts moves, etc. etc.

Exercise Imaging: Stair climber, treadmill, jump rope, rowing machine, seated hand cranking, seated bicycling, etc.

Isometrics & Isotonics: This is where we exert muscular force against immoveable and yielding resistances respectively. For example, pushing your hand together would be an isometric exercise if no movement occurred. Gradually moving your hand through a range of motion, against the yielding resistance of the other hand, would be an isotonic exercise.

Physical Challenges: Examples would be linking the hands together behind the back, knee dips, heel clicks, touching the knee to the forehead, touching the toe to the nose, balancing high on the toes with the eyes closed, jumping up and doing a 180^0, jumping up and doing a 270^0.

Self-Selecting (The Don Hellison Approach): Once the students have had experience doing different exercises you might try allowing them to self-select their own preferred activity to do. Everyone simply does his/her own activity (takes self-responsibility). You might want to set some parameters such as everyone needs to elevate their heart rate or feel themselves breathing deeply.

Storytime: Start the activity with an introduction like the beginning of a story e.g., "Once upon a time…" or "Let's begin our journey." Here's one I made up:
HIKING THROUGH THE WOODS
WAKE-UP: Stretch, put on hat for sun protection
HIT THE TRAIL: walking, power walking
FEELING GOOD: skipping, spinning around, clicking heels
BRUSH, LIMBS & LOGS: swing arms through brush, ducking under limbs, stepping over logs
APPLE TREE (5-a-Day, fiber and 50 cal): reach, reach and jump, climb & stretch
LAKE: skipping stones, rowing old boat, practicing swim strokes
BEAR ON THE TRAIL: walking, running, sprinting, leaping rocks
BACK ON THE TRAIL: walking
TRAILS END (Met hour a day mod/vig activity guideline): few stretches and 6 deep breaths
<u>Variation</u>: this might be a good activity to assign student leaders.

U Can Two Can Workout: The students need two canned goods (10-16 oz). They perform various exercises. Example exercises are arm circles, arm curls, shadow boxing, military press, butterflies, trunk twists, lat pulls and rowing the boat.
Variation: Good music possibilities would be "Locomotion" or "Crocodile Rock."

Poetry in Motion: Select poems and chants that have a clear rhythm, then set some motion to it. For the example below I have had the students marching in place and reaching their arms up and down. I recite a line, they repeat it, and we just keep moving through the poem.
The Antiseptic Baby and the Prophylactic Pup

Were playing in the garden when the Bunny gamboled up;
They looked upon the Creature with a loathing undisguised,
It wasn't disinfected and it wasn't Sterilized.
They said it was a Microbe and a Hotbed of Disease;
They steamed it in a vapor of a thousand-odd degrees,
They froze it in a freezer that was cold as Banished Hope
And washed it in permanganate with carbolated soap.
In sulphurated hydrogen they steeped its wiggly ears,
They trimmed its frisky whiskers with a pair of hard-boiled shears;
They donned their rubber mittens and they took it by the hand
And elected it a member of the Fumigated Band.
There's not a Micrococcus in the garden where they play;
They bathe in pure iodoform a dozen times a day,
And each imbibes his rations from a hygienic cup.
The Bunny and the Baby and the Prophylactic Pup."

Variation: To the above example everyone could pretend that they were jumping rope and doing tricks to the cadence.

Father Abraham: You probably have done this or other sing-a-longs. They all usually work great. I like to put on a false-face and do Father Abraham as follows.

Everyone sings: "Father Abraham, had seven sons, seven sons had Father Abraham, and they never laughed, and they never cried, all they did was go like this."

"With a left" – everyone gets his/her left arm pumping
"And the right" – everyone get both arms pumping
"And the left" – the left leg is added
"And the right" ___ the right leg is added
"And the hips" – the hips are added
"And the head" – the head is added
"And the tongue" – the tongue is added

Invisible Jump Rope: (review basic counting, addition and subtraction)
- teacher calls number and the children jump and count up to…
- start at 20 and count and jump backwards
- "Two, four, six, eight, staying healthy's really great! While you jump count by two up to 20 then your're through! Ready go!"
- count by 5's up to 100

Using music is always a great way to energize movement and make it more fun. Below I have provided some start-up ideas. One of the schools I work with went ahead and burned CDs for all their teachers.

Mod Marches: This is one of a number of CDs that have fun songs for children to move to. It is so easy to make up movements to do. I have used the "It's a Small World" cut and had the students pretend that they are marching and playing the instruments.

Chicken Dance: We all already know this one. We make beak movements, flap wings, etc.

Mirroring: The students pair up. One person leads the other. When the teacher calls switch, the other person becomes the leader. When the teacher calls "Find someone new," they quickly pair with someone else and begin anew. This is fun to do with music. It can also be done in small groups.

Shoe Aerobics: Have the students take their shoes off and put them on their hands. Put on any music with a fun beat and go for it. It is fun to be clapping the shoes together over their head, under their legs, etc.

Four-Wall Game: Signs are put on the four walls. Although any fast music should work, I have done it using the song "A Whole Lotta Shaking Going On. "Wall one sign said "Arms, "wall two sign said "Knees", wall three sign said "Hips," wall four said "Whole body." Throughout the song I would call out the different numbers and the students would have to quickly turn to face that wall and do the prescribed shaking movement.

Let's Get Ready to Rumble: This is great up-beat music to do any vigorous movements. I have had the students use a sheet of paper as a prop. We wave it, shake it, twist it, wad it up and toss it, stomp on it, even tear it up and toss it up in the air for a finale.

Macarena: Simply have the students does the Macarena hand movements as they step in place (walk, jog, skip). The music I have increases in tempo as it goes and makes for a good challenge to keep up.

Surfing: Use the song "Wipe Out." When the drums are playing, the students imitate a drummer. Or you can have them swing their arms vertically in front of them, swinging up above the head and down to the waist. Encourage them to stay to the beat and tempo of the drums. When the music changes (drums stop-), the students imitate a surfer, bending at the knees and moving up and down. "Bend low and get into the tube. Stand up and put your 10 toes over the front of the board and lean backwards using the arms for balance and "Hang Ten!"

Shake It Up: The students need a 3 liter soda bottle filled with maybe 2" – 3" of colored water (glitter, small objects can also be added). Turn on "Twist and Shout" and

let the students shake the bottle as much as they want. Encourage students to shake the bottle high, low, right, left, two hands, one hand, under the leg, away from the body, etc.
Variation: Have students come up with routines with a partner.

COOL-DOWNS

Electricity: Two lines sit facing each other, hands joined with their teammates on both sides. I start the message at one end by simultaneously squeezing the hand of the head person of each line. The students relay a hand squeeze down their line. When the last person in the line has his/her hand squeezed, he/she attempts to pick-up a ball or other object that is placed directly between them. It is a race to see which line can produce the fastest current. A rule is that everyone's eyes must be on the ball so as not to anticipate the coming message. False messages due to nervous twitches result in "short circuits" and points for the other team.

AC-DC: A hand squeeze message is sent around a circle of seated people in any direction. A person can relay the message to continue it in the same direction or he/she can reverse it back towards the sender. The "it" person in the center tries to locate who has the message. Set a short time limit so no one gets stuck in the center for an embarrassing length of time. A good variation is to have someone in the circle "who's the leader." That person is doing an activity which everyone else in the circle duplicates. The leader keeps trying to change the activity without being identified by "it." If this variation was being used as a cool-down you might have everyone in the circle seated, for more vigorousness they could be standing and doing things like jumping jacks and jogging in place.

Killer: Everyone mills around shaking hands with people they meet. One person has been secretly appointed the "killer." The killer winks at people he/she wishes to kill. Those killed do not die instantaneously but after a few seconds die a horrible shrieking death and drop to the floor. If someone thinks he/she knows who the killer is, he/she says "I have an accusation to make." If someone else says "I second it," both people count 1-2-3 and simultaneously point at the suspect. If they both point to the true killer the game is over. If they point to different people or to a non-killer, they must die the death of ignominious false accusers and the game continues. It is fun when everyone has been killed and you have a complete cool-down.

Sculpturing: Students are paired and one is designated the sculptor and the other the clay. The task of the sculptor is to gently bend the clay into an interesting shape.

Activities to Help You Start

The task of the clay is to be pliable and to hold the positions as best as possible. It works well to have slow music playing and to frequently give a command for role reversal and partner switching. At the very end you might have everyone step back and have the sculptors judge which are the most interesting shapes.

COOPERATIVE/NEW GAMES

Levitations: The entire class lies down on their backs with their heads on a line. The direction in which they are oriented is alternated so that if the first child has his/her feet in a northern direction and next child's feet are to the south. This results in people being ear to ear in what I call a zipper formation. The first command is to have all the lying down students extend their arms into the air to form a row of supporting hands. At one end of the line I have a volunteer whom I will gently place on those hands. That levitated person will be rigid, facing toward the ceiling, and prepared to be passed head first down the row of hands. I will move to the other end of the line to receive the child when the passing nears completion.

I have seen a number of variations to this game. Sometimes instead of lying down the students are seated in a row. They are all close together, facing the same direction with their hands above their heads. The levitated person is passed in the same manner but of course is somewhat higher above the ground. Because of the greater height there should be a spotter walking on each side of the column. Then, to take this game to yet new heights it is possible to have the class standing close together instead of sitting. This can be exciting in the extreme but might necessitate that there are more than one strong spotter on each side of the floating child.

Levitations can also be played with the children lying on their backs in a circle, their heads together and legs radiating outwards spoke fashion. After the levitating child is positioned on their circle of hands, they attempt to produce a rotating motion. Sometimes it is possible to get a fairly rapid ride.

Lap Game: Begin by having the class stand in a circle. Everyone is facing the same direction, either clockwise or counter-clockwise. They are close enough together so that they can easily place their hands on the waist of the person in front of them. The instructor gives the command, "On my knees, please." On "please" everyone is to sit down on the thighs of whoever is behind them. If all do it together it will work. If someone hesitates you are likely to have a laughing collapse. When there has not been a collapse I will ask for the releasing of hips and the waving of hands. An almost sure way to end in a pile is to have everyone attempt to make three small, synchronized steps backwards.

Knots: This game works best with about 8 to 10 students per group. Everyone stands in a small circle and puts his/her hands into the center. Hands are joined with others. The only stipulation is that (1) you must not hold both hands of another person nor (2) can you be holding one of the hands of a person immediately on your left or right. After this positioning has been accomplished the group's task is to untangle themselves without letting go of hands. It usually is not easy but it should always be possible to make it into a circle or two links of a chain.

Blind Run: Form two parallel lines facing each other, about 6 feet apart. Players stand in their lines at least two arms' lengths apart (forming a lane of about 25 feet is good). Once the lines are formed and people are paying attention, a person on one end of the lines runs between the lines from one end to the other with his/her eyes closed. The two people at the end where the runner winds up take care to let the runner know they have come to the end of the line by gently tapping on the shoulder or hip, and, if the runner continues, with the word "stop." The end people should not try to forcibly stop the runner. For a second or third turn, runners can spin around before running and periodically during the whole run.

Touch My Can: The concept is simple but it can be challenging when you have a class of thirty or more students. Two people support a pop can between them by each pushing against it with one of his/her fingertips. The rest on the class join in with their fingertips. The objective is for everyone to be touching the can but without touching anyone else in the class.

Body Surfing: The entire class, except for one surfer, lies face down in a line, shoulder to shoulder. When the instructor yells "surfs up!" everyone begins continuously rolling in the same direction. It is imperative that everyone remains close together so as to avoid gaps. With the current flowing the surfer gently extends onto the waves and is transported along in prone position. The surfer needs to follow a path near the shoulder level of the students and not slide down to the legs and feet.

If you felt it best to reduce the amount of body contact, a small gymnastic mat could be used as a surfboard.

Around the Clock: The class joins hands in a circle. From here on all that is involved is having the group locomotor around the circle. For example, everyone slides once around and back, or jogs twice around and twice back. Challenges can be introduced by timing how long it takes them to jog around a back, three times. The game requires cooperation because some children will be slower than others and thus some must learn to moderate their pace if others are not to be pulled down or become unattached.

DANCE

Golden Oldies

There are many oldies but goodies that should not be forgotten. It is tough to beat *The Twist, YMCA, Limbo, Electric slide, The Stroll.*, etc. Here are a couple of my favorites.

Bunny Hop: You have been deprived if you haven't already done this in your salad days. The basic step is an easily learned one for probably third graders on. Two hopping side-touches are made with the right foot, two hopping side-touches are made with the left foot, then a jump is made forward (a jump is performed with both feet), a jump made backward, and then three forward jumps. I like to initiate the dance with everyone doing it on their own. Then, as the dance progresses people can start hooking together by grasping the waist of someone else. In the end you might have an interesting snake line. I have an Elvis Presly "I'm All Shook Up" tape that works great.

Hand Jive: Here is the way I learned it.
   Clap both hands to thighs twice
   Clap hands together twice
   Wave R hand twice over the L hand
   Wave L hand twice over the R hand
   Hit the R fist on top of the L fist twice
   Hit the L fist on top of the R fist twice
   Hitchhike the R thumb over your shoulder twice
   Hitchhike the L thumb over your shoulder twice

Folk Dance

I like to adapt folk dances to match the developmental needs of the children. That means I feel free to change the skills involved to make them simpler, or more complex, or more physically demanding. Also, I like to get the activity initiated right away with little worry about all the slowing organizational aspects such as boy-girl pairings, group formations, and highly specific sequences of steps. Here is how you can do that with a couple of fun folk dances (music and complete instructions for these could be easily obtained where folk and children's music is sold).

Mexican Hat Dance (La Raspa): The basic step is called a "bleeking" step. This is where you jump up and place your right foot out in front of you with the heel touching the floor. Then you reverse and do the same with your left. The basic rhythm is easily established by the music: three bleeking steps (R,L,R), followed by a pause, three more "bleeking" steps (R,L,R), followed by a pause, etc.

To get immediate action, everyone attempts this step to the music (If first and second graders cannot do it you might see if they can simply jump up and down to the music's rhythm.). When the "bleeking" segment of the music is over the children could individually jog or skip randomly around until you cue them that the "bleeking" segment is about to begin again. If time and the skills of the children permit you can begin the expansion process: two quick hand claps can be added during the pause between the "bleeking" steps. During the locomotoring phase everyone can find the closest person for a partner to skip beside in a big, two-by-two class circle. During the next locomotoring phase you might ask for right and left elbow turns with partners.

You can see that the above procedure gradually leads to an approximation of the "official" dance. Sometimes it might be educational to get to a culturally correct version of the dance, but that does not always have to be the goal. I have taught a conditioning variation of this dance where all movements were done in crab position.

Troika (three horses): This is a popular Russian folk dance. The music has a good running tempo that gradually increases to a challenging speed. In the "official" dance everyone is in a big circle with groups of threes running counter-clockwise together. Sixteen counts of running is followed by some dishrag movements, a circling of the 3s with grapevine steps and stomping.

An effective progressive instructional approach is to have the children running solo to the music. Beginning variations might consist of directional changes, stomping during the easily recognizable ending beats, running with one or two partners. Slightly more complex elements might be added later: circling of groups of threes, dishrag movement in groups of three, grapevine circling of groups of threes, etc.

Macarena: I like to teach the macarena movements and then see if the students can do them while performing various locomotor skills: walking, jogging, skipping, sliding, galloping, cariocaing. Okay, if that is a piece of cake, add to the challenge with a muscular strength and/or muscular endurance version in a curl-up or push-up position.

    R palm down, L palm down
    R palm up, L palm up
    R hand to L shoulder, L hand to R shoulder
    R hand to head, L hand to head
    R hand to L waist, L hand to R waist
    R hand to R hip, L hand to L hip
    Stand still and hula, hula, hula, clap

Square Dance

Scatter square dance is application of the same instantly active organizational progressions used in the other dances. The children dance their way through an expanding list of square dance skills that are intermixed with fun cooperative stunts and imitations (see Figure 11.1). To teach scatter square dance three things are needed. (1) A listing of activities on a large poster. This displayed referral list will make your calling easy and will help the rehearsal of the children. (2) A lengthy compilation of music. This can be either traditional square dance music or more popular country tunes. (3) A microphone system. This activity will work beautifully if your calls can be heard, but confusion worse than death will ensue if your voice is overcome by the music and the sounds of the stomping-clapping children.

You will find that calling scatter square dance is not difficult and can be delightful. Experience, and the children's input, will quickly suggest improvements and additions to your list. Having the children keep repeating the skill over and over until you decide what next to call helps them learn it better and provides you time to think what next to call.

Figure 12.1 Scatter Square Dance Calls & Descriptors

1. Keep time to the music	head, shoulders, elbows, hips, knees, toes, walking in place
2. Hit the lonesome trial	moving in all different directions in time with the music
3. Wave to those you pass	
4. Say "Hi to you"	
5. Do Si Do a partner	arms are folded and partners walk around each other right shoulder to right shoulder
6. Turn a partner	right elbows hooked**
7. Sasha a partner	join hands and slide
8. Circle up two with someone new	partner circles are done with two hands
9. Turn one by yourself	make some turns - don't let this one continue too long or dizziness results
10. Honor your partner	bows and curtsies - if this is too old fashion. I suppose you could substitute something more hip
11. Find a friend and promenade	moving with a partner hand in hand
12. Horse & rider	one person put hands on shoulders of another and rides his/her horse
13. Circle up 3, go back the other way	circle out direction and then the other
14. Hook up a horse & buggy	two people hook elbows and a third, with hands on their shoulders, drives
15. Right hand star	partners touch right hands in a raised position and walk forward around
16. Left hand star	partners touch left hands in a raised position and walk forward around
17. Shoot that star	from a star position the hands are pushed against each other and both sent away
18. Back up that star	walking backward
19. Birdie in a cage (duck, frog, etc.)	three people join hands in a circle around a fourth- that person is a bird, duck, frog, etc. and acts the part
20. Dive for the oyster	form a group of four, two partners stoop under the arms of the other pair and come back out
21. Dig for the clam	same dive for the oyster action by the other pair

Activities to Help You Start

22. Four leaf clover	two partners stoop under the arms of the other pair and then turn away from each other to end the group in a wrapped clover pattern
23. Follow the wagon trail behind _ & _	partners are promenading in a line behind a designated pair
24. Circle up that wagon train	everyone promenading in a circle
25. Follow the wagon train, make a tunnel, others go through	lead couple makes an arch which the others pass under
26. Circle up wagon train, all join hands in one big ring	
27. Circle to the left (and right)	
28. Go into the middle and come back out	
29. Go in once again, come back out with a great big grin	
30. Now into the middle and give a little shout	
31. Circle wagon train with your partner	
32. Inside person move up one	by moving in front of partners a single file circle should result
33. Face your partner, join right hands	you have set the stage for the Grand right & left
34. Grand right & left	pass your partner, left hand to next person on your way, right to next, etc. until home
35. Weave	same as Grand right & left but with arms folded and passing shoulders
36. When home Do Si Do and	remind them of this as they are in route about the circle

** I began by saying "swing" a partner but soon discovered that swings suggested a too vigorous action to the energetically disposed.

GENERAL GAMES

Rainbow Run: This game is relatively complicated so it will be necessary to sit everyone down and carefully teach all the rules. It basically is a scavenger hunt type game. A wall chart is made so that small groups of children are working through differing sequences of colors. For instance, the first color for group A might be red. This would mean that the group members must run and look under the many cones spread over the gym or playing field. Under one of the cones is hidden a red magic marker which they use to check a recording card that everyone carries. After this, they run to an exercise wall where they perform the prescribed activity on the red sign. Finally, they return to the original wall chart to see what their next color assignment is and the whole process is repeated.

You could play the game until all groups had finished or you could cut the activity off at a set time limit. One important detail is that the markers must never be removed from their cones because that would make it impossible for the other groups to complete their assignments (I have known some teachers to tie the markers to the cones as an anchoring precaution). This game certainly has great possibilities for interesting variations. Colors could be just one of many coding systems (animals, geometric shapes, numbers, planets, etc.).

Card Game: The class is divided into small groups. Each group has a stack of playing cards. The cards have been shuffled but each group has the same number of cards. The game is played by attempting to get through your cards as quickly as possible; each card has a designated activity that must be done before moving to the next. The activity possibilities are unlimited but I have provided a cooperative activities version below. Notice that some groups might be luckier than others in the card numbers they draw. This tends to increase the excitement and the more skilled students are not always the winners.

- Face cards
    - Aces: run two laps around the cones, hands joined
    - Kings: race walk around the cones, hands joined
    - Queens: one lap around the cones joined together in train fashion
    - Jacks: slide one lap round the cones, hands joined
    - Joker: everyone does 10 shoe juggles

- Hearts: that number of partner push-ups (one partner has feet on the shoulders of the other as they both do push-ups)

- Spades: that number of people through a push-up tunnel (the squad is in push-up position shoulder to shoulder, the end person crawls through, followed by the next, etc.)

Diamonds	that number of partner dips and curl-ups (one partner is in curl-up position, the other is in dip position with his/her hands on the knees of the curl-up performer)
Clubs	that number of around the clocks (the squad standing in a circle with hands joined, they run around the circle and back as quickly as they can)

Bird's Nest: The class is divided in small groups. Each group has a "bird's nest" which might be represented by a cone with a hula-hoop around it. Nine or so bins are located throughout the play space. Different objects are in the different bins (bean bags in one, nerf balls in another, jump ropes another, etc.). Each bin should have the same number of equipment pieces as there are total students.

The game simply has all the students running at once. Each student's assignment is to retrieve all nine objects, one at a time, and place them in his/her "nest."

Daytona Speedway: The class stands around the perimeter of a square about 30 feet per side. The game is progressive in nature. To begin, two of the opposing lines walk across the square and back without touching anyone (this speed is first gear). Then the other two lines follow suit. Next the activity is repeated at a slow jog (second gear) and finally at a fast but controlled speed (third gear).

When these levels have been demonstrated without crashes and fender benders the entire progressive process is repeated with all four lines going at once.

Partner variations of this game can be fun. One child can drive his/her partner stock car fashion. The child playing the car might have his/her hand up as protective bumpers. Possibilities involve motorcycle events, Mac Truck races (groups of 4), or nighttime driving in which the vehicles have their eyes closed. Of course, nighttime events must be done in first gear.

Indianapolis Speedway: This is a circular relay race. The class is divided into teams (pit crews or grease monkeys) who remain on the infield of a racetrack. When the race is started with a green flag one member from each team races counter-clockwise around the track to tag a teammate who then becomes the racing car. The teams are responsible for keeping count of the number of laps their team has completed. The race will have been set at 10 or 15 laps. When they have achieved this number they are to sit in a straight line and raise their hands.

To add further spice to the atmosphere the teacher introduces commands like "flat tires" "blow outs" and "crash & burns". When "flat tire" is called all the children in racing car mode must stop and do five jumping jacks before continuing onward. "Blow out" means three push-ups are needed. "Crash & burn" is yet more serious. The car crashes to the ground and their pit-crew rushes to their aid. They pick-up or drag the disabled car back to the pit-stop and then send the next car on its way.

I also like to further build upon the *anticipatory set* by playing race music, waving a checked flag, and having victory laps to cool down the engines.

HULA-HOOP ACTIVITIES

As with ropes or other implements, the number of games and activities that can be done is limited only by our creativity and that of the children. I like to begin with each child having a hoop to warm-up around, over, and through. A good *home position* for hoops is on the floor with the student standing inside it.

Spinning: The easiest spinning is around the wrist and forearm. With practice the non-dominant arm can be used, it can be transferred back and forth from arm to arm. Different locomotor skills can be done at the same time. Perhaps they can learn to pass the hoop from their arm to that of another, while they are skipping.

Spinning can also be done around the neck, waist, and ankle.

Hoop Imaginings: The younger children especially like to pretend. Here are some ideas: hoops above heads - angels, hoops in front of face - mirrors, hoops hanging on ears - world's largest ear-ring, hoops in front - race car steering wheels, hoops around necks - plow horses, hoops around waist - zooming, swooping spaceships.

Twirling: The hoop is set on end and is given a vigorous wrist snap so that it twirls on end for a period of time. All the children will be able to do this to some degree. While the hoop is twirling the children can see how many jumping jacks or push-ups they can do. They can locomotor around it: running, sliding facing in, sliding facing out, etc. Partners can start their twirls at the same time and run around each other's hoops. The whole class can start on command and see if they can give high 10s to five different people and still get back home to catch their hoop before it stops wobbling.

If a child waits until the hoop starts to wobble toward the floor, he/she can jump into the hoop and out again without being "bit" by it. A goal might be to see how many times you can enter and exit before it stops.

Rover: Producing a "Rover" hoop will be difficult for many students but there will be others who can learn it. In this trick you are throwing the hoop out ahead of you with a wrist snap that imparts backspin to it. If enough spin has been applied the hoop will come back home to you like the good dog Rover being called. If some of the students can get hoops rolling like this they and others can practice running beside and around it, straddle jumping over it, or even diving through it. I have had some students diving back and forth through one as many as eight times before it stopped.

Musical Hoops: This game is much like the old familiar musical chairs. The hoops are lying about the floor as the children weave about them to music. When the music stops everyone scrambles to get inside a hoop. If you like you can remove a couple of hoops so that two students will be caught without a hoop. Adhering to our rule of not eliminating people from activities I would suggest merely giving them a point and then letting them continue in the action. There are a variety of positions which might be assumed in the hoops: one foot balance, crab position, two body parts touching inside the hoop and two outside, three in and one out, etc. It is also fun to call numbers indicating how many people are to swiftly get inside of one hoop.

Hoop Drills: Squads of about six children each are lined up. In front of each squad is a row of six or seven hoops, spaced approximately six inches to a foot apart. The challenge is to traverse through the hoops in a variety of ways without stepping on the hoops. For example, the squad leader might leap through all the hoops so that he/she is stepping only inside each hoop. His/her squad members follow immediately behind. It works best if the leader has traveled some distance beyond the last hoop to permit room for the following students to finish their leaps. When they have been given this much room you can have the last student turn around and lead the same activity back through with the squad now in reverse order.

Besides leaping through the hoops the assignment might be to: slide, skip, weave, or follow some hop-scotch pattern (one, two, one, two; one, two, three, one, two, three). Connecting the squads together increases the challenge: sliding with hands joined, train fashion with hands on hips, train fashion while weaving about the hoops, etc.).

Of course these drills can be turned into relay races in which the teams compete against their own times or the other squads. Generally, with enough variety, it will not be necessary to add this competitive element. Also, I have found that racing through the hoops greatly increases the chance of someone tripping. Taping the hoops to the floor or using floor markings would be the more prudent and safe thing to do.

Poison Hoops: This game can be played in a whole class circle or in separate squads. When in a squad formation everyone is in a line with his/her hands joined. A pile of hoops are lying in front of the first person. The leader picks-up one hoop with his/her free hand and wiggles the hoop through his/her body to the next person. The next person, without the use of hands wiggles and sends it on down the line. The group's task is to convey all the hoops from the head person to the last person, and back again.

I have also heard of this game being played where everybody is lined up facing the same direction. They are connected by reaching one of their hands backwards between their legs and the other hand forward to grasp the hand coming from between the legs of the person in front of them. Oh what a tangled web we weave...

MUSIC ACTIVITIES

Shoe Aerobics: This is your basic aerobics class led by an instructor but with one difference, everybody has their shoes on their hands. With strongly beating music can you not imagine all the slapping of the soles together, over-the-head, behind the back, under the legs, crab walking, hands and knees, etc. It is not hard to think of things to do once you get started.

Any prop will do. *The Paper dance* is simply playing with some energizing music and a piece of paper. For example, how about putting on the fast paced "Let's Get Ready to Rumble" and then waving, swinging, fanning, turning, folding, wadding, tossing, and stomping the paper.

Shape museum: One half of the class assumes original static shapes and hold them. The rest of the students jog around and through the museum of shapes. When a moving child finds an interesting shape he/she stops and creates a new shape in front of that person. That person says "thank you" and is unfrozen to join the joggers. The game continues in this fashion with half the class always posed in shapes and half the class moving. Mellow music generally works well.

A more vigorous variation of this game is called the *Dynamic shape museum*. The difference here is that the shapes are moving in place, jogging in place, jumping jacks, twisting, bending, and so on. More up-tempo music can be used.

Act-React: The teacher does a movement for a set number of counts (maybe 8 or 16) and then stops. As soon as the teacher stops, the class then mimics what they saw. As soon as they are done the teacher executes another movement segment and the game continues back and forth. Stationary movements such as jumping jacks and arm circles are the easiest with which to begin. Next, side-to-side and back-and-forth movements can be incorporated.

I have known dance instructors to progress to much more intricate movement skills and to increase their segments lengths to 32 or 64 counts. Also, they may even eliminate the lag time to create continuous leader and student movement. In other words, the instructor never stops moving and the followers replicate everything while remaining a set number of counts behind. You can see how this would be a good test of attention abilities.

Four-Wall Game: It doesn't get much simpler than this and still be exciting. Signs are posted on the four walls. One day's example might be (1) head & shoulders, (2) arms, (3) hips & knees, and (4) whole body jump & bounce. When the leader shouts "one" the students turn as fast as possible to face that wall and begin moving their head & shoulders creatively in time with the music. When another number is called they quickly rotate to it and move the prescribed body part(s). Up-beat music should be used; "Whole Lota Shakin" is a good one that comes to mind.

Criss-Cross Game: Groups of children are at the four corners of a square. One group leads with an activity across the center of the floor. They may be individually sliding, skipping or crawling; or they may be hooked together as a team as they do some locomotor skill. When the opposite group sees what the approaching group is doing they duplicate it by weaving through them in route to the vacated corner. As soon as these groups have cleared out of the center the side groups follow suit.

The game continues in this manner with the children thinking up new movements and patterns. After one group has led the activities for five or six times the other groups should be given their chance at leadership. I have known this game to flow for an extended period of time. In introducing this game there is one point that may be worth making to the students; tell them that a considerate activity selection would be one that everyone in the class should be able to perform. For instance, leading with a handspring would be inappropriate because there will be some who cannot do it and maybe someone would be injured in making an attempt.

Me and My Shadow: Everyone is moving in a line following whatever actions the head person initiates. When anyone wishes to begin a new activity he/she can separate from the line and begin a new activity. Followers can stick with the same leader, follow the new or chart their own course. This game usually results in a good mix of followers and leaders. I have learned that if you don't want a group always tagging after you the initiation of something akin to one-handed push-ups will result in a winged dispersal.

Partner Mirroring is a similar game in which one partner faces and mirrors the actions of the leader. The command is frequently given to change leaders and to quickly find someone new to continue the game. *Small group mirroring* is the same game but with a group of about four students in a circle. They are numbered one through four and take turns being the leader. *Creative circle* is simply having the entire class in a circle with each child in turn assuming directorship. This game seems to work better after the children have had some leadership experiences in the less intimidating partner or small group versions.

PARACHUTE ACTIVITIES

I strongly encourage you to consider getting a parachute. There are endless everyone-active activities you can do with them. The students love playing with it and it lends itself to a managed environment because everyone is holding on to a designated position. To gain access I suggest first checking with your physical education specialist. If you need to purchase one they are not expensive and last for many years. The catalog references I listed in chapter 7 will have them in various sizes. Small ones big enough for six people will be 15-20 dollars while extra large ones with 36 handles will be approximately 350 dollars.

Merry-Go-Round: Everyone holds with L or R hand and walk, hop, slide, gallop, run, etc. Run while holding the chute like a kite.

Ocean Waves: Everyone holds the chute with both hands and shakes it. They will gladly do it and it will not take long for them to tire their arms. They can do this while moving also.

Circle the Ball: Place a playground ball on the raised chute. Make the ball roll around the chute in a clockwise or counter-clockwise direction. Try it with two balls, a large beach ball, or cage ball.

Popcorn: Place a number of bean-bags (6-10) on the chute. Shake the chute to make them rise like popping corn. When I do the same thing with jump ropes I call it *Poison Snakes*.

Team Ball: Divide the chute players in half, so each team defends half of the chute. Using two to six balls, and variety, try to bounce the balls off the opponent's side.

Umbrella: Everyone holds the chute with both hands and raises their arms in unison. Then, a moment later, they lower their arms (remaining in position).

Mushroom: Everyone raises the chute and walks forward; everyone lowers the chute and returns.

Fly Away: With the chute inflated, youngsters take one step forward. On command, they release the chute and it remains suspended in the air for several seconds. On command the class reaches for the ribs again. Care must be taken that the chute is not released too soon.

Ghost Town: Starting in the forward bend position, youngsters inflate the chute on command. They take three steps toward the center, stand still, leave go of the chute, and allow it to settle down on them.

Face Museum: Make an umbrella, pull it to the ground with everyone putting his/her head inside. It is fun to make faces. I have called this a *Rogue's Gallery* but may be you will not want to.

Amusement Ride: Make an umbrella, pull it to the ground with everyone sitting on the edge inside of the chute. Make it into an amusement or space ship ride by rocking forwards, backwards, and sideward.

Mountain of Air: Youngsters umbrella the chute and then quickly bring the edges to the floor to trap the air (this time they are remaining on the outside). Students whose number has been called then crawl across the top until the air is all out.

Circular Dribble: Each child has a ball. The object is to run in circular fashion counter clockwise, holding onto the chute with the L hand and dribbling with the R hand. The dribble should be started first, then on signal, each starts to run. If a ball is lost, the child must recover the ball and try to hook on at his or her original place.

Run for It: Have the children around the chute and count off by fours. Start them running, holding the chute in one hand. Call out one of the numbers. Children holding the number immediately release their grip on the chute and run forward to the next vacated place. This means that they must put on a burst of speed.

Passing Under: Children have numbers. When called they run, hop, skip, etc. under the chute to a new vacated position. In addition to numbers it is fun to designate movers on the basis of things like hair color, white socks, shorts, handedness, or everyone with two ears.
   * *Individual stunts:* go under and do 5 jumping-jacks, 2 push-ups, or may be both the jumping-jacks and push-ups.
   * *Cooperative activities:* go under and shake hands with 2 people, or jumping high 10s with 3 people, or a patty-cake sequence.
   * *Stunts with props:* go under and do 3 jump ropes, or hula-hoop three revolutions (this results in some hoop collisions), or dribble behind your back, or pick up 5 bean-bags.

Tug-Of-War: Divide class into two equal teams. On signal, they pull against each other and try to reach a restraining line. Another tug-of-war that is often more enjoyable for primary-age children is an individual pull, where all children tug in any direction they desire.

Horse and Jockey: Youngsters are paired off and standing evenly around the chute with the "horse" holding the chute waist high and legs in a straddle position. The "jockey" is in a squat position facing the "horse." On a signal all jockeys scramble between the horses' legs and speed away to the right running all the way around the chute and back to their horse. In the meantime, the horses have inflated the chute and then placed themselves on all fours, still holding the chute so the "jockeys" can mount their "horse" as they return back to the starting place. The first jockey to run around the chute and mount his horse is declared the winner. Partners can then exchange places.

Jaws: This makes for a good culminating game because it is a favorite and everyone ends up in a big laughing pile. The game begins with everyone sitting with the chute pulled tightly up to his/her chin. One person, the shark, swims about under the chute in search of prey. When the shark grabs some unfortunate's leg he/she gives a scream and is drug beneath the surface. Now there are two sharks and the waters become more and more dangerous.

Air Conditioning: This makes for a good cool down. Some of the children lay down under the chute and the rest of the fans them with air by repeating umbrellas.

The Big Sleep: This is the ultimate cool down. Everyone lays down under the chute with the edge pull up to his/her chin. I guarantee you will hear some snores.

Rhythms: Since many rhythms are by nature in a circular formation, the parachute lends itself very well to rhythms adaptations. In some instances it helps to overcome the stigma of "dancing" since the outcome seems to appear very different. Old standbys are things like the Hokey Pokey and Green Sleeves. Blow I have described two simple, well-known folkdances. By doing these I think you will see how easy it would be to do with others.

    * *Pop! Goes the Weasel:*
- count off by 2's; hold parachute in R hand
- walk 12 steps then make umbrella
- 1's pop under and move ahead one person
- REPEAT

    * *La Raspa (Mexican Hat Dance)*
- Chorus
    Hop on L with R heel forward
    Hop on R with L heel forward
    Hop on L with R heel forward
    REPEAT 8 times
- Umbrella up for 8 counts; umbrella down for 8 counts (REPEAT)
- Chorus

- Umbrella up of 8 counts; umbrella down for 8 counts (1's run under and exchange positions)
- Umbrella up of 8 counts; umbrella down for 8 counts (2's run under and exchange positions)
- Chorus
- 16 count gallops with R hand on the parachute
- 16 count gallops with L hand on the parachute
- Chorus
- Ripples (32 counts)
- Chorus
- 16 count gallops with R hand on the parachute
- 8 count-put parachute to the ground

RELAYS

Here are a few suggestions for relays. (1) Be a good official. If you are keeping track of times or comparing team performances, you must ensure that the skills are being done according to specifications. (2) Keep the finishing lines well away from walls so as to afford safe stopping distance. (3) Have a discernible finishing position. Sitting in a straight line with their hands up would serve well. (4) I prefer relays in which more than one person goes at a time and thus the amount of cooperation and on-task time is increased.

Train Relay: The squads hook together in a straight line, hands on the waist of the person in front of them. They must not become disconnected throughout the race. At the turnaround on a down and back course it is best to simply turn around so that their order is reversed on the return trip (this avoids a dangerous whip cracking effect).

Circle-of-Friends Relay: The squads form circle-of-friends by joining hands around one of their teammates. The object is to race in this formation, taking the inner person down and back the course. This is then repeated for each member of the squad being given the escort.

Shuttle Relay: The squads are lined-up, hands joined, with the center persons straddling a centerline. When the race begins the lines run or slide in one direction and then the other in a designated pattern. On a basketball court a good sequence is back and forth from foul line to foul line, baseline to baseline, foul line to foul line, and then back to center position.

Rescue Relay: The object here is to move the squad from one location to another. The squad leaders are positioned at the opposite end of the play area. The race begins with the leaders running to their squad, grabbing the first member by the hand and taking them back to the other area. The squad leaders' task is done and they remain there. The first transported member goes back to get member number two and takes them back. This repeats itself until everyone has been transposed to the new location. To further increase activity and teamwork *Accumulative rescue relay* can be played. In this version the leader takes the first member back in the same fashion but then returns with the first member to pick-up the second member, and third member, etc. Clearly the squad leaders earn their running stars.

Reindeer Relay: The squads are arraigned with one member sitting on a carpet or blanket holding one end of a rope (this is Santa). The other team members hold onto the other end of the rope (they are reindeer). The task of each Santa is to deliver, one at a time, a number of objects (gifts) to a bucket at the other end of the gym. Rotating Santas and reindeer after each trip is fun. Keep the anticipatory set rolling with Christmas music and sleigh bells.

ROPE ACTIVITIES

Ropes offer many options for enjoyable challenges for individuals and groups. It should not be too difficult to get individual ropes for each child (the best fit is when stood on the rope will come up to the armpits), a number of Double-Dutch length ropes (these are about 8 to 10 feet), and a big long, heavy duty one (about 25 to 30 feet). Before beginning to handle the ropes a good warm-up procedures is to have everyone lay their rope in a circle on the floor. Endless exercises can be done around and through them. Many similar things can be done when lain in a straight line. When the ropes are picked-up and being used, a good *home position* is for everyone to stand on the center of the rope.

Individual jump-rope challenges: The idea here is to make a sizable list of stunts for the children in work on, both in class and at home and recess. To meet the needs of all the students, the list should include easier stunts as well as advanced ones (Figure 12.2). Incentives can be provided for demonstrated improvements. For example, they could qualify for a "Skipper's Club" or participate in a jump routine. I do not favor charting each student's progress on a publicly displayed chart. Although such a procedure will be motivating to some students, the lesser skilled can find it disheartening. I would rather everyone had a chart in his/her own portfolio and learned to focus primarily on self-improvement as opposed to social comparison.

Figure 12.2. Individual Jump Rope Challenges

Stunts
1. _____ Basic 1/2 time jumping of rope swung by others (50 times)
    (1/2 time jumping is a slow jump with a small bounce in-between)
2. _____ Basic 1/2 time jumping self-swung (50 times)
3. _____ Basic full-time jumping of rope swung by others (50 times)
4. _____ Basic full-time jumping self-swung (50 times)
5. _____ One foot jumping (50 times)
6. _____ Boxer step (50 times)
    (hopping on right foot twice, left foot twice, etc.)
7. _____ Bleeking step (50 times)
    (Bleeking is alternating heel touches)
8. _____ Running in place (50 times)
9. _____ Basic backwards spin (50)
10. _____ Criss-crosses (10 times)
11. _____ Consecutive criss-crosses (10 times)
12. _____ Double twirls (10 times)
13. _____ Consecutive double twirls (10 times)
14. _____ Consecutive under the legs (10 times)
15. _____ Egg beater jumping (20 times)
16. _____ Double Dutch jumping (20 times)

Conditioning Challenges
17. _____ Running one lap around the gym
18. _____ Running 5 laps around the gym
19. _____ Skipping one lap around the gym
20. _____ 2 minute basic jumping
21. _____ 5 minute basic jumping
22. _____ 10 minute basic jumping

Jump routines: This is where you choreograph the children's jumping skills to music. For a beginning level group an effective formation is to have two lines facing each other. For the first 16 counts or so, the members of the lead line do a step to the music (maybe the basic jumping in place). For the following 16 counts they stop while the other line follows their suite. The routine continues back and forth in this alternating manner. The advantage of this procedure is that it gives the lines time to rest and an opportunity to plan the next step. The skills can be kept fairly simple such as running in place, one foot jumping, or the boxer step. If some children have mastered only one or two skills there is no reason they cannot be assigned more fundamental movements than their teammates. When higher levels of skills are possessed the skills and patterns can be made as demanding as you wish. The skills of cross-overs and double jumps can be add; patterns where the teams exchange positions and simultaneously travel in circles can be instituted.

Cooperative task assignments: A variety of partner and small group challenges can be designed. What is nice about this is that the different groupings of children can work at their own rate on different skills. Different skills can be added to those of rope jumping. For instance, a ball can be dribbled, passed, and shot at baskets. I usually set ten or fifteen jumps as being the criterion that is necessary before a skill is considered accomplished.

Double-Dutch: Even if you are not an experienced Double-Dutcher it might be possible to involve your class in this exciting challenge. Very likely there will be some students in your class, or the older grades, who both know how and would be eager to help with instruction. Another, simpler way of jumping duel ropes is the *egg-beater*. Two swingers hold a Double-Dutch length rope and two other swingers have their rope at a right angle to them, so that the ropes are crossed in the center. If the two groups begin swinging at the same time the egg-beater effect is achieved and one or multiple children can dare to enter the center for jumping. It looks harder than it actually is.

Long Rope Jumping: There are many things that can be done with a long rope. *Run throughs* are where the rope is swung and one child after another runs into and immediately exits on the opposite side. I like to have everyone continue jogging around so that the entire class creates a non-stop jogging circle. See how many laps can be completed.

Doing *paired run throughs* demands more cooperation and it also dictates that the pace of the joggers be increased. They will have to go twice as fast as the singles did if they expect to maintain a continuous flow through the rope. Because the outside partners have to run much faster than their partners I sometimes specify a figure 8 pattern; if a clockwise turn is followed on the first run through a counter-clockwise path will be taken on the next. To moderate the faster pace of the partner format, the skill can be changed to require the execution of one jump before the partners escape.

Addition jumping is having someone jumping the long swinging rope and then others keep joining in. The object is to see how many can be jumping at once. I have seen whole classes of elementary children doing it with the instructor jumping with a small

Activities to Help You Start

child on his shoulders. What do you think to be the maximum number of elementary age jumpers? Would you believe 230 children did 13 jumps?

Jumping the Shot: This game also makes use of the extra long rope but it does so in a much different manner. A heavy rubber ball or a number of bean-bags are placed in a sock which in turn is tied to the end of the rope. The instructor or instructor's aid kneels in the center of the floor and begins to swing the rope over his/her head much like a cowboy lariat. Gradually more rope is let out so that the end of the rope with the sock is traveling close to the ground. The children who are positioned beyond the circumference move in until they must start jumping over the rope as it swings past. If most everyone is being too hesitant I have required that they join hands in a circle around the swinger. This draws everyone into the action and maybe you will be able to have the whole class jumping in wave fashion.

With more skill and daring students can intersperse tricks in between the jumps (touching the floor, hitting the deck, 3 jumping jacks, etc.).

It is also possible to *run against the current* or *run with the current*. *Running against the current* means the student(s) run inside the circle in direction opposite the spinning rope. Frequent leaps are necessary. *Running with the current* might sound easier but is actually harder. You have to be really fast to get around and out before the rope catches you and if you don't make it in time the timing of your leap is more difficult.

STUNTS (INDIVIDUAL CHALLENGES)

Ski Boogying: Everyone stands next to a line. On command they begin to jump from side to side over the line as quickly as possible. I usually challenge them to do their maximum in one minute. Jumping 145 times is considered simmering, 160 warm, 175 cooking, and 185 hot stuff. Slanty rope challenges can be created by providing wider lines or objects to jump over.

Fish Hawk Dive: Everyone is given a piece of paper that they fold lengthwise in half. They place the paper on the floor, standing on end. Then they balance in front of the paper on one knee and foot. The task is to dip forward and pick the paper up with one's mouth; balance must be maintained even after the paper has been raised.

While others continue to practice, those who have achieved the skill are next required to lay the paper on its side and thus must dip lower to reach it. Beyond that, there is a standing variation called the *Crane dive*. This is tough but can be done by some.

Crazy Walk: This is a task in which the children walk forward, but with a catch. The catch being that the free foot must come forward from around behind the support leg. With proper shifting of weight it is possible to place the swing foot ahead of the other and thus make slow but consistent transit. After some practice *crazy walk* races can be fun. One foot must remain on the ground at all times.

Blind Stand: The task is simply or not so simply this. Stand on your toes, extend your arms out in front, close your eyes, and then hold that position. I consider 15 seconds simmering, 20 warm, 25 cooking, and 30 hot-stuff. Try the one-foot version.

Human Tops: Attempt to jump and spin halfway around (180 degrees) and land in good balance. Challenge them to do it in both directions. More advanced progressions would be 270s, 360s and one foot variants of them.

Foot Drills: Place markings on the floor using tape or poly spots. All sorts of configurations can be laid out: circle, seven, Z, eight, triangle, etc. The task is to as quickly as possible do repeated, two footed jumps around the circle, up and down the seven, up the Z and back, etc. The spots need to be only about a foot apart and it is fun to keep the distances standardized so that self-improvement goals can be set and realized.

STUNTS (PARTNER CHALLENGES)

Scooter: Two children sit facing each other. The feet of each are underneath the others bottom. They reach forward and place their hands on their partner's shoulders. After this positional unit has been achieved they attempt to begin rocking back and forth so that one's bottom and then the other's come off of the ground. If this can be done, one of the children must learn to slightly extend his/her legs when the other's weight is lifted and shifted backwards. With practice they will gradually get the feel of being able to progress across the floor. Eventually they might be ready for scooter races.

Pop-Ups: Person 1 is in push up position. Person 2 crawls under the bridge formed by person 1 and stands up. Person 1 now flattens out on his/her stomach and person 2 jumps over the top of person 1. The progression continues and the idea is to see how many pop-ups the partners can do in a set time.

Partner-Lean: Partners side by side with a partner. Each person's feet are together and as close to the other's as possible. Their inside hands are tightly clasped. The task is for them to lean away from each other until their joined arms are completely straightened. If the children do not slowly and cooperatively work against one another balance will be lost. When a fully extended position is held the instructor or another student should be able to pass between them.

Double Top: Partners literally stand toe to toe. They tightly clasp one another's hands and in slow unison lean away from each other. After they have achieved a fully extended lean they are to begin to take tiny steps around each other. If a good lean has been established a fast marry-go-round spinning action is producible. Make sure they know to not let go of their partner, and make sure the grouping are well spaced so there is not a chance of them crashing into other human tops.

Seated Cycling: Two children sit facing each other. They raise their legs so as to put the soles of their feet together. Next they attempt to establish a cycling leg motion, slow at first and then more rapidly. A good expansion of this skill is to add the hands so that they are maintaining both the hands and feet in a coordinated cadence.

Up and At 'em: From a standing position, partners hold a ball in between their foreheads. The challenge is to lower their bodies to a push-up and then prone position without touching the ball with their hands or dropping it. And then of course, the process must be reversed to a standing position again. *Partner ball carries* are also fun. Students attempt to move from one location to another. Negotiating obstacles can add excitement. Also, the ball carries do not need to be restricted to the head-to-head position. Consider head-to-back, back-to-back, shoulder-to-shoulder, etc. (Group carries are also great, five people carrying four balls, etc.)

TAG GAMES

Here are a few guidelines it is good to keep in mind when playing any tag game. (1) Have more than one person it. If only one person is it he/she may not be able to catch anyone and thus is placed in an embarrassing position. (2) Make sure boundaries are established and enforced. Without them the children will run far away and into dangerous areas. (3) Make sure the "it" people are easily identifiable to avoid confusion. Pennies, hats or large balls make for good distinguishing markers. (4) I also have a rule of *killing it before it dies*. That means I do not need to feel that the game must be played until the last person is tagged. After the children have had good exercise, but before their interest has waned, I terminate the game. By so doing the children will be eager to play the game another day.

Walking Tag: Everyone has a partner. Within each pair one is designated the initial chaser (perhaps the taller of the pair, the one with the cleanest shoes, etc.). At the beginning command the "its" must spin once around before beginning the chase. As indicated by the name, walking is how everyone locomotors. When touched the tagged person spins around once and assumes the role of chaser.

The idea behind the spinning around is that it gives the fleeing person a chance to get a small lead. Requiring walking is also a good initial rule for minimizing collisions while still requiring a lot of activity.

Two good variations of this game are *couple tag* and *monster tag*. In *couple tag* pairs of students with hooked elbows play other pairs. Before initiating the chase the partners much pivot around in hooked elbow position. The chaser is the monster in *monster tag*. In this game I let the children reverse roles at anytime they wish. This role switching can be done by the fleeing student suddenly pivoting about and letting out a scream. This means he/she has metamorphosed into the monster. "Monster Mash" music goes well with all the screaming of the class.

Variants of Basic Tag: The format of basic tag has a few "it" people (as designated by balls, pennies, etc.) trying to tag any of the non-"it" people. When someone is tagged he/she is never long eliminated from the action. There are two concepts for accomplishing his/her re-entry.

Unfreezing oneself concept: *Jumping jack tag* or *push-up tag* would be examples. After being tagged, five jumping jacks or three push-ups will respectively get you back in the game. *Circuit tag* would see the tagged persons running outside the tag area where a circuit has been set-up. After navigating themselves through the circuit they flow back into the tag activity. *Samurai warrior tag* is an exciting one for the younger children. The teacher is the Samurai warrior, replete with robe and sword. Those who have been tagged go to the warrior to be saved. The warrior strikes the sword to the ground and simultaneously yells "Samurai warrior will save you!" Then the sword is swung over the heads and under the legs of those children, carefully of course. The children duck and jump and then return to tag.

Unfreezing others concept: Tagged people assume a stationary position signaling that they have been tagged and need to be rescued. In *tunnel tag* they stand with their legs apart and if some non-"it" person crawls through their legs they are enabled to re-join the game. In *shake-and-bump tag* the tagged individuals stand with their right arms out in front of them. They are unfrozen when someone comes by, gives their hand a shake and bumps hips with them.

Variants of Everyone It Tag: In its simplest form everyone is "it" and tries to run about tagging everyone else. No one is eliminated, if you are tagged it only means that that person scored a point. There is much high intensity activity when everyone is "it" so usually the games will need to be stopped within a minute or so.

Beanbag tag is the same as everyone it tag except now the students score points by throwing their bean bags to hit somebody's foot. Requiring the beanbags to be slid or bowled is a good variation. *Bum tag* is the same as beanbag tag but now nerf or yarn-balls are thrown at the backsides of others. *First aid tag* has everyone "it" at the start. When someone is tagged he/she is wounded and must hold that body part with one hand. He/she can still tag others with the free hand. When tagged a second time that wound also must be held. With no hands available for tagging those people are incapable of further tagging but are yet alive and can continue to run about. A third tag brings death.

Variants of Multiplying "Its" Tag: These tag games begin with one or two people being "it" (remember the danger of having a slower student being it by him/herself). *One-arm bandit tag* has the "it" person chasing everyone else. He/she is identifiable because one arm is held behind his/her back. When anyone is tagged that person puts one arm behind him/her and also becomes a bandit. *Snake-pit tag* is a favorite of younger students. The snake pit is the area within the boundaries of the tag game. The boundaries are made more confined than normal because the "it" person is a snake and thus can only crawl and slither about. When someone has been touched (bitten) by the snake, he/she joins the snakehood. In *Home-on-the-range tag* the "it" is a pair of hand-in-hand students. The "it" pair represents a horse and rider. All else are steers out on the range valuing their liberty. When the horse and rider tags a steer they take it back to a corral area. After a second steer has been added to the corral the two steers form a horse and rider and join the round-up.

WALK/RUN ACTIVITIES

Conversational Jogging: This is the official name of the activity but I have also called it RUNNING AT THE MOUTH. Students are asked to find a friend and to begin jogging (this works great as a walking activity as well). As they complete a lap or so the teacher holds up a sign indicating a topic of conversation: "your favorite book", "what I'm doing for the holidays", "my favorite animal", "my best sport's experience", etc.). Following the activity is a good time to talk to the students about the run or walk. Hopefully some students can be made to realize that these activities can be made enjoyable by conversation and that the time went rapidly

Time Estimation Run: The perimeter of a full size basketball court equals 288 feet; therefore 18.33 laps equals 1 mile; 9.16 laps = 1/2 mile. Everyone initially estimates how long it will take him or her to run a mile (or whatever distance selected). They keep track of their laps and tell the teacher when they reach the finish line. He/she whispers the time to them. As they are cooling down they must calculate the number of seconds between their estimated and the actual time. When everyone has finished the instructor surveys to see how well everyone paced themselves.

I have done this run at Halloween and called it the PUMPKIN RUN. The students with the closest estimates won pumpkins.

Nature Walk: I am amazed at how little most children, and even adults, know about the natural environment around them. Ahead of time, all or some of the students are given a specific topic that they are to learn to identify. They must also find out some interesting information pertaining to it. These topics are natural things that will be likely encountered on the hike you have selected. Possibilities in your neighborhood park might be an oak tree, lilac bush, house sparrow, starling, crab grass, basalt rock, and ladybug. If the student sees his/her assigned subject on the walk, the student stops the class and tells some interesting fact about it. Sometimes it might be fun to take along binoculars or even a camera.

Another nature option would be to take along a checklist and see how many different birds, trees, mammals, insects, or flowers could be identified.

Good Citizen Clean-Up Walk: I am also amazed that many children are careless about dropping wrappers, cups, etc. When I go for a walk I generally make it a habit to pick-up at least one bit of litter. It seems to me a good environmental lesson to have the kids do the same. A garbage bag and some plastic gloves would be good to take along.

Card Run: Children are to run a course, maybe for 15 minutes. Each time they pass the teacher they get a playing card. A figure 8 shaped course works well because the students pass the teacher more frequently and thus accumulate more cards. After the time is up and everyone is cooling down, some games may be played with the cards: anyone with three of a kind gets a reward, anyone with two pairs gets a reward, etc. You can see that the more cards someone has earned the better he/she is likely to do in the card games.

Alphabet Walks: Students try to spot objects whose first letter spells out the 26 letters of the alphabet. Students should report them in alphabetical order and actually see them. Can you or your team go from A to Z in 20 – 30 minutes?

Walk Across America: Keep a map on your classroom wall and plot your daily progress using your classes' total miles. Using your daily averages, how many days would it take to walk across America? Where would you be by a certain date such as Memorial Day? Could you do it in 80 days?

If 30 of your children averaged about 10 minutes of walking daily (a half mile each), then by the end of the school year your class would have totaled 3,000 miles walking – the distance from Independence Hall in Philadelphia, Pennsylvania to The Space Needle in Seattle, Washington. And all along the way you could be discussing our nation's geography, history and culture while practicing mileage addition.

Walk With the Principal: Each week one of the students in the school is rewarded for doing something good. The reward is the privilege of walking with the Principle on Friday afternoon.

I read were an elementary school principal had a policy of inviting two students outside at lunch for long walking conversations every day. It was an offer her students could not refuse. After several weeks, she selected two new children to accompany her. This rotation would go on throughout the school year. Everyone got a chance to walk. Being selected was not a punishment either. It was simply this principal's way of controlling her weight and finding out what was really going on in her school.

While I think it would be great if you could get your principal to participate in this way, an alternative might be to schedule it yourself, WALK WITH THE P.E. TEACHER.

The Calorie Run: In preparation for this run, you need to list a variety of foods, determine the calorie content of each food, and figure out how far your average student would have to run to burn off the calories in each food. You can use a burn rate of 20-25 calories per quarter mile to estimate distance. Write each food name, calorie content, and distance on a separate card, and put all the cards in a box. Each student draws a card and then runs the required distance to burn the calories. Once students understand the assignment, you may hear them say they want an apple or orange instead of a candy bar!

pat of butter	45	calories	1 tablespoon of mayonnaise	99	calories
orange	64	calories	10 French fries (3 1/2")	214	calories
banana	101	calories	baked potato	145	calories
carrot (7 1/2")	15	calories	potato chips (10)	114	calories
raised doughnut	124	calories	broccoli (1/2 cup)	20	calories

Mixed-Up Walk: For limited amounts of time, add some walking variations (e.g., backward; sideways slide with a left shoulder lead, then a right shoulder lead; skipping; galloping; marching). For example, have students start with backward walking for one minute, then regular walking for one minute, then skipping for one minute, then regular walking, and so on. Tasks assigned can be different types of movement or varying challenges such as,

Cross-Country Walking: Set up a cross-country walking race between two or more teams from your class. Try to balance the teams as evenly as possible in terms of athletic students versus sedentary students. Design a safe course with a nice variety of walking areas, such as through a park, beside a pond, etc. Draw and distribute a map of the course and discuss it with students to make sure they understand the route. Ideally, walk the route with the class prior to the competition. During the race, students walk as quickly as possible along the route. At the finish line, they receive a number indicating their place. The team with the lowest number of points is the winner. This is a competitive activity, but it can be approached in a positive and fun manner.

The Straw Walk: Challenge your students to walk at their fastest maintainable pace on a 1/4-mile track. Reward students with one soda straw for every lap they complete. After 15 minutes, whistle everyone to stop. Have all walkers measure their heart rates, then record their own straw walk scores (the number of straws collected plus any fractional lap, e.g. 4 straws + 1/2 lap = 4.5 straw walk score = 4.5 mph pace). Every straw represents 1 mph in speed because everyone is moving on a 1/4-mile track for 1/4 hour.

The Little Straw Walk: The primary purpose of The Little Straw Walk is to get children moving at their fastest aerobic walking pace for a sustained period of time. The course can be built on a fairly small playground area. Make a circular or oblong track using 10 cones. The cones are placed 17 1/2 yards apart to that you end up with a 175-yard or 1/10th of a mile course.

Line the kids up at the starting line. Blow a whistle and start your stopwatch. Reward them with straws each time they complete a lap. Blow a final, 6-minute whistle to freeze everyone in place. Since The Little Straw Walk is a 1/10th-hour walk on a 1/10th-mile loop, the score turns out to be your exact mile-per-hour walking pace. Thus, if Johnny is standing next to the 5th cone on the course with 3 straws in his hand when the whistle blows, that means Johnny is a 3.5-mph walker.

How Fit Are Your Little Walkers?

	3 Straws	3 1/2 Straws	4 Straws	4 1/2 Straws	5 Straws
Kindergarten	G	VG	E	O	O
1st grade	G	VG	E	E	O
2nd grade	F	G	VG	E	

The PACER: The PACER (Progressive Aerobic Cardiovascular Endurance Run) is an aerobic running challenge for K on up. The objective is keep up with the music. The children run back and forth across a 20-meter distance. The music is slow to start with but it gradually gets faster and faster. To do this one you will need to order the tape, but it is not expensive and would be worth the effort. The children will love it and you will be able to use it many times. (The FITNESSGRAM, developed by The Cooper Institute for Aerobics Research, Dallas, TX. 75230, (214) 701-8001).

Walk to School: Children who walk to school accumulate an average of 2,000 more steps per day than children who are transported. So, it's not surprising that many organizations have developed programs encouraging children to walk to school. Perhaps the best known is *Kidswalk* which was developed by the Centers for Disease Control and Prevention. Materials, PowerPoint presentations, and training guides are available at the website.

Landmark Orienteering: Students may be given 15 minutes to get to as many control points as possible. With a partner (joined at the wrist) they are to locate each control point as described below. When reaching each control point they are to identify the appropriate information in the space provided and then move on to the next point. A 1-minute grace period to return to the staring point will be given.
1. What is the street number on the building to the West of the school building?

_____ 10 pts

2. How many windows are there on the front of the school building?

_____ 5 pts

3. What is the inscription on the softball fields backstop?

_____ 20 pts

4. How many trees are in the field next to the soccer field?

_____ 10pts

5. What color is the door of the utility shed next to the playground equipment?

_____ 5pts

Cross Country Orienteering: Each student is given a marker and his/her own copy of a map of the area. A number of checkpoints have been marked on it. The task is to find all of the checkpoints as quickly as possible. Each checkpoint has attached to it a small plastic bag with a cardboard model of one item (symbol, anima, vegetable). The student records the item and returns to the starting point.

Kids Marathon: Kids run a marathon? Yes, but not all at once: Here's how it works: The Seattle Kids Marathon is a non-competitive running or walking event. Maybe you could use some of their ideas to create something.
　*Establish a measured safe, route that is easily accessible to participant
　*Participants run, or walk, the course to total 25 miles within a 6-week period
　*Students keep journal entries of their training experience
　*Students who complete the 25 miles qualify for the culminating event

*The event is a 1.2 mile run or walk to the Finish Line of the Seattle Marathon
*Students receive milepost awards, a certificate and a T-shirt
For more specifics: http:///www.seattlemarathon.org/kids.asp

Ironkids Triathlon: Another way to spice up a running program would be to tie it in with biking or even swimming. This obviously would require some significant organization but it could be great fun. The basics of the National IronKids Triathlon are listed below to give you some ideas. The competition is divided between boys and girls, and then by age. The kids can get friends and compete as a relay team so that everyone does not have to do each event. Although I think it would be great to have swimming as part of the event, organizing a Biathlon would be more feasible compromise.

Age: 7-10 years
    Swim: 100 meters
    Cycle: 5 km/3.1 miles
    Run: 1 km/ .6 miles

Age: 11-14 years
    Swim: 200 meters
    Cycle: 10 km/ 6.2 miles
    Run: 2 km/ 1.2 miles

WARM-UPS

One Behind: This is a good simple one to do in your classroom as an activity break. You or a student leader does a series of exercises at the front of the class. The class follows suit but the trick is that they stay one exercise behind the leader. When the leader starts to do exercise two the class begin on exercise one. Stretches, isometrics, and calisthenics all work fine. I have not tried it yet but it might be fun to have the class delayed by two activities, or half the class behind one while the other half is two behind.

Astronaut Drill: Everyone is locomotoring in a circle. It could be walking, walking with arm circles, walking with arm windmills, jogging, bear walking. Periodically groups are identified to go to the center of the circle and do a prescribed activity. The identified groups could be left-handers, those wearing shorts, those with birthdays in months which begin with a J, etc.

Partner Warm-Up: Partners stand back-to-back, one facing into the circle, the other facing out. The outside people jog a counterclockwise lap while the inside people do a prescribed activity such as curl-ups, lateral stretch, treadmills, sit and reach, rope skipping. When a jogger gets back home the roles are reversed.

High-Tens: Students move around the gym in different directions to music. When the music stops, they give as many high-tens to as many different people as possible. They start locomotoring again when the music begins. Something like a five or ten second music break works well. Of course, activities other than high-tens could be specified (low fives, hand shake variations, foot-fives, etc.).

Over-Unders: Half of the class is scattered about in push-up or crab positions. The other half of the class will be traveling over and under. When a person goes under a bridge, the bridge flips over into the crab position. When a person goes over a crab, the crab flips over into the bridge position. Give the class a set amount of time to see how many bridges and crabs they can go over and under.

Hall of the Mountain King: "In the Hall of the Mountain King" is a segment from the *Peer Gynt Suite* by Edvard Grieg. The music starts with a very slow tempo and gradually increases until it is extremely fast. The children are lined-up in the center of the gym and are to begin walking slowly in step with the beat. They first go forward 16 counts to the music and then backwards 16 counts. Their task is to keep up as long as possible to the increasing speed. Sometimes falls occur when going fast backwards. To avoid this problem and to create variety you can have them pivoting so that they are always moving forwards. Sliding to the left and right also works well.

I suggest you keep your ears attuned for other music that has an increasing tempo (Bolero, Cotton-Eye Joe, Dueling Banjos, etc.)

[ANNOTATED RESOURCES]

This is a core of the resources that I have found to be especially useful. Many of them have been referred to in the text but there are others that have not. The list has been kept brief so that these important ones do not get lost in a crowd. Of course, most of these references have linkages if you wish to research further.

Web Sites

www.pecentral.org
This is the largest and most used web site for health and physical education teachers. It has just about everything you will want: lesson ideas of all kinds, assessment ideas, preschool physical education, instructional resources, health and physical education products, books and music, top web site links, and much more.

www.pelinks4u.org
This site is a smaller version of pecentral.org but can be particularly useful to those teaching in the State of Washington. It is located in Central Washington University and hence can keep people updated on conferences, workshops, and state political happenings.

www.fns.usda.gov/tn
This is where you will find the USDAs "Team Nutrition" Program. They have all kinds of ways to help you teach sound nutrition to kindergarten through high school. They have lots of free resources, lesson plans for different grades, overheads, posters, student workbooks, etc.

www.pbs.org/teachersource/health.
This site it called the PBS Teacher Source. It is a more general site with lessons and activities in all fields. Besides Health and Fitness there are the areas of Arts and Literature, Science and Technology, Social Studies, and Early Childhood. They are all worth a visit.

www.aahperd.org
This is the home of *the American Alliance of Health, Physical Education, Recreation and Dance (AAHPERD)*. This is a big organization with an extensive web site. Here you will have a wealth of information in such areas as coaching, recreation, health,

physical education, adaptive physical education. This is where you will find all the particulars of the *Fitnessgram* and *Activitygram*. Also, they will have interesting information such as position statements on things as diverse as "activity recommendations for toddlers and preschoolers" and "the proscription of dodgeball" and "a code of ethics for coaches."

www.wahperd.com
The Washington Alliance of Health, Physical Education, Recreation and Dance (WAHPERD) is the state level of *AAHPERD* organization. It can be primarily helpful in keeping you aware of events happening within the state. *Jump Rope for Heart* and *Hoops for Heart* programs are examples. This organization also puts on an annual state conference that has much to offer.

Books

Dejager, D. & Humberg, C. *Adventure Racing Activities for Fun and Fitness*, Human Kinetics, 2008.
Adventure racing is becoming a increasingly popular activity. These authors present many modifications that be used in activity classes on the school grounds.

Hammett, C.T. *Movement Activities for Early Childhood*, Human Kinetics, 1992.

Hellison, D. *Teaching Responsibility Through Physical Activity*, Human Kinetics, 1995. (1 800 747-4457)
Don Hellison teaches students with behavioral problems. From his experiences he developed the *Personal and Social Responsibility Model (PSRM)*. It has been proven to be an effective guide for teaching affective behaviors.

Launder, A.G. *Play Practice: The Games Approach to Teaching and Coaching Sports*, Human Kinetics, 2001. (1 800 747 4457)
This book introduces many fun and effective drills and game modifications. A large range of sports is covered. I especially recommend this book for coaches of team sports.

McCall, R. M. & Craft, D. H. *Moving With A Purpose: Developing Programs for Preschoolers of All Abilities*. Human Kinetics, 20000.
Simply a great number of great ideas for preschooler activities.

Pangrazi, R., Beighle, A. & Pangrazi, D. *Promoting Physical Activity and Health in the Classroom*. Benjamin Cummings, 2009.
This book contains many excellent classroom activity ideas that are well organized for immediate use. It also is particularly strong on management and discipline techniques.

Siedentop, D., Hastie, P.A., & van der Mars, H. (2004) *Complete Guide to Sport Education* (2nd ed.). Champaign, IL: Human Kinetics.
This book gives ideas how to modify sports to make them more educational. It also explains how to use the contextual aspects of sports to make the sports experience more challenging and fun. Practical experiences of teachers at a variety of grade levels, with a wide variety of sports, are offered.

Sweetgall, R. *Pedometer Walking*, Creative Walking, Inc. (2001)
This book, and others by Rob Sweetgall, provides good ideas for fun walking activities and lessons. Visit his web site (www.creataivewalking.com) for pedometer ideas and other resources. I also liked his older book *Walking for Little Children*.

LeFevre, D.N. *Best New Games*, Human Kinetics, 2002 (1 800 747-4457)
If you like the concept of new games this is a good resource with which to start.

Carnes, C. *Teacher's Guide for Awesome Elementary School Physical Education Activities*, The Education Company, 1990.
Cliff Canes' book simply has a lot of good everyone-active games for elementary children. If you like them you might want to check out his *Awesome Jump Rope Activities Book*.

Catalogs

Human Kinetic Publishers (www.humankinetics.com)
This is the world's largest publisher in the area of coaching and physical activity. They have an impressive list of materials for all sports and aspects of coaching. Free catalogs are available upon request.

SPORTTIME, 1 Sportime Way, Atlanta, GA, USA 30340 (1 800 444-5700)
They have endless physical education and coaching supplies and equipment. Also things like music tapes and CDs.

WOVERINE Sports, 745 State Circle, Box 1941, Ann Arbor, MI 48106 (1 800 521-2832)
They have endless physical education and coaching supplies and equipment. Also things like music tapes and CDs.

THINGS FROM BELL, P.O. Box 135, East Troy, WI 53120, (1 800 432 2842)
They have endless physical education and coaching supplies and equipment. Also things like music tapes and CDs.

NASCO, 4825 Stoddard Rd., Modesto, CA 95356-9318 (1 800 558-9595)
They have endless physical education and coaching supplies and equipment. Also things like music tapes and CDs.

Journals

Journal of Health, Physical Education, Recreation and Dance (www.humankinetics.com)
This is an AAHPERD publication. Its purpose is to promote high-quality programs in health, physical education, recreation, dance and sport. It has articles on what is happening in these areas.

Strategies: A Journal for Physical and Sport Educator
(www.humankinetics.com)
This is another AAHPERD publication. It strives to share "best practices" of field professionals in sport and physical education. It offers many practical activity and teaching/coaching methods ideas.

Teaching Elementary Physical Education: The Independent Voice of Elementary and Middle School Physical Educators (www.humankinetics.com)
This resource provides many practical activity and teaching methods specifically designed for elementary and middle schoolteachers.

Nutritive Value of Selected Foods and Fast Foods

This section presents nutritional information about a wide array of foods, including many fast foods. Values are given for calories, protein, carbohydrates, fiber, fat, saturated fat, and cholesterol for common foods and serving sizes. Use this information to assess your diet and make improvements. This is only a sampling of the most common foods. See the MyDietAnalysis database for a more extensive list of foods.

MDA Code	Food Name	Amt	Wt (g)	Ener (kcal)	Prot (g)	Carb (g)	Fiber (g)	Fat (g)	Sat (g)	Chol (g)
Beverages										
Alcoholic Beverages										
22831	Beer	12 fl. oz	360	157	1	13		0	0	
34053	Beer, light	12 fl. oz	353	105	1	5	0	0	0	
22606	Beer, nonalcoholic	12 fl. oz	353	73	1	14	0	0	0	
22884	Wine, red	1 fl. oz	29	24	0	1		0	0	
22861	Wine, white	1 fl. oz	29.3	24	0	1		0	0	
22514	Gin, 80 proof	1 fl. oz	27.8	64	0	0	0	0	0	
22593	Rum, 80 proof	1 fl. oz	27.8	64	0	0	0	0	0	
22515	Tequila, 80 proof	1 fl. oz	27.8	64	0	0	0	0	0	
22594	Vodka, 80 proof	1 fl. oz	27.8	64	0	0	0	0	0	
22670	Whiskey, 80 proof	1 fl. oz	27.8	64	0	0	0	0	0	
Coffee, Tea, and Dairy Drink Mixes										
20012	Coffee, brewed	1 cup	237	2	0	0	0	0	0	0
20686	Coffee, decaffeinated, brewed	1 cup	237	0	0	0	0	0	0	0
20439	Coffee, espresso	1 cup	237	5	0	0	0	0	0.2	0
20402	Coffee, from mix, French vanilla, sugar & fat free	1 ea	7	25	0	5	0	0	0.1	0
85	Chocolate milk, prepared w/syrup	1 cup	282	254	9	36	1	8	4.7	25
46	Hot cocoa, w/aspartame, sodium, vitamin A, prepared w/water	1 cup	256	74	3	14	1	1	0	0
48	Hot cocoa, prep from dry mix with water	1 cup	275	151	2	32	1	2	0.9	3
166	Hot cocoa, w/marshmallows, from dry packet	1 ea	28	112	1	24	1	1	0.4	2
39	Chocolate flavor, dry mix, prepared w/milk	1 cup	266	226	9	32	1	9	4.9	24
41	Strawberry flavor, dry mix, prepared w/milk	1 cup	266	234	8	33	0	8	5.1	32
20014	Tea, brewed	1 cup	237	2	0	1	0	0	0	0
20036	Tea, herbal (not chamomile) brewed	1 cup	237	2	0	0	0	0	0	0

Ener = energy (kilocalories), **Prot** = protein, **Carb** = carbohydrate, **Fiber** = dietary fiber, **Fat** = total fat, **Sat** = saturated fat, **Chol** = cholesterol

*This food composition table has been prepared for Pearson Education, Inc. and is copyrighted by ESHA Research in Salem, Oregon, the developer of the MyDietAnalysis software program.

MDA Code	Food Name	Amt	Wt (g)	Ener (kcal)	Prot (g)	Carb (g)	Fiber (g)	Fat (g)	Sat (g)	Chol (g)
Fruit and Vegetable Beverages and Juices										
71080	Apple juice, canned or bottled, unsweetened	1 ea	262	123	0	31	0	0	0	0
20277	Capri Sun All Natural Juice Drink, Fruit Punch	1 ea	210	99	0	26	0	0	0	0
5226	Carrot juice, canned	1 cup	236	94	2	22	2	0	0.1	0
3042	Cranberry juice cocktail	1 cup	253	137	0	34	0	0	0	0
20024	Fruit punch, canned	1 cup	248	117	0	30	0	0	0	0
20035	Fruit punch, from frozen concentrate	1 cup	247	114	0	29	0	0	0	0
20101	Grape drink, canned	1 cup	250	153	0	39	0	0	0	0
3053	Grapefruit juice, from frozen concentrate, unsweetened	1 cup	247	101	1	24	0	0	0	0
20045	Lemonade flavor drink, from dry mix	1 cup	266	112	0	29	0	0	0	0
20047	Lemonade w/aspartame, low kcal, from dry mix	1 cup	237	5	0	1	0	0	0	0
20070	Orange drink, canned	1 cup	248	122	0	31	0	0	0	0
20004	Orange flavor drink, from dry mix	1 cup	248	122	0	31	0	0	0	0
71108	Orange juice, canned, unsweetened	1 ea	263	110	2	26	1	0	0	0
3090	Orange juice, fresh	1 cup	248	112	2	26	0	0	0.1	0
3091	Orange juice, from frozen concentrate, unsweetened	1 cup	249	112	2	27	0	0	0	0
5397	Tomato juice, canned w/o salt	1 cup	243	41	2	10	1	0	0	0
20849	Vegetable and fruit, mixed juice drink	4 oz	113	55	0	8	0	0	0	0
20080	Vegetable juice cocktail, canned	1 cup	242	46	2	11	2	0	0	0
Soft Drinks										
20006	Club soda	1 cup	237	0	0	0	0	0	0	0
20685	Low-calorie cola, with aspartame, caffeine free	12 fl. oz	355	4	0	1	0	0	0	0
20845	Cola, with higher caffeine	12 fl. oz	370	152	0	39	0	0	0	0
20008	Ginger ale	1 cup	244	83	0	21	0	0	0	0
20032	Lemon-lime soft drink	1 cup	246	98	0	25	0	0	0	0
20027	Pepper-type soft drink	1 cup	246	101	0	26	0	0	0.2	0
20009	Root beer	1 cup	246	101	0	26	0	0	0	0
Other										
20033	Soy milk	1 cup	245	127	11	12	3	5	0.6	0
20041	Water, tap	1 cup	237	0	0	0	0	0	0	0
Breakfast Cereals										
40095	All-Bran/Kellogg	0.5 cup	30	78	4	22	9	1	0.2	0
40032	Cap'n Crunch/Quaker	0.75 cup	27	108	1	23	1	2	0.4	0
40297	Cheerios/Gen Mills	1 cup	30	111	4	22	4	2	0.4	0
40126	Cinnamon Toast Crunch/Gen Mills	0.75 cup	30	127	2	24	1	3	0.5	0
40195	Corn Flakes/Kellogg	1 cup	28	101	2	24	1	0	0.1	0
40089	Corn Grits, instant, plain, prepared/Quaker	1 pkg	137	93	2	21	1	0	0	0
40206	Corn Pops/Kellogg	1 cup	31	117	1	28	0	0	0.1	0
40179	Cream of Rice, prepared w/salt	1 cup	244	127	2	28	0	0	0	0
40182	Cream of Wheat, instant, prepared w/salt	1 cup	241	149	4	32	1	1	0.1	0
40104	Crispix/Kellogg	1 cup	29	109	2	25	0	0	0.1	0

MDA Code	Food Name	Amt	Wt (g)	Ener (kcal)	Prot (g)	Carb (g)	Fiber (g)	Fat (g)	Sat (g)	Chol (g)
40218	Froot Loops/Kellogg	1 cup	30	118	2	26	1	1	0.5	0
40217	Frosted Flakes/Kellogg	0.75 cup	31	114	1	28	1	0	0	0
11916	Frosted Mini-Wheats, bite size/Kellogg	1 cup	55	189	6	45	6	1	0.2	0
40209	Raisin Bran/Kellogg	1 cup	61	195	5	47	7	2	0.3	0
40210	Rice Krispies/Kellogg	1.25 cup	33	128	2	28	0	0	0.1	0
60887	Shredded wheat, large biscuit	2 ea	37.8	127	4	30	5	1	0.2	0
40211	Special K/Kellogg	1 cup	31	117	7	22	1	0	0.1	0

Dairy and Cheese

500	Cream, half & half	2 Tbs	30	39	1	1	0	3	2.1	11
11	Milk, condensed, sweetened, canned	2 Tbs	38.2	123	3	21	0	3	2.1	13
19	Milk, lowfat, 1% fat, chocolate	1 cup	250	158	8	26	1	2	1.5	8
218	Milk, 2%, w/added vitamins A & D	1 cup	245	130	8	13	0	5	3	
6	Milk, nonfat/skim, w/added vitamin A	1 cup	245	83	8	12	0	0	0.1	5
1	Milk, whole, 3.25%	1 cup	244	146	8	11	0	8	4.6	24
20	Milk, whole, chocolate	1 cup	250	208	8	26	2	8	5.3	30
72088	Yogurt, fruit variety, nonfat	1 cup	245	230	11	47	0	0	0.3	5
1287	American cheese, nonfat slices	1 pce	21.3	32	5	2	0	0	0.1	3
13349	Cheez Whiz cheese sauce/Kraft	2 Tbs	33	91	4	3	0	7	4.3	25
1014	Cottage cheese, 2% fat	0.5 cup	113	102	16	4	0	2	1.4	9
1015	Cream cheese	2 Tbs	29	101	2	1	0	10	6.4	32
1452	Cream cheese, fat free	2 Tbs	29	28	4	2	0	0	0.3	2
1016	Feta, crumbled	0.25 cup	37.5	99	5	2	0	8	5.6	33
47887	Mozzarella, whole milk, slice	1 ea	34	102	8	1	0	8	4.5	27
1075	Parmesan, grated	1 Tbs	5	22	2	0	0	1	0.9	4
1024	Ricotta, part skim	0.25 cup	62	86	7	3	0	5	3.1	19
1064	Ricotta, whole milk	0.25 cup	62	108	7	2	0	8	5.1	32

Eggs and Egg Substitutes

19525	Egg substitute, liquid	0.25 cup	62.8	53	8	0	0	2	0.4	1
19506	Egg, white, raw	1 ea	33.4	17	4	0	0	0	0	0
19509	Egg, whole, fried	1 ea	46	92	6	0	0	7	2	210
19515	Egg, whole, hard boiled	1 ea	37	57	5	0	0	4	1.2	157
19521	Egg, whole, poached	1 ea	37	54	5	0	0	4	1.1	156
19516	Egg, whole, scrambled	1 ea	61	101	7	1	0	7	2.2	215
19508	Egg, yolk, raw, fresh	1 ea	16.6	53	3	1	0	4	1.6	205

Fruit

72101	Apricots, canned, heavy syrup, drained	1 cup	182	151	1	39	5	0	0	0
3164	Fruit cocktail canned in juice	1 cup	237	109	1	28	2	0	0	0
71079	Apple w/skin, raw	1 cup	125	65	0	17	3	0	0	0
3331	w/added vitamin C	0.5 cup	128	97	0	25	2	0	0	0
3657	Apricot, raw	1 cup	165	79	2	18	3	1	0	0
3210	Avocado, California, peeled, raw	1 ea	173	289	3	15	12	27	3.7	0
71082	Banana, peeled, raw	1 ea	81	72	1	19	2	0	0.1	0
71976	Grapefruit, fresh	0.5 ea	154	60	1	16	6	0	0	0
3055	Grapes, Thompson seedless, fresh	0.5 cup	80	55	1	14	1	0	0	4
3642	Melon, fresh, wedge	1 pce	69	23	1	6	1	0	0	5
3168	Mixed fruit (prune, apricot, & pear) dried	1 oz	28.4	69	1	18	2	0	0	0

HEALTH RESOURCES H-11

Nutritive Value of Selected Foods and Fast Foods

MDA Code	Food Name	Amt	Wt (g)	Ener (kcal)	Prot (g)	Carb (g)	Fiber (g)	Fat (g)	Sat (g)	Chol (g)
3216	Nectarine, raw	1 cup	138	61	1	15	2	0	0	0
3726	Peach, peeled, raw	1 ea	79	31	1	8	1	0	0	0
3106	Pear, raw	1 ea	209	121	1	32	6	0	0	0
3766	Raisins, seedless	50 ea	26	78	1	21	1	0	0	0
72113	Pineapple, fresh, slice	1 pce	84	38	0	10		0		5
3085	Orange, fresh	1 ea	184	86	2	22	4	0	0	
3135	Strawberries, halves/slices, raw	1 cup	166	53	1	13	3	0	0	0

Grain Products

Breads, Rolls, and Bread Crumbs

71170	Bagel, cinnamon-raisin	1 ea	26	71	3	14	1	0	0.1	0
71167	Bagel, egg	1 ea	26	72	3	14	1	1	0.1	6
71152	Bagel, plain/onion/poppy/sesame, enriched	1 ea	26	67	3	13	1	0	0.1	0
42433	Biscuit, w/butter	1 ea	82	280	5	27	0	17	4	0
71192	Biscuit, Plain or Buttermilk, refrig dough, baked, reduced fat	1 ea	21	63	2	12	0	1	0.3	0
42004	Bread crumbs, dry, plain, grated	1 Tbs	6.8	27	1	5	0	0	0.1	0
49144	Bread, crusty Italian w/garlic	1 pce	50	186	4	21	10	2.4	6	
70964	Bread, garlic, frozen/Campione	1 pce	28	101	2	12	1	5	0.8	
42069	Bread, oat bran	1 pce	30	71	3	12	1	1	0.2	0
42095	Bread, wheat, reduced kcal	1 pce	23	46	2	10	3	1	0.1	0
71247	Bread, white, commercially prepared, crumbs/cubes/slices	1 pce	9	24	1	5	0	0	0.1	0
42084	Bread, white, reduced kcal	1 pce	23	48	2	10	2	1	0.1	0
26561	Buns, hamburger, Wonder	1 ea	43	117	3	22	1	2	0.4	
42021	Hamburger/hot dog bun, plain	1 ea	43	120	4	21	1	2	0.5	0
42115	Cornbread, prepared from dry mix	1 pce	60	188	4	29	1	6	1.6	37
71227	Pita bread, white, enriched	1 ea	28	77	3	16	1	0	0	0
71228	Pita bread, whole wheat	1 ea	28	74	3	15	2	1	0.1	0
71368	Roll, dinner, plain, homemade w/reduced fat (2%) milk	1 ea	43	136	4	23	1	3	0.8	15
42161	Roll, French	1 ea	38	105	3	19	1	2	0.4	0
71056	Roll, hard/kaiser	1 ea	57	167	6	30	1	2	0.3	0
42297	Tortilla, corn, w/o salt, ready to cook	1 ea	26	58	1	12	1	1	0.1	0
90645	Taco shell, baked	1 ea	5	23	0	3	0	1	0.2	0

Crackers

71451	Cheez-its/Goldfish crackers, low sodium	55 pce	33	166	3	19	1	8	3.2	4
43507	Oyster/soda/soup crackers	1 cup	45	193	4	32	1	5	0.7	0
70963	Ritz crackers/Nabisco	5 ea	16	79	1	10	0	4	0.6	0
43587	Saltine crackers, original premium/Nabisco	5 ea	14	59	2	10	0	1	0.3	0
43545	Sandwich crackers, cheese filled	4 ea	28	134	3	17	1	6	1.7	1
43546	Sandwich crackers, peanut butter filled	4 ea	28	138	3	16	1	7	1.4	0
44677	Snackwell Wheat Cracker/Nabisco	1 ea	15	62	1	12	1	2		
43581	Wheat Thins, baked/Nabisco	16 ea	29	136	2	20	1	6	0.9	0
43508	Whole wheat cracker	4 ea	32	142	3	22	3	6	1.1	0

MDA Code	Food Name	Amt	Wt (g)	Ener (kcal)	Prot (g)	Carb (g)	Fiber (g)	Fat (g)	Sat (g)	Chol (g)
Muffins and Baked Goods										
42723	English muffin, plain	1 ea	57	132	5	26		1	0.2	
62916	Muffin, blueberry, commercially prepared	1 ea	11	30	1	5	0	1	0.2	3
44521	Muffin, corn, commercially prepared	1 ea	57	174	3	29	2	5	0.8	15
44514	Muffin, oatbran	1 ea	57	154	4	28	3	4	0.6	0
44518	Toaster muffin, blueberry	1 ea	33	103	2	18	1	3	0.5	2
Noodles and Pasta										
38048	Chow mein noodles, dry	1 cup	45	237	4	26	2	14	2	0
38047	Egg noodles, enriched, cooked	0.5 cup	80	110	4	20	1	2	0.3	23
38060	Spaghetti, whole wheat, cooked	1 cup	140	174	7	37	6	1	0.1	0
38251	Egg noodles, enriched, cooked w/salt	0.5 cup	80	110	4	20	1	2	0.3	
38102	Macaroni noodles, enriched, cooked	1 cup	140	221	8	43	3	1	0.2	
38118	Spaghetti noodles, enriched, cooked	0.5 cup	70	111	4	22	1	1	0.1	4
Grains										
38076	Couscous, cooked	0.5 cup	78.5	88	3	18	1	0	0	0
38080	Oats	0.25 cup	39	152	7	26	4	3	0.5	0
38010	Rice, brown, long grain, cooked	1 cup	195	216	5	45	4	2	0.4	0
38256	Rice, white, long grain, enriched, cooked w/salt	1 cup	158	205	4	45	1	0	0.1	0
38019	Rice, white, long grain, instant, enriched, cooked	1 cup	165	193	4	41	1	1	0	0
Pancakes, French Toast, and Waffles										
42156	French toast, homemade, w/reduced fat (2%) milk	1 pce	65	149	5	16	1	7	1.8	75
45192	Pancake/waffle, buttermilk/ Eggo/Kellogg	1 ea	42.5	99	3	16	0	3	0.6	5
45117	Pancakes, plain, homemade	1 ea	77	175	5	22	1	7	1.6	45
45193	Waffle, lowfat, homestyle, frozen	1 ea	35	83	2	15	0	1	0.3	9
Meat and Meat Substitutes										
Beef										
10093	Beef, average of all cuts, lean & fat (1/4" trim), cooked	3 oz	85.1	260	22	0	0	18	7.3	75
10705	Beef, average of all cuts, lean (1/4" trim), cooked	3 oz	85.1	184	25	0	0	8	3.2	73
10133	Beef, whole rib, roasted, 1/4" trim	3 oz	85.1	305	19	0	0	25	10	71
58129	Ground beef (hamburger), 25% fat, cooked, pan-browned	3 oz	85.1	236	22	0	0	15	6	76
58119	Ground beef (hamburger), 15% fat, cooked, pan-browned	3 oz	85.1	218	24	0	0	13	5	77
58109	Ground beef (hamburger), 5% fat, cooked, pan-browned	3 oz	85.1	164	25	0	0	6	2.9	76
10791	Porterhouse steak, lean & fat (1/4" trim), broiled	3 oz	85.1	280	19	0	0	22	8.7	61
58257	Rib eye steak, small end (ribs 10–12), 0" trim, broiled	3 oz	85.1	210	23	0	0	13	4.9	94

MDA Code	Food Name	Amt	Wt (g)	Ener (kcal)	Prot (g)	Carb (g)	Fiber (g)	Fat (g)	Sat (g)	Chol (g)
58094	Skirt steak, trimmed to 0" fat, broiled	3 oz	85.1	187	22	0	0	10	4	51
58328	Strip steak, top loin, 1/8" trim, broiled	3 oz	85.1	171	25	0	0	7	2.7	67
10805	T-Bone steak, lean & fat (1/4" trim), broiled	3 oz	85.1	260	20	0	0	19	7.6	55
11531	Veal, average of all cuts, cooked	3 oz	85.1	197	26	0	0	10	3.6	97
Chicken										
15057	Chicken breast, w/o skin, fried	3 oz	85.1	159	28	0	0	4	1.1	77
15080	Chicken, dark meat, w/skin, roasted	3 oz	85.1	215	22	0	0	13	3.7	77
15026	Chicken, dark meat, w/o skin, fried	3 oz	85.1	203	25	2	0	10	2.7	82
15042	Chicken drumstick, w/o skin, fried	3 oz	85.1	166	24	0	0	7	1.8	80
15048	Chicken, wing, w/o skin, fried	3 oz	85.1	180	26	0	0	8	2.1	71
15059	Chicken, wing, w/o skin, roasted	3 oz	85.1	173	26	0	0	7	1.9	72
Turkey										
51151	Turkey bacon, cooked	1 oz	28.4	108	8	1	0	8	2.4	28
51098	Turkey patty, breaded, fried	1 ea	42	119	6	7	0	8	2	26
16110	Turkey breast w/skin, roasted	3 oz	85.1	130	25	0	0	3	0.7	77
16038	Turkey breast, no skin, roasted	3 oz	85.1	115	26	0	0	1	0.2	71
16101	Turkey, dark meat w/skin, roasted	3 oz	85.1	155	24	0	0	6	1.8	100
16003	Turkey, ground, cooked	1 ea	82	193	22	0	0	11	2.8	84
Lamb										
13604	Lamb, average of all cuts (1/4" trim), cooked	3 oz	85.1	250	21	0	0	18	7.5	83
13616	Lamb, average of all cuts, lean (1/4" trim), cooked	3 oz	85.1	175	24	0	0	8	2.9	78
Pork										
12000	Bacon, broiled, pan-fried, or roasted	3 pcs	19	103	7	0	0	8	2.6	21
28143	Canadian bacon	1 pce	56	68	9	1	3	1	2.7	
12211	Ham, cured, boneless, regular fat (11% fat), roasted	1 cup	140	249	32	0	0	13	4.4	83
12309	Pork, average of retail cuts, cooked	3 oz	85.1	232	23	0	0	15	5.3	77
12097	Pork, ribs, backribs, roasted	3 oz	85.1	315	21	0	0	25	9.4	100
12099	Pork, ground, cooked	3 oz	85.1	253	22	0	0	18	6.6	80
Lunchmeats										
13000	Beef, thin slices	1 oz	28.4	42	5	0	0	2	0.8	20
58275	Bologna, beef and pork, low fat	1 ea	14	32	2	0	0	3	1	5
13157	Chicken breast, oven roasted deluxe	1 oz	28.4	29	5	1	0	1	0.2	14
13306	Corned beef, cooked, chopped, pressed	1 ea	71	101	14	1	0	5	2	46
13264	Ham, slices, regular (11% fat)	1 cup	135	220	22	5	2	12	4	77
13101	Pastrami, beef, cured	1 oz	28.4	41	6	0	0	2	0.8	19
13215	Salami, beef, cotto	1 oz	28.4	59	4	1	0	4	1.9	24
16160	Turkey breast slice	1 pce	21	22	4	1	0	0	0.1	9
58279	Turkey ham, sliced, extra lean, prepackaged or deli-sliced	1 cup	138	163	27	2	0	5	1.8	92

MDA Code	Food Name	Amt	Wt (g)	Ener (kcal)	Prot (g)	Carb (g)	Fiber (g)	Fat (g)	Sat (g)	Chol (g)
Sausage										
13070	Chorizo, pork & beef	1 ea	60	273	14	1	0	23	8.6	53
57877	Frankfurter, beef	1 ea	45	148	5	2	0	13	5.3	24
13012	Frankfurter, turkey	1 ea	45	102	6	1	0	8	2.7	48
57890	Italian sausage, pork, cooked	1 ea	83	286	16	4	0	23	7.9	47
13021	Pepperoni sausage	1 pce	5.5	26	1	0	0	2	0.9	6
13185	Pork sausage links, cooked	2 ea	48	165	8	0	0	15	5.1	37
58227	Sausage, pork, precooked	3 oz	85	321	12	0	0	30	9.9	63
58007	Turkey sausage, breakfast links, mild	2 ea	56	132	9	1	0	10	4.4	34
Meat Substitutes										
7509	Bacon substitute, vegetarian, strips	3 ea	15	46	2	1	0	4	0.7	0
7722	Garden patties, frozen/ Worthington, Morningstar	1 ea	67	119	11	10	4	4	0.5	1
7674	Harvest burger, original flavor, vegetable protein patty	1 ea	90	138	18	7	6	4	1	0
90626	Sausage, vegetarian, meatless	1 ea	28	72	5	3	1	5	0.8	0
7726	Spicy Black Bean Burger/ Worthington, Morningstar	1 ea	78	115	12	15	5	1	0.2	1
Nuts										
4519	Cashews, dry roasted w/salt	0.25 cup	34.2	196	5	11	1	16	3.1	0
4728	Macadamia nuts, dry roasted, unsalted	1 cup	134	962	10	18	11	102	16	0
4592	Mixed nuts, w/peanuts, dry roasted, salted	0.25 cup	34.2	203	6	9	3	18	2.4	0
4626	Peanut butter, chunky w/salt	2 Tbs	32	188	8	7	3	16	2.6	0
4756	Peanuts, dry roasted w/o salt	30 ea	30	176	7	6	2	15	2.1	0
4696	Peanuts, raw	0.25 cup	36.5	207	9	6	3	18	2.5	0
4540	Pistachio nuts, dry roasted, salted	0.25 cup	32	182	7	9	3	15	1.8	0
Seafood										
17029	Bass, freshwater, cooked w/dry heat	3 oz	85.1	124	21	0	0	4	0.9	74
17037	Cod, Atlantic, baked/broiled (dry heat)	3 oz	85.1	89	19	0	0	1	0.1	47
19036	Crab, Alaskan King, boiled/ steamed	3 oz	85.1	83	16	0	0	1	0.1	45
17090	Haddock, baked or broiled (dry heat)	3 oz	85.1	95	21	0	0	1	0.1	63
17291	Halibut, Atlantic & Pacific, baked or broiled (dry heat)	3 oz	85.1	119	23	0	0	3	0.4	35
17181	Salmon, Atlantic, farmed, cooked w/dry heat	3 oz	85.1	175	19	0	0	11	2.1	54
17099	Salmon, Sockeye, baked or broiled (dry heat)	3 oz	85.1	184	23	0	0	9	1.6	74
71707	Squid, fried	3 oz	85.1	149	15	7	0	6	1.6	221
17066	Swordfish, baked or broiled (dry heat)	3 oz	85.1	132	22	0	0	4	1.2	43
56007	Tuna salad, lunchmeat spread	2 Tbs	25.6	48	4	2	0	2	0.4	3
17151	White tuna, canned in H₂O, drained	3 oz	85.1	109	20	0	0	3	0.7	36
17083	White tuna, canned in oil, drained	3 oz	85.1	158	23	0	0	7	1.1	26

Nutritive Value of Selected Foods and Fast Foods

MDA Code	Food Name	Amt	Wt (g)	Ener (kcal)	Prot (g)	Carb (g)	Fiber (g)	Fat (g)	Sat (g)	Chol (g)
Vegetables and Legumes										
Beans										
7038	Baked beans, plain or vegetarian, canned	1 cup	254	239	12	54	10	1	0.2	0
5197	Bean sprouts, mung, canned, drained	1 cup	125	15	2	3	1	0	0	0
7012	Black beans, boiled w/o salt	1 cup	172	227	15	41	15	1	0.2	0
5862	Beets, boiled w/salt, drained	0.5 cup	85	37	1	8	2	0	0	0
90018	Cowpeas, cooked w/salt	1 cup	171	198	13	35	11	1	0.2	0
7081	Hummus, garbanzo or chickpea spread, homemade	1 Tbs	15.4	27	1	3	1	1	0.2	0
7087	Kidney beans, canned	1 cup	256	210	13	37	11	2	0.2	0
7006	Lentils, boiled w/o salt	1 cup	198	230	18	40	16	1	0.1	0
7051	Pinto beans, canned	1 cup	240	206	12	37	11	2	0.4	0
6748	Snap green beans, raw	10 ea	55	17	1	4	2	0	0	0
5320	Snap yellow beans, raw	0.5 cup	55	17	1	4	2	0	0	0
90026	Split peas, boiled w/salt	0.5 cup	98	116	8	21	8	0	0.1	0
7054	White beans, canned	1 cup	262	307	19	57	13	1	0.2	0
Fresh Vegetables										
9577	Artichokes (globe or French) boiled w/salt, drained	1 ea	20	10	1	2	1	0	0	0
6033	Arugula/roquette, raw	1 cup	20	5	1	1	0	0	0	0
90406	Asparagus, raw	10 ea	35	7	1	1	1	0	0	0
5558	Broccoli stalks, raw	1 ea	114	32	3	6	4	0	0.1	0
5036	Cabbage, raw	1 cup	70	17	1	4	2	0	0	0
90605	Carrots, baby, raw	1 ea	15	5	0	1	0	0	0	0
5049	Cauliflower, raw	0.5 cup	50	12	1	3	1	0	0	0
90436	Celery, raw	1 ea	17	2	0	1	0	0	0	0
7202	Corn, white, sweet, ears, raw	1 ea	73	63	2	14	2	1	0.1	0
5900	Corn, yellow, sweet, boiled w/salt, drained	0.5 cup	82	89	3	21	2	1	0.2	0
5908	Eggplant (brinjal) boiled w/salt, drained	1 cup	99	35	1	9	2	0	0	0
5087	Lettuce, looseleaf, raw	2 pcs	20	3	0	1	0	0	0	0
51069	Mushrooms, brown, Italian, or crimini, raw	2 ea	28	6	1	1	0	0	0	0
90472	Onions, chopped, raw	1 ea	70	29	1	7	1	0	0	0
5116	Peas, green, raw	1 cup	145	117	8	21	7	1	0.1	0
7932	Peppers, jalapeno, raw	1 cup	90	27	1	5	2	1	0.1	0
90493	Peppers, sweet green, chopped/sliced, raw	10 pcs	27	5	0	1	0	0	0	0
6990	Pepper, sweet red, raw	1 ea	10	3	0	1	0	0	0	0
9251	Potatoes, red, flesh and skin, baked	1 ea	138	123	3	27	2	0	0	0
9245	Potatoes, russet, flesh and skin, baked	1 ea	138	134	4	30	3	0	0	0
5146	Spinach, raw	1 cup	30	7	1	1	1	0	0	0
90525	Squash, zucchini w/skin, slices, raw	1 ea	118	19	1	4	1	0	0	0
6924	Sweet potato, baked in skin w/salt	0.5 cup	100	90	2	21	3	0	0.1	0
5180	Tomato sauce, canned	0.5 cup	123	39	2	9	2	0	0	0
90532	Tomato, red, ripe, whole, raw	1 pce	15	3	0	1	0	0	0	0
5306	Yam, peeled, raw	0.5 cup	75	88	1	21	3	0	0	0

MDA Code	Food Name	Amt	Wt (g)	Ener (kcal)	Prot (g)	Carb (g)	Fiber (g)	Fat (g)	Sat (g)	Chol (g)
Soy and Soy Products										
7564	Tempeh	0.5 cup	83	160	15	8	9	1.8	0	
7015	Soybeans, cooked	1 cup	172	298	29	17	10	15	2.2	0
7542	Tofu, firm, silken, 1" slice	3 oz	85.1	53	6	2	0	2	0.3	0
Meals and Dishes										
92216	Tortellini with cheese filling	1 cup	108	332	15	51	2	8	3.9	45
57658	Chili con carne w/beans, canned entree	1 cup	222	269	16	25	9	12	3.9	29
57703	Chili, vegetarian chili w/beans, canned entree/Hormel	1 cup	247	205	12	38	10	1	0.1	0
57068	Macaroni and cheese, unprepared/Kraft	1 ea	70	259	11	48	1	3	1.3	10
70958	Stir fry, rice & vegetables, w/soy sauce/Hanover	1 cup	137	130	5	27	2	0		
70943	Beef & bean burrito/Las Campanas	1 ea	114	296	9	38	1	12	4.2	13
16195	Chicken & vegetables/Lean Cuisine	1 ea	297	252	19	32	5	6	1	24
70917	Hot Pockets, beef & cheddar, frozen	1 ea	142	403	16	39		20	8.8	53
70918	Hot Pockets, croissant pocket w/chicken, broccoli, & cheddar, frozen	1 ea	128	301	11	39	1	11	3.4	37
56757	Lasagna w/meat sauce/Stouffer's	1 ea	215	277	19	26	3	11	4.7	41
11029	Macaroni & beef in tomato sauce/Lean Cuisine	1 ea	283	249	14	37	3	5	1.6	23
5587	Mashed potatoes, from granules w/milk, prep w/water & margarine	0.5 cup	105	122	2	17	1	5	1.3	2
70898	Pizza, pepperoni, frozen	1 ea	146	432	16	42	3	22	7.1	22
56703	Spaghetti w/meat sauce/Lean Cuisine	1 ea	326	313	14	51	6	6	1.4	13
Snack Foods										
10051	Beef jerky	1 pce	19.8	81	7	2	0	5	2.1	10
63331	Breakfast bars, oats, sugar, raisins, coconut	1 ea	43	200	4	29	1	8	5.5	0
61251	Cheese puffs and twists, corn based, low fat	1 oz	28.4	123	2	21	3	3	0.6	0
44032	Chex snack mix	1 cup	42.5	181	5	28	2	7	2.4	0
23059	Granola bar, hard, plain	1 ea	24.5	115	2	16	1	5	0.6	0
23104	Granola bar, soft, plain	1 ea	28.4	126	2	19	1	5	2.1	0
44012	Popcorn, air-popped	1 cup	8	31	1	6	1	0	0.1	0
44076	Potato chips, plain, no salt	1 oz	28.4	152	2	15	1	10	3.1	0
5437	Potato chips, sour cream & onion	1 oz	28.4	151	2	15	1	10	2.5	2
44015	Pretzels, hard	5 pcs	30	114	3	24	1	1	0.1	0
44021	Rice cake, brown rice, plain, salted	1 ea	9	35	1	7	0	0	0.1	0
44058	Trail mix, regular	0.25 cup	37.5	173	5	17	2	11	2.1	0
Soups										
50398	Beef barley, canned/Progresso Healthy Classics	1 cup	241	142	11	20	3	2	0.7	19
50081	Chicken noodle, chunky, canned	1 cup	240	175	13	17	4	6	1.4	19

MDA Code	Food Name	Amt	Wt (g)	Ener (kcal)	Prot (g)	Carb (g)	Fiber (g)	Fat (g)	Sat (g)	Chol (g)
50085	Chicken rice, chunky, ready to eat, canned	1 cup	240	127	12	13	1	3	1	12
50088	Chicken vegetable, chunky, canned	1 cup	240	166	12	19	0	5	1.4	17
90238	Chicken, chunky, canned	1 cup	240	170	12	17	1	6	1.9	29
50697	Cup of Noodles, ramen, chicken flavor, dry/Nissin	1 ea	64	296	6	37	14	6.3		
50009	Minestrone, canned, made w/water	1 cup	241	82	4	11	1	3	0.6	2
92163	Ramen noodle, any flavor, dehydrated, dry	0.5 cup	38	172	4	25	1	6	2.9	0
50043	Tomato vegetable, from dry mix, made w/water	1 cup	253	56	2	10	1	1	0.4	0
50028	Tomato, canned, made w/water	1 cup	244	85	2	17	0	2	0.4	0
50014	Vegetable beef, canned, made w/water	1 cup	244	78	6	10	0	2	0.9	5
50013	Vegetarian vegetable, canned, made w/water	1 cup	241	72	2	12	0	2	0.3	0

Desserts

MDA Code	Food Name	Amt	Wt (g)	Ener (kcal)	Prot (g)	Carb (g)	Fiber (g)	Fat (g)	Sat (g)	Chol (g)
62904	Brownie, commercially prepared, square, lrg, 2-3/4" x 7/8"	1 ea	56	227	3	36	1	9	2.4	10
46062	Cake, chocolate, homemade, w/o icing	1 pce	95	340	5	51	2	14	5.2	55
46091	Cake, yellow, homemade, w/o icing	1 pce	68	245	4	36	0	10	2.7	37
71337	Doughnut, cake, w/chocolate icing, lrg, 3 1/2"	1 ea	57	270	3	27	1	18	4.6	35
45525	Doughnut, cake, glazed/sugared, med, 3"	1 ea	45	192	2	23	1	10	2.7	14
47026	Animal crackers/Arrowroot/Tea Biscuits	10 ea	12.5	56	1	9	0	2	0.4	0
90636	Chocolate chip cookie, commercially prepared 3.5" to 4"	1 ea	40	196	2	26	1	10	3.1	0
47006	Chocolate sandwich cookie, creme filled	3 ea	30	140	2	21	1	6	1.1	0
62905	Fig bar, 2 oz	1 ea	56.7	197	2	40	3	4	0.6	0
90640	Oatmeal cookie, commercially prepared, 3-1/2" to 4"	1 ea	25	112	2	17	1	5	1.1	0
47010	Peanut butter cookie, homemade, 3"	1 ea	20	95	2	12	0	5	0.9	6
62907	Sugar cookie, refrigerated dough, baked	1 ea	23	111	1	15	0	5	1.4	7
57894	Pudding, chocolate, ready to eat	1 ea	113	158	3	26	1	5	0.8	3
2612	Pudding, vanilla, ready to eat	1 ea	113	147	3	25	0	4	1.7	8
2651	Rice pudding, ready to eat	1 ea	142	231	3	31	0	11	1.7	1
57902	Tapioca pudding, ready to eat	1 ea	113	135	2	22	0	4	1.1	1
71819	Frozen yogurts, chocolate, nonfat	1 cup	186	199	8	37	2	1	0.9	7
72124	Frozen yogurts, flavors other than chocolate	1 cup	174	221	5	38	0	6	4	23
2010	Ice cream, light, vanilla, soft serve	0.5 cup	88	111	4	19	0	2	1.4	11
90723	Ice popsicle	1 ea	59	47	0	11	0	0	0	0
42264	Cinnamon rolls w/icing, refrigerated dough/Pillsbury	1 ea	44	150	2	24	5	1.2		

MDA Code	Food Name	Amt	Wt (g)	Ener (kcal)	Prot (g)	Carb (g)	Fiber (g)	Fat (g)	Sat (g)	Chol (g)
71299	Croissant, butter	1 ea	67	272	5	31	2	14	7.8	45
45572	Danish, cheese	1 ea	71	266	6	26	1	16	4.8	11
45593	Toaster pastry, Pop Tart, apple-cinnamon/Kellogg	1 ea	52	205	2	37	1	5	0.9	0
23014	Chocolate syrup, fudge-type	2 Tbs	38	133	2	24	1	3	1.5	1
510	Whipped cream topping, pressurized	2 Tbs	7.5	19	0	1	0	2	1	6
54387	Whipped topping, frozen, low fat	2 Tbs	9.4	21	0	2	0	1	1.1	0

Fats, Oils, and Condiments

MDA Code	Food Name	Amt	Wt (g)	Ener (kcal)	Prot (g)	Carb (g)	Fiber (g)	Fat (g)	Sat (g)	Chol (g)
90210	Butter, unsalted	1 Tbs	14	100	0	0	0	11	7.2	30
8084	Oil, vegetable, canola	1 Tbs	14	124	0	0	0	14	1	0
8008	Oil, olive, salad or cooking	1 Tbs	13.5	119	0	0	0	14	1.9	0
8111	Oil, safflower, salad or cooking greater than 70% oleic	1 Tbs	13.6	120	0	0	0	14	0.8	0
44483	Shortening, household	1 Tbs	12.8	113	0	0	0	13	2.6	0
1708	Barbecue sauce, original	2 Tbs	36	63	0	15	0			
27001	Catsup	1 ea	6	6	0	2	0	0	0	0
53523	Cheese sauce, ready to eat	0.25 cup	63	110	4	4	0	8	3.8	18
54388	Cream substitute, powdered, light	1 Tbs	5.9	25	0	4	0	1	0.2	0
50939	Gravy, brown, homestyle, canned	0.25 cup	60	25	1	3	1	0.3	2	
23003	Jelly	1 Tbs	19	51	0	13	0	0	0	0
25002	Maple syrup	1 Tbs	20	52	0	13	0	0	0	0
44476	Margarine, regular, 80% fat, with salt	1 Tbs	14.2	102	0	0	0	11	1.8	0
8145	Mayonnaise, safflower/soybean oil	1 Tbs	13.8	99	0	0	0	11	1.2	8
8502	Miracle Whip, light/Kraft	1 Tbs	16	37	0	2	0	3	0.5	4
435	Mustard, yellow	1 tsp	5	3	0	0	0	0	0	0
23042	Pancake syrup	1 Tbs	20	47	0	12	0	0	0	0
23172	Pancake syrup, reduced kcal	1 Tbs	15	25	0	7	0	0	0	0
53524	Pasta sauce, spaghetti/marinara	0.5 cup	125	92	2	14	1	3	0.4	0
53646	Salsa picante, mild	2 Tbs	30.5	8	0	1	0	0		0
504	Sour cream, cultured	2 Tbs	28.8	62	1	1	0	6	3.8	13
53063	Soy sauce	1 Tbs	18	11	2	1	0	0	0	0
53652	Taco sauce, red, mild	1 Tbs	15.7	7	0	1	0	0		0
53004	Teriyaki sauce	1 Tbs	18	15	1	3	0	0	0	0
8024	1000 Island, regular	1 Tbs	15.6	58	0	2	0	5	0.8	4
8013	Blue/Roquefort cheese, regular	2 Tbs	30.6	154	1	2	0	16	3	5
90232	French, regular	1 Tbs	12.3	56	0	2	0	6	0.7	0
44498	Italian, fat-free	1 Tbs	14	7	0	1	0	0	0	0
44696	Ranch, reduced fat	1 Tbs	15	33	0	2	0	3	0.2	3
8035	Vinegar & oil, homemade	2 Tbs	31.2	140	0	1	0	16	2.8	0

Fast Food

MDA Code	Food Name	Amt	Wt (g)	Ener (kcal)	Prot (g)	Carb (g)	Fiber (g)	Fat (g)	Sat (g)	Chol (g)
6177	Baked potato, topped w/cheese sauce	1 ea	296	474	15	47		29	10.6	18
56629	Burrito w/beans & cheese	1 ea	93	189	8	27		6	3.4	14
66023	Burrito w/beans, cheese, & beef	1 ea	102	165	7	20	2	7	3.6	62
66024	Burrito w/beef	1 ea	110	262	13	29	1	10	5.2	32
56600	Biscuit w/egg sandwich	1 ea	136	373	12	32	1	22	4.7	245
66029	Biscuit w/egg, cheese, & bacon sandwich	1 ea	144	477	16	33	0	31	11.4	261

MDA Code	Food Name	Amt	Wt (g)	Ener (kcal)	Prot (g)	Carb (g)	Fiber (g)	Fat (g)	Sat (g)	Chol (g)
66013	Cheeseburger, double, condiments & vegetables	1 ea	166	417	21	35		21	8.7	60
56649	Cheeseburger, large, one meat patty w/condiments & vegetables	1 ea	219	563	28	38		33	15	88
15063	Chicken, breaded, fried, dark meat (drumstick or thigh)	3 oz	85.1	248	17	9	1	15	4.1	95
15064	Chicken, breaded, fried, light meat (breast or wing)	3 oz	85.1	258	19	10	1	15	4.1	77
56000	Chicken filet, plain	1 ea	182	515	24	39		29	8.5	60
56635	Chimichanga w/beef & cheese	1 ea	183	443	20	39		23	11.2	51
5461	Cole slaw	0.75 cup	99	147	1	13		11	1.6	5
56606	Croissant w/egg & cheese sandwich	1 ea	127	368	13	24		25	14.1	216
56607	Croissant w/egg, cheese, & bacon sandwich	1 ea	129	413	16	24		28	15.4	215
66021	Enchilada w/cheese	1 ea	163	319	10	29		19	10.6	44
66020	Enchirito w/cheese, beef, & beans	1 ea	193	344	18	34		16	7.9	50
66031	English muffin w/cheese & sausage sandwich	1 ea	115	393	15	29	1	24	9.9	59
66010	Fish sandwich w/tartar sauce	1 ea	158	431	17	41	0	23	5.2	55
90736	French fries fried in vegetable oil, medium	1 ea	134	427	5	50	5	23	5.3	0
56638	Frijoles (beans) w/cheese	0.5 cup	83.5	113	6	14		4	2	18
56664	Ham & cheese sandwich	1 ea	146	352	21	33		15	6.4	58
56662	Hamburger, large, double, w/condiments & vegetables	1 ea	226	540	34	40		27	10.5	122
56659	Hamburger, one patty w/condiments & vegetables	1 ea	110	279	13	27		13	4.1	26
66007	Hamburger, plain	1 ea	90	274	12	31		12	4.1	35
5463	Hash browns	0.5 cup	72	151	2	16		9	4.3	9
66004	Hot dog, plain	1 ea	98	242	10	18		15	5.1	44
2032	Ice cream sundae, hot fudge	1 ea	158	284	6	48	0	9	5	21
6185	Mashed potatoes	0.5 cup	121	100	3	20		1	0.6	2
56639	Nachos w/cheese	7 pcs	113	346	9	36		19	7.8	18
6176	Onion rings, breaded, fried	8 pcs	78.1	259	3	29		15	6.5	13
6173	Potato salad	0.333 cup	95	108	1	13		6	1	57
56619	Pizza w/pepperoni 12" or 1/8	1 pce	108	275	15	30		11	3.4	22
66003	Roast beef sandwich, plain	1 ea	139	346	22	33		14	3.6	51
56671	Submarine sandwich, cold cuts	1 ea	228	456	22	51	2	19	6.8	36
57531	Taco		171	369	21	27		21	11.4	56
71129	Shake, chocolate, 12 fl. oz	1 ea	250	317	8	51	5	9	5.8	32
71132	Shake, vanilla, 12 fl. oz	1 ea	250	369	8	49	2	16	9.9	57

[ABOUT THE AUTHOR]

Scott Melville was born and raised in Western Pennsylvania. He majored in Health and Physical Education at Slippery Rock State College, played on the baseball and basketball teams, and graduated in 1969. After a few years as an elementary physical education teacher in the public schools he began his graduate studies, eventually earning a Ph.D. in Motor Learning from the University of Iowa in 1976. Following community college and small college teaching and coaching experiences he moved to Spokane and began his career at Eastern Washington University in 1980. His primary teaching assignments have been Elementary Health and Physical Education Methods, Motor Learning, and Coaching Education.

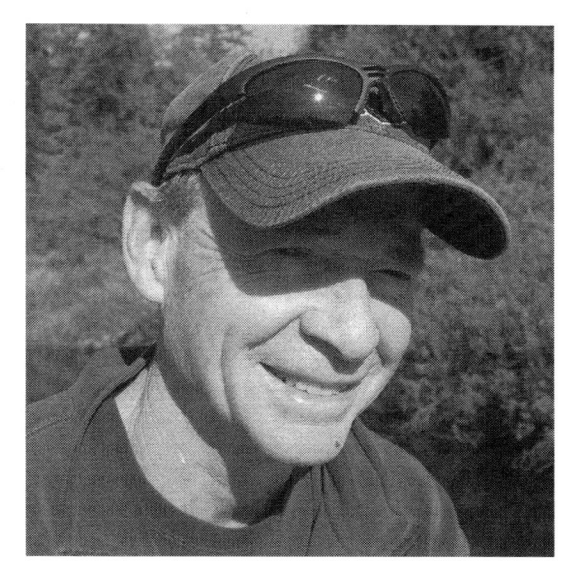

His chief hobbies are reading (non-fiction and poetic writings), painting (watercolors and egg-tempera) and physical activities (running, swimming, bicycling), He lives happily with his wife Julie (a school teacher) in Spokane. Students and all others are invited to visit their art gallery at 1915 S Grand Boulevard.

Made in the USA
Charleston, SC
03 April 2010